A Brief History of Epidemic and Pestilential Diseases: With the Principal Phenomena of the Physical World, Which Precede and Accompany Them, and Observations Deduced From the Facts Stated : in two Volumes

A BRIEF

HISTORY

OF

EPIDEMIC AND PESTILENTIAL DISEASES;

WITH THE

PRINCIPAL PHENOMENA OF THE PHYSICAL
WORLD, WHICH PRECEDE AND AC-
COMPANY THEM,

AND

OBSERVATIONS DEDUCED FROM THE
FACTS STATED.

IN TWO VOLUMES.

By NOAH WEBSTER,

Author of Differtations on the English Language and feveral other Works—Member of the Connecticut Academy of Arts and Sciences—of the Society for the Promotion of Agriculture, Arts and Manufactures, in the State of New-York—of the American Academy of Arts and Sciences, and correfponding Member of the Hiftorical Society in Maffachufetts.

VOL. I.

HARTFORD:

PRINTED BY HUDSON & GOODWIN.

1799.

[*PUBLISHED ACCORDING TO ACT OF CONGRESS.*]

ADVERTISEMENT.

THE work quoted under the title of "Magdeburgh History," is a compilation of Ecclesiastical History made by several writers at Magdeburgh, and divided into centuries.

The work quoted under the title of "Hist. August." is a collection of the histories of the Roman affairs under the Emperors.

The work cited under the title of "Angl. Script," is a collection of the early historians of England.

The work cited under the title of "Germ. Script," is a collection of the ancient histories of Germany, by Pistorius.

In a few instances, authors are cited without the page or chapter. This has arisen from the manner in which my materials were obtained—which was to transcribe passages from books wherever I found them, in public or private libraries, and sometimes, when books fell in my way by accident, without the intention of using them as authorities. The instances however are not numerous, and the passages may generally be found with ease by the index or chronological order of the work. Since I have had it in view to publish this treatise, and especially since discovering a disposition in some persons to decry this attempt to investigate truth, by charging me with a design to collect facts for the purpose of supporting preconceived opinions, I have been more careful to note my authorities. This must be my apology for citing so many authorities, which might otherwise appear like affectation.

CONTENTS of the FIRST VOLUME.

Introduction, - - - - Page v.

SECTION I.
Of the diversity of opinions respecting the cause and origin of pestilence. - - - - - - - 9.

SECTION II.
Historical view of pestilential epidemics, and the phenomena in the physical world which precede, attend or follow them, from the earliest accounts to the Christian era, - - - 24.

SECTION III.
Historical view of pestilential epidemics, from the Christian era, to the year 1347, - - - - - - 65.

SECTION IV.
Historical view of pestilential epidemics, from the year 1347 to 1500, - - - - - - - 133.

SECTION V.
Historical view of pestilential epidemics from the year 1500 to 1600. 151.

SECTION VI.
Historical view of pestilential epidemics from the year 1600 to the close of the year 1700, - - - - 171.

SECTION VII.
Historical view of pestilential epidemics from the year 1701, to the year 1788, - - - - - - 216.

SECTION VIII.
Historical view of pestilential epidemics from the year 1788 to the year 1799, including the last epidemic period, - 283.

ERRORS.

PAGE 37, line 9, from bottom, read *ficculi's*
    44, line 10, read *metu*.
    76, line 16, read *Lampridius*.
    87, line 3, from bottom, after *cold*, place a comma
    104, line 22, read *dea.on*
    106, line 2, read *inguinaria*.
    156, line 9, read *Alemar*, also in page 174, line 12
    169, line 4, from bottom, read *Penrith*.
    204, line 18, after *petechial*, read *fever*.
    241, line 3, read 1750.
    260, line 18, for *of* read *or*.

IN page 255 a fact is stated which contradicts the statement respecting the planet Mars in page 241. There is an error in one of the statements, and I leave astronomers to determin by calculations which of the authorities, Ames' Almanac for 1750, or the Annual Register, is wrong The error is not material to my subject The only question of confequence, is, whether the near approach of Mars had any influence, in producing the extreme heat of 1749 and 1766—a question I pretend not to determin.

INTRODUCTION.

A PUBLICATION on the subject of diseases, from the pen of a man who has never before turned his attention to medical science or to chymistry, is a circumstance, which, if it does not require an apology, demands at least an explanation.

The prevalence of the catarrh, commonly called influenza, in the years 1789 and 90, first awakened my curiosity on the subject of epidemic diseases. A journey which I made in October 1789, from Hartford to Boston; and another in March 1790 from Hartford to Albany; led me to observe the *progressiveness* of that disease, with its other phenomena.

The appearance of the scarlatina anginosa in 1793 revived my curiosity, and a similar circumstance, a journey from Hartford to New-York in April of that year, led me to observe a progression in that disease from West to East. A slight attack which my own children suffered, in May following, together with a similar attack of many other children in Hartford, and its more violent effects some months after, convinced me that the epidemic was *progressive* in *malignancy*, as well as in regard to *place*.

Had no other epidemic appeared, my curiosity would probably have subsided and been extinguished. The malignant fever in New-York in 1791, had excited alarm in that city, and was a subject of notice in Hartford where I then refided; but no idea had been conceived, that it was connected with a peftilential ftate of the air, in the United States, which was afterwards to produce more ferious and general calamities.

In autumn 1793 however that peftilential ftate of air arrived to its crifis in Philadelphia, where the mortality occafioned by the yellow fever, fpread deftruction and difmay, from Auguft to November. The fatality of the difeafe fpread confternation thro the United States, and excited apprehenfions in Europe.

No American citizen could be indifferent to the prevalence of this difeafe in his own country. Still it was conceived that the diftemper might have been produced from imported infection, and that a more rigid execution of the laws relating to quarantine, might prevent a repetition of the calamity. Here refted apprehenfion and enquiry.

But this tranquillity was of fhort duration. The appearance of the fame difeafe in New-Haven in 1794, and in New-York, Baltimore and Norfolk in 1795, revived my curiofity, with double zeal to fearch out the caufes of thefe phenomena, fo unufual in this country. The facts which had come to my knowledge, relating to the origin and propagation of this difeafe, led me to fufpect the common theory of *infection* to be ill-founded. But as a preliminary to all other enquiries, it appeared neceffary to fettle the controverfy relative to the *imported* or *domeftic* fources of the diftemper; for without a decifion of this queftion, legiflative and police-regulations, for preventing a return of the evil, or mitigating its severity, would probably be fruitless. The question appeared to be extremely important, and the differences of opinion on the subject, among medical gentlemen, seemed to preclude the possibility of a decision among them, that should silence doubts in the public mind.

In this situation of the controversy, I resolved to make an effort to obtain evidence which might decide the point, in one way or the other; and as facts only can be relied on as a sure basis of principles and theory, I determined to make a collection of facts, from all parts of the United States, where the yellow fever, or other malignant fevers had prevailed, during the preceding years. For this purpose, on the 31st of October 1795, I addressed a circular letter to the physicians of Philadelphia, New-York, Baltimore, Norfolk, New-Haven, and in general, throughout the United States, requesting them to communicate to me whatever facts had come within their observation, which could throw light on the question of the foreign or domestic origin of the yellow fever. In consequence of which I received a number of communications, which were published in 1796, and to which is prefixed my circular letter.

These communications, tho less numerous and satisfactory than were desirable, united with a multitude of facts within my own observation, *convinced* me of the fallacy of the vulgar opinion, respecting the origin of the yellow fever in the United States, from imported sources. I found repeatedly that the reports of persons taken ill, in consequence of intercourse with vessels from the

West-Indies, or with diseased seamen, infected cotton or clothing, or the like causes, were mere idle tales, raised by the ignorant or interested, and wholly unsupported by evidence. Scarcely an instance could be found, in which the evidence of the propagation of disease, from imported infection, was sufficient to render the fact even probable.

On the other hand, the evidence of the origination of the disease in New-York, Baltimore, Norfolk, Newburyport, Boston and Charleston, appeared to be clear and satisfactory. In most of those places, the fact has never been questioned.

When the same disease appeared in Philadelphia in 1797; the question of importation or domestic origin, again agitated the faculty and the public. The revival of the discussion, and particularly, certain publications of Dr. William Currie, in the Philadelphia prints, called forth my exertions to unite opinions and save the citizens of this country from the distraction of measures, which must necessarily follow a division of opinions. I considered and still consider the question as resting principally on fact, and not on medical skill; therefore proper to be investigated and discussed by any man who has leisure and means, as well as by physicians.

These considerations gave rise to the observations which I addressed to Dr. Currie, thro the medium of the public papers, in the months of October, November and December 1797. The design of these observations was originally limited to the purpose of proving the yellow fever of our country to be generated by local and domestic causes, by laying together the facts which I had collected from various parts of the United States, without any intention of examining the hiftory and phenomena of peftilential difeafes in other countries, and other periods of the world.

In purfuing this object however, I was led infenfibly to examin all the books I could find, on the fubject of the plague; and the fubject being new, I found too much pleafure in profecuting it, readily to abandon the purfuit. Facts which were new to me were daily prefenting themfelves to my mind; and after three months inveftigation, I was perfuaded that thofe facts are of too much importance to philofophy, to medicin and to human happinefs, not to merit publication. Such is the origin of the prefent treatife.

When I began my enquiries into the origin of the yellow fever, in 1795, I had no preconceived fyftem to maintain. My view was to collect facts and from them to deduce TRUTH. It is not my intention to advance theory over fact; but as far as juft philofophy and found logic will permit, draw theory from facts, and if poffible, by fair reafoning, from the uniform operations of nature, to arrive at fixed principles. If conjectures fhould in any inftance be advanced, they will be offered as fuch, and not as the bafis of practice.

As there is a difference of opinion in regard to the caufes of the plague, and other peftilential difeafes, as well as in regard to the identity of the yellow fever and plague, I fhall define my manner of ufing certain terms, which will often occur in the following work.

That pestilential disease which usually, in the Levant, produces swellings in the glands, as buboes, I shall call the *glandular* or *inguinal* plague.

The pestilential disease which has afflicted some of the cities in America, and is usually called yellow fever, I shall denominate, the *bilious* or *American plague*.

In the Levant plague, swellings in the groin, in the arm-pits, and behind the ears, do not, in every case, appear; but they are the general distinguishing marks of the true pestis or plague.

In the yellow fever, the skin is not, in every case, marked by a yellow color; but it is generally the fact, and therefore this form of pestilence may very well take its denomination from that circumstance of its bilious appearance.

Whether these are disease specifically distinct, or only the same disease varied and modified by climate, season or other circumstances, is a question that belongs to the faculty. It is sufficient for my purpose to observe, that in most of the symptoms, they agree—that they are pestilential and greatly to be dreaded by mankind. I shall therefore treat them as different forms of the same disease. There may be some cause for believing that the moisture of a country, abounding with woods, and marshy grounds, may occasion the difference in the color of bodies which fall victims to pestilence.

The words *infection* and *contagion*, are used by medical writers and in popular custom, as synonymous, and their etymologies warrant the practice. But I conceive there are distinctions in this quality or power of diseases, of communicating themselves by contact or near approach, which require to have each its appropriate language.

That quality of a difeafe which communicates it from a fick to á well perfon, on fimply inhaling the breath or effluvia from the perfon of the difeafed, at any time and in any place, may be called *fpecific contagion*. Such is the contagion of the fmall-pox and the meafles, which are therefore called *contagious* difeafes.

That quality of a difeafe which, tho infalutary will not communicate it, without the aid of other caufes, as warm weather, or peculiar fituation and habit of body, and which requires the healthful perfon to be a confiderable time, under its influence, to give it effect, may be called *infection*. Such is the quality of the plague, in all its forms, dyfentery, and all typhus fevers. It may perhaps be poffible for the effluvia of thofe who have thefe difeafes, to be fo concentrated and virulent, as to communicate them to a perfon in health, by a fingle infpiration of air into the lungs. But if fuch can be the cafe in any inftance, it is not the ordinary ftate of thofe difeafes. Even in the plague, many attendants on the fick never receive the difeafe at all; and in moft cafes, healthful perfons may, for hours, breathe the air of the rooms where the patients are, without any injury.

Hence infection is capable of all degrees of activity and force, from a flight impurity of air, which affects no perfon in health, to that virulent ftate of air, which will produce vomiting in a perfon fuddenly expofed to it. *Infection* is ufually rendered inactive by fevere cold; *fpecific contagion* is never deftroyed, but often rendered more active by cold. Hence the winter in northern latitudes ufually puts an end to the plague, but makes no favorable alteration in the fmall-pox. There are fome exceptions to this remark, as it regards the plague, which will be noticed in the following work.

Thefe diftinctions, which will appear, in the courfe of this treatife to be well founded, have never been defined or ufed by European phyficians, fo far as my information extends, and to the want of them, are to be afcribed many errors and abfurdities in opinion, as well as warm controverfies in regard to the contagion of the plague.

That ftate of our atmofphere which produces difeafe, or difpofes the body to difeafe, independent of other caufes, I call *general* or *primary* contagion. Synonymous with thefe phrafes, will be ufed a peftilential ftate or conftitution of the air.

The word *peftilence* may be ufed as fynonymous with plague; or as expreffing all kinds of contagious and infectious epidemics. I have ufed it in both fenfes; and often to exprefs an idea of that feries of epidemics which are clofely connected with the plague.

Whether thefe diftinctions are juft or not, is not very material; it is fufficient that they will exprefs my ideas in the following treatife.

SECTION I.

Of the diversity of opinions respecting the cause and origin of pestilence.

FROM the date of the earliest historical records, the opinions of men have been divided on the subject of the causes and origin of pestilential diseases. All enquiries of the philosopher and the physician have hitherto been baffled, and investigations, often repeated, have ended without leading to satisfactory conclusions.

In the history of opinions on this mysterious subject, there is a remarkable distinction between the ancients and moderns. The ancients derived most of their knowledge and science from personal observation, as they had very few books and little aid from the improvements of their predecessors. The philosophers of antiquity, attentive to changes in the seasons and to the revolutions of the heavenly bodies, attempted to trace pestilential diseases to extraordinary vicissitudes in the weather, and to the aspects of the planets. Modern philosophers and physicians, on the other hand, unable to account for pestilence on the principle of extraordinary seasons, and disdaining to admit the influence of the planets to be the cause, have resorted to invisible animalculæ, and to infection concealed in bales of goods or old clothes, transported from Egypt or Constantinople, and let loose, at certain periods, to scourge mankind and desolate the earth.

In both periods of the world, the common mass of people, usually ignorant and always inclined to believe in the marvellous, have cut the Gordian knot of difficulty, by afcribing peftilence to the immediate exercife of divine power; under the impreffion that the plague is one of the judgments which God, in his wrath, inflicts on mankind to punifh them for their iniquities.

Without deciding on the comparative merit of thefe refpective opinions, it is fufficient to obferve, that they are all probably incorrect; and thofe of the philofophers, altogether inadequate to explain the origin of peftilential Epidemics.

It may however be of ufe to infert, in this place, the explanations of the caufe of peftilence, given by fome of the principal writers on the fubject.

Hippocrates, the father of medical fcience, and a man of very acute obfervation, confidered peftilence as the effect of particular feafons and winds. A peftilential ftate or conftitution of air he defcribes, as occafioned by a continuation of foutherly winds, and a warm, humid, clouded atmofphere.

De morbis vulgaribus, lib 3.

Galen followed the fame theory. He fays that peftilent difeafes arife from a putridity of the air; and in another place, *a cœli flatu*, from the ftate of the air or weather.

p. 627, in Hippoc.—

It will at once occur to an intelligent reader, that a particular defcription of weather, producing peftilence, muft be principally calculated for a particular country or latitude. The ftate of feafons which Hippocrates calls *peftilential*, is evidently calculated to produce or augment autumnal difeafes in temperate latitudes; and is precifely the ftate of weather which exifted in the United States in 1795, when the bilious plague prevailed in the cities of New-York, Baltimore and Norfolk. But it does not correfpond with the feafon in 1793, when the fame difeafe raged in Philadelphia; for that was exceffively dry, nor with the fummer of 1797, which was temperate, in refpect to heat, cold and moifture.

Hippocrates indeed feems to have been aware that the feafons alone were not fufficient to account for peftilence, for he fpeaks of *to theion*, fome divine principle in the air, by which modern writers of celebrity suppose to be intended what is now called an *epidemic conflitution*, refulting from changes in the atmofphere produced by unknown caufes. Ariftotle prob. 1. relates that a hot and dry fouth wind will produce peftilence.

The philofophical warrior and hiftorian, Ammianus Marcellinus, after mentioning a plague which broke out in Amida, a city of Perfia, when befieged by Sapor A. D. 359, from the corruption of numerous dead bodies which lay unburied in the ftreets, proceeds to unfold the caufes of peftilential diftempers, in the following manner.

" Philofophers and eminent phyficians have taught that peftilence is produced by excefs of heat or cold, of drouth or moifture. Whence it is that thofe who live near wet and marfhy places are fubject to coughs, difeafes of the eyes and the like. Thofe, on the other hand, who refide where the heat is great, are troubled with febrile complaints; and in proportion as the matter of fire is more active, drouth is more rapid in deftroying life. Hence, during the war of ten years in Greece, this fpecies of difeafe prevailed, and it was faid that men perifhed by the *weapons of Apollo*, by which was fuppofed to be meant, the *heat of the fun*. And, according to Thucydides, the mortality among the Athenians, in the beginning of the Peloponnefian war, was occafioned by an acute difeafe, which proceeded from the fervid regions of Ethiopia, and gradually extended to Attica.

" Others are of opinion that air, like water, vitiated by the effluvia of dead bodies, or fimilar fubftances, is deprived of its falubrity; or at leaft that a fudden change of air will produce the more flight complaints. Some alfo affirm that the air, rendered grofs by a denfer vapor from the earth, clofing the pores of the body and checking perfpiration, becomes fatal to the lives of fome; for which reafon, other animals than man, which are continually bending towards the earth, are the firft victims to peftilence, as Homer teftifies, and which is proved by many examples, during the prevalence of peftilential difeafes.

" The firft fpecies of plague is called *pandemic*, and this afflicts moft feverely thofe who are fubject to exceffive heat, in hot regions. The fecond is denominated *epidemic*, which when it rages, obscures the sight and excites dangerous humors. The third Lamodes, which is temporary, but produces sudden death."

Lib 19

The historian has here explained the causes of ordinary diseases, occasioned by extremes of weather, marsh effluvia, vitiated air, and the direct action of violent heat, or stroke of the sun. No person will dispute the justness of his remarks, for the same causes, at this day, produce the same effects. But the causes assigned are not adequate to all the effects, which we wish to explain. They do not uniformly occasion pestilence ; and on th other hand, pestilence sometimes rages without the influence of those causes.

Ætius, an eminent physician, about the close of the 5th century, compiled the opinions and methods of cure practised by the most celebrated of his predecessors. In this compilation, entitled " Tetrabibios," chap. ix. we find the following paragraph on the subject of Epidemic diseases.

" Those are called popular or epidemic diseases, which spring from a common cause, as bad food or water, immoderate grief or want of customary exercise, hunger or repletion, especially when abundance succeeds extreme want. But the nature of the country often causes epidemic diseases : the air we breathe being vitiated by the evaporation from putrid substances. These substances are multitudes of dead bodies after battles, marshes or stagnant water in the vicinity, which emit poisonous and fetid vapours.—This cause is in continual operation. And the air which surrounds us, always changes its temperament, when it becomes immoderately hot or cold, dry or humid. To other causes we are not all equally exposed, nor at all times ; but the circumambient air, when we are abroad, surrounds us all alike, and is inhaled with the breath.

" Sometimes the surrounding air, becoming unusually humid and hot, induces a pestilential constitution ; and as humors, tending to putrefaction, are collected in the body by eating unwholesome food, this air becomes the source of a pestilential fever. Therefore if a person takes moderate exercise, and is temperate and regular in his diet [victu modesto ac castigato] he wholly escapes all affections of this kind."

Such were the opinions of the physicians and philosophers of antiquity. No distinction appears to have been made by them, between the plague and other pestilential diseases. All were ascribed to the same causes.

At what time the distinction between *Pestis* and *Pestilentia* was first made, has not occurred to my enquiries. But I find it in the writings of Prosper Alpinus, a Venetian physician, who wrote about the close of the 16th century, and who had been, for some years, a practitioner in Egypt. This author maintains that pestilent fevers are occasioned by local causes, as vitiated air, and by peculiarities of season, as extreme heat and humidity. But he asserts that the plague in Egypt rarely proceeds from corrupted air, and never, except after an unusual overflowing of the Nile, when that river has exceeded its common bounds. He contends that if this disease was produced by noxious exhalations from putrid and stagnant water, and marshy places, it would occur every year. He therefore concludes for certain that the plague is usually imported from Greece, Syria, Barbary, or Turkey. " Plerumque igitur id genus morbi ibi contagio ex aliis locis asportari solet." The contagion of the plague is usually imported from other countries.

Rerum Egypt vol. 2, p. 73, vol. 3, 61, and vol 4, 299

The same author asserts that the plague brought from Barbary is more malignant and of longer duration, than when brought from Greece or Syria.

Diemerbroeck, an eminent Dutch physician of the last century, has recorded an account of a violent plague in Nemueguen in 1636, and subjoined to it the best treatise on the origin of that disease, which I have been able to find, tho in one or two particulars, his ideas are very inaccurate. This author, whose treatise, I am surprised to find, is little known in this country, assigns three causes of the pestis or true plague. First, the just anger of heaven, provoked by the exhalations from the sinks of our sins and abominable deeds. Secondly, a most malignant, poisonous, and to human nature, deadly pestilent germ, [seminarium,] like a fubtle fermentum or leaven, fent from heaven, in a very fmall quantity, diffufing itfelf through the air like a fubtle gas, and rendering it impure. This gas, he fuppofes to fpread over many regions its numerous particles, and to imprefs on the air an infection like poifon, which often affects not only many perfons, but almoft the whole world.

However whimfical we may think this author's explanation of the peftilent principle; that fome fuch general caufe exifts in the atmofphere, at certain periods, will be rendered very probable, if not certain, by the facts hereafter to be related.

The "feminarium e cœlo demiffum" of Diemerbroeck feems to be the *to theion* of Hippocrates. In what the effence of this principle confifts, is not known; but there muft be an alteration in the chymical properties of the atmofphere to folve the difficulties that attend our inquiries into the caufe of peftilence.—That this alteration is the effect of a poifon, " e cœlo demiffum," is an hypothefis unfupported by facts and wholly incredible.

The third caufe of peftilence, mentioned by this author, is infection.

Diemerbroeck alfo maintains the diftinction between *peftis* and *peftilentia*. The latter is fuppofed to proceed from foul exhalations, intemperate feafons and the like. But the plague, he contends, cannot be occafioned by thofe caufes, tho thefe may aid the feminarium or general caufe.

Van Helmont, a Flemifh writer of fome celebrity, in the laft century, maintains that the plague cannot be afcribed to the "importunate and unfeafonable changes of times, nor to putrefaction;" that the "poifon of the plague is a far fecret one from any other;" that the "matter of that difeafe is a wild fpirit tinged with poifon, exhaling from a difeafed perfon, or drawn inwards from a gas of the earth putrified by continuance, and receiving internally an appropriate ferment, and by degrees attaining a peftilent poifon in us." "The remote, crude and firft occafional matter of the peftilence, is an air putrified thro' continuance, or rather a hoary putrified gas, which putrefaction of the air, hath not the 8200th part of its feminal body." This explanation feems to be hardly intelligible.

Works, Lond. Edit. 1662, p. 1085, 1090, 1102, 1125.

This author contends that " the peft is not fent down from heaven, but that popular plagues do draw their firft occafional matter from an earthquake, and from the confequences of camps and fieges."

p. 1125.

Hodges, who wrote a treatife on the great plague in London in 1665, obferves that the air fuffers fome effential alteration which is neceffary to favor the propagation of peftilence. The nitro-aerial principle, which caufes or invigorates vegetable and animal life, fometimes becomes imperfect, degenerate or corrupt, being tainted with fomething pernicious to vitality. He calls it poifonous, and obferves that it proves injurious to trees and cattle, as well as to man. He fuppofes the corrupting principle to be a fubtle aura or vapor extricated from the bowels of the earth. To this caufe alfo he afcribes the death of fifh during periods of peftilence. At the fame time he contends that the infecting principle is generated in Africa or Afia, and conveyed to other countries. The feat of the difeafe he fuppofes to be in the animal fpirits.

Van Swieten maintains that the caufe of Epidemics is in the hidden qualities of the air, and inexplicable. He fuppofes it not impoffible that exhalations in earthquakes may augment or leffen the deleterious quality of the air in peftilence.

Com vol 16, 47.

Sydenham not only agrees with Diemerbroeck, Van Swieten, and others, in afcribing peftilence to occult qualities in the air, but has entered into the fubject of explaining the peculiar fymptoms of difeafes by the influence of an Epidemic conftitution of the air. His *occult qualities* have been ridiculed by later phyficians, and fo far as his theory, in this refpect, has been neglected, the fcience of medicin has degenerated. If I miftake not, it can be made evident, that one of the moft important, as well as moft difficult branches of medical fcience, is to afcertain the effect of the reigning conftitution of air, on prevailing difeafes, and to apply that knowledge to the cure of thofe difeafes.

Dr. Mead's treatife on the plague has been much admired and celebrated; yet I will affert, that next to the " Traitè de la peste," a treatise in quarto on the plague of Marseilles, published by royal permission, it is the weakest and least valuable performance on that subject now extant. The author acknowledges he had never seen the disease of which he wrote; and therefore must have formed his opinions on the observations of others.

His essay is intended to demonstrate that the plague is propagated by specific contagion only, and he attempts to prove that this disease, like the small-pox and measles, has been bred in Egypt or Ethiopia, and thence propagated and entailed on Europe.

Works, p 242 & 3

In support of this theory he even goes so far as to call in question the unanimous testimony of historians, who relate that the terrible plague of 1347, 8, 9, and 50, began in Cathay, China. In opposition to which he " questions not," that that pestilence originated in Egypt. He alledges that we must seek the cause of plague in Egypt and *no where else*.

p 246.

He ascribes the plague to the putrefaction of animal substances and unseasonable moisture, heats and want of winds; but says " no kind of putrefaction in European countries is ever heightened to a degree capable of producing the true plague."

p 247 & 8.

This author assigns three causes of plague. 1st. Diseased persons: 2d. goods transported from infected places. 3d. a corrupted state of air.

p 250.

He thinks the causes mentioned so obvious that he wonders at authors who resort to hidden qualities, such as malignant influences of the heavens, arsenical, bituminous or other mineral effluvia, with the like imaginary or uncertain agents.

p 249

He does not however deny all latent disorders in the air, but considers them as secondary causes only, increasing and promoting the disease when once bred, but he thinks infection to be the means of its propagation. In this he differs widely from Diemerbroeck who utterly denies that the disease is originally derived from infection, although he agrees that it may be afterwards communicated from person to person by contact or near approach. Diemerbroeck alfo maintains the latent qualities of the air to be the *principal* caufe of the plague; or caufe *fine qua non*—a point which the facts to be hereafter detailed will moſt clearly demonſtrate.

Dr. Mead fays, " the plague is never originally bred with us, but is always brought accidentally from abroad."
p 261.

The fame opinion is afferted moſt pofitively in James' Medical Dictionary, and in moſt modern publications on the fubject. The compilers of the Encyclopedia fay, " the plague, as *is generally agreed*, is never bred or propagated in Britain, but always imported from abroad, efpecially from the Levant, Leffer Afia or Egypt where it is very common." Such alfo was the opinion of the celebrated Cullen.
Encyclop art. plague and medicine no 221.

The following fentence in Dr. Mead is very exceptionable, as it is calculated to check a fpirit of free enquiry—a fpirit to which mankind are greatly indebted for improvements in fcience.

" It may be juſtly cenfured in thofe writers that they ſhould undertake to determine the fpecific nature of thefe fecret changes and alterations which we have no means at all of difcovering," alluding to changes in the air.
p 249

In oppofition to all thefe great authorities, it will probably be proved, that the plague generally, if not always originates, in the country where it exiſts as an epidemic. The common opinion of the propagation of peſtilence folely by infection, has had a moſt calamitous effect on medicin and on human happinefs. It has prevented the refearches of acute modern philofophers and phyficians, who might have been able, by diligence and a comprehenfive view of the fubject, to trace peſtilence to its real caufes, and to fuggeſt the true means of avoiding this terrible fcourge.

Thompfon who travelled in Egypt about the year 1734, and whofe account of that country has not been mended by modern travellers, obferves, " The coming and going of the plague are two things not eafily to be accounted for, notwithſtanding we are assured of the facts in a most unquestionable manner. That the infection is propagated in the air, and thereby transferred from place to place, seems to be a matter out of dispute; but how it is generated therein, we are much at a loss to determine." He proceeds to state, like many others, " that the plague is generally brought into Egypt from Constantinople or by Caravans from the southern countries." And on the whole he thinks it rarely generated in that country.

Travels, vol 2, p. 194 & 5.

In the Monthly Review vol. 33, there is an account of the plague in Constantinople, by Dr. Mackenzie, in which are some passages worthy of notice. After asserting his opinion that this distemper can be communicated only by the touch or near approach, he adds, " that both here and at Smyrna, the plague breaks out, in some years, when it is not possible to trace whence it is conveyed." He supposes the disease to proceed from " venomous moleculæ lodged in wool, cotton, hair, leather and skins," in houses not well cleansed after pestilence; but that the plague from this source is not so fatal as when it comes from abroad. The air he thinks no otherwise concerned in producing the disease, than as " a vehicle to convey the venomous particles from one body to another."

Dr. Chandler, in his account of a plague in Smyrna, has nearly the same idea, as Mackenzie, with respect to the origin of the disease. He says " the plague might perhaps be truly defined, a disease arising from certain animalculæ, probably invisible, which burrow and form their nidus in the human body These whether generated in Egypt or elsewhere, subsist always in some places suited to their nature. *They are imported almost annually into Smyrra*, and this species is commonly destroyed by intense heat They are least fatal at the beginning and latter end of the season. If they arrive early in the spring, they are weak; but gather strength, multiply and then perish The pores of the skin, opened by the weather, readily admit them."

Baron de Tott in his memoirs observes " The researches I have carefully made concerning the plague, which I once believed to originate in Egypt, have convinced me, that it would not be so much as known there, were not the seeds of it conveyed thither by the commercial intercourse between Constantinople and Alexandria. It is in this last city that it always begins to appear. It rarely reaches Cairo, though no precaution is taken to prevent it, and when it does, it is presently extirpated by the heats, and prevented from arriving as far as the Said. It is likewise well known that the penetrating dews, which fall in Egypt about midsummer, destroy, even in Alexandria, all remains of this distemper."

Vol 4 page 70.

In vol 1, p. 38 he says, " that the researches into the nature of this distemper have only produced opinions which are self contradictory or unsupported by facts "—" There is no difficulty with respect to the causes which preserve and propagate it. Both the one and the other may be referred to the *dealers in old clothes in Constantinople*."

Du Pauw, in his Philosophical Dissertations on the Egyptians and Chinese, speaks of the plague as a disease of Egypt; and supposes the plague at Vienna in 1680, to have been imported from that country.—" Egypt is the hot bed of the plague—this disorder is not produced by famin—by exact annotations continued during twenty-eight years, we find that it raged five times, without being preceded by any scarcity of food, and contrary to what I once suspected, unrestricted to a periodical course."

Vol 1 p 87, 89.

Savary alledges, in opposition to the last mentioned author, that the pestilence is *not* native in Egypt, and that he consulted Egyptians and physicians who had lived there 20 years, who *informed* him that the plague was brought thither by the Turks. He supposes Constantinople to be now the residence of this dreadful affliction, which is preserved in existence by means of old clothes, which, after a plague has ceased, are distributed and sold very low by the Jews, and thus the disease is propagated.

Dr. Alexander Russel has given an account of the plague in Aleppo in 1742 and 3, and endeavored to ascertain from what quarter the disease originated and invaded that city. He seems to think, it always appears first at Tripoli, Sidon, or on the Sea Coast. It was asserted that the great plague of 1719 came from the northward; but as this fact does not suit his theory, he, like

Dr. Mead, in the case before mentioned, gives no credit to the assertion, but adheres to his opinion that all plagues originate in Egypt.—At the same time he is puzzled to trace the disease, in any instance, to that country.

See his hist of Aleppo.

Dr. Patrick Russel has published a quarto volume on the plague of Aleppo in 1760, and the subject of quarantine. In this work, he has preserved a number of important facts, but without understanding the subject sufficiently to apply them to useful purposes. All his theory and practical remarks are founded on the vulgar supposition of the origin of that disease in one or two cities only, and its propagation by specific contagion—a supposition totally unfounded; his treatise of course will be found of little value, in this respect.

Mr Volney, with all his philosophy and several months residence in Egypt, furnishes no additional light, on the subject of the origin of pestilence. He says, " some persons have attempted to establish an opinion, that the plague originates in Egypt; but this supposition, *founded on vague prejudices*, seems to be disproved by facts." This is an extraordinary assertion for a man who has the character of a philosopher. And on what authority does it rest? Simply on the declaration of European Merchants who have been settled for many years at Alexandria, and of the Egyptians, who say that the disease first appears in Alexandria, and that it is invariably preceded by an arrival from Smyrna or Constantinople. Therefore this philosopher concludes, " that the disease certainly originates from Constantinople, where it is perpetuated by the absurd negligence of the Turks, who publicly sell the effects of persons who die of that distemper." Here we have another great man ascribing this vast effect, an epidemic pestilence, to so trifling a cause, as infection preserved in furs, woolens, and old clothes!

What is still more astonishing, the same author adopts the ideas of the Egyptians, which Prosper Alpinus had adopted before him and which he has evidently copied from Alpinus, that a plague coming from one country is less malignant than when it comes from another, as tho there could be a difference in the *specific* contagion of the disease, when produced in different countries. Volney says "when brought from the Archipelago, or even from Damietta, into the harbours of Latakia, Saide or Acre, it *will not spread;* it rather chufes preliminary circumftances, and a more complex route; but when it paffes directly from Cairo to Damafcus, all Syria is fure to be infected."

Travels in Egypt and Syria vol 1. 253 et feq

It is really furprifing that, if the fact is well evidenced, that a plague proceeding from one country is more malignant than one proceeding from another, men of extenfive erudition and obfervation fhould not undertake to affign fome rational caufe for the phenomenon, rather than to propagate the vulgar tales and opinions of the Egyptians.

From this lengthy ftatement of opinions in regard to the origin and caufes of peftilence; opinions weak, contradictory, abfurd or inaccurate, what conclufion fhall be drawn. This, moft evidently, that the *fubject is not underftood.* Perhaps it never will be underftood. But furely a fubject fo interefting to the life and happinefs of man, deferves moft critical and laborious enquiry. A fubject which concerns the lives of millions of the human race ought not to be abandoned by the man of fcience, until every effort to find the truth fhall have been exhaufted. Yet ftrange as it may appear, even a hiftory of peftilence that all devouring fcourge which has fwept away a large portion of the human race in every age, is yet a defideratum in our libraries.

To fupply in part this defect, and to ftimulate further refearches into the origin of this frequent and formidable calamity, I will recite fuch hiftorical accounts of the plague, as an imperfect examination of authors has enabled me to collect. And as the moft accurate obfervers of the operations of nature, have fuggefted the probability that peftilential epidemics are caufed by fome occult qualities in the air, or by vapor from the internal parts of the earth, or by planetary influence, it is abfolutely neceffary to enquire how far fuch fuggeftions are fupported by facts. For this purpofe, I fhall note, as I proceed, any extraordinary occurrence or phenomena in the phyfical world, as earthquakes, eruptions of volcanoes, appearance of comets, violent tempefts, unufual feafons, and other fingular events and circumftances, which may appear to be connected with peftilence, either as caufe or effect, or as the effect of a common caufe.

The refult of this procefs will probably be a refutation of fome of the foregoing opinions, and the eftablifhment of fuch as are more rational and philofophical.

It is proper however to premife, that this inveftigation, which has been purfued but a few months only, amidft other occupations, has been fubjected to inconveniences peculiar to the United States. No man can find in this country *all* the books neceffary for a complete examination of a hiftorical or fcientific fubject. The public libraries in New-York and New-Haven, tho very valuable, are deficient. Thofe of Harvard College and Philadelphia, are more extenfive, but incomplete I have examined them all, tho in fome of them I could fpend but little time; yet in none of them could I find all the authorities which it was my wifh and intention to confult.

It is further to be premifed, that I have, as far as it could be done, reforted to original hiftorians for my facts and authorities. This is certainly the only fafe method for a compiler; but in the United States, it cannot be purfued with complete fuccefs, for want of the original writers of the local hiftories of countries. Moft of the Greek and Roman authors are to be obtained in our public or private libraries; but fome of the beft hiftorians of Italy, Germany, the Baltic nations and Spain, who have lived within the laft four or five centuries, are not to be found; others are in the original languages, which I do not underftand.

As to the modern hiftorical compilations in my native language, they are almoft ufelefs on this fubject. The moft able and celebrated of them, Hume, Robertfon, Smollet, Rapin and Gibbon, have paffed over moft of the plagues which have defolated cities and countries, without notice, or with fome general remarks which afford little light on the fubject of their origin.

Moft modern writers appear to think every thing beneath their notice, except war and political intrigues. They detail, with difgufting minutenefs, whatever relates to the deftruction or annoyance of mankind by the ambition of princes and demagogues;

while they omit or flightly mention whatever regards the civil and domestic economy, the private manners and habits, the arts, the health, and the focial happiness of nations. To this defcription, Dr. Henry's Hiftory of England, is an exception.

Nor have modern travellers furnifhed us with many valuable materials to fupply the defects of our hiftories. They pafs from country to country; examin and defcribe a few external objects, fuch as cities, buildings, paintings and ftatues, but leave more ufeful fubjects unexamined, and return home with a book of vulgar tales and errors.

In refpect to ufeful hiftory, the ancient authors have the preference over the modern. Modern compilers appear to have written for fame or for money, rather than for the fake of unfolding and diffufing truth. Hence they have principally attended to thofe animated periods of the world, which were diftinguifhed for great achievments; or thofe prominent events, a defcription of which would intereft the paffions of their readers. Or they have felected for defcription fuch parts of the hiftory of nations as would enable them to adorn their works with an elevated ftyle; omitting a multitude of fubordinate facts, as below the dignity of hiftory. Others appear to have undertaken hiftorical compilation, folely or principally to fupport fome preconceived fyftem of government or religion; and have ftudied to bend the evidence of facts, to the accomplifhment of that purpofe.

Thefe obfervations have arifen out of my enquiries, relative to peftilential difeafes. I have difcovered that many of the hiftories or rather abridgements and compilations which are almoft the only authorities confulted by American readers in general, are very incomplete, and no man who relies on them only, and neglects original writers, can acquire an accurate and comprehenfive knowledge of hiftory.

SECTION II.

Historical view of pestilential epidemics, and the phenomena in the physical world, which precede, attend or follow them, from the earliest accounts, to the Christian era.

IT is an agreed point that the five books of Moses are the most ancient authentic history now extant. In the very threshhold of this genuine history, we meet with accounts of the plague in Egypt. In the fifth chapter of Exodus, the pestilence is mentioned as a formidable calamity.

It is remarkable, that throughout the history of the Jews, and in the prophets, *pestilence*, *famin* and *the sword* are often mentioned in connection with each other, and described as the most dreadful calamities that can befal mankind. It will probably appear that famin and pestilential diseases do at times reciprocally produce each other, and that war not unfrequently occasions both. But there is ground to believe that famin and pestilence are usually the effects of one common cause. In the Bible, as in other ancient writings, no distinction is made between general pestilence which spreads over whole countries, and those autumnal epidemics, which are evidently produced by powerful local causes. There are however many passages in scripture that corroborate the principles respecting pestilence, which are still observed, and which doubtless depend on established laws of nature.

When David was summoned to receive his punishment for numbering the children of Israel, he was permitted to elect one of the three calamities, famin, the sword or pestilence. For a pious reason, he preferred pestilence, and seventy thousand of his subjects perished.

2 Sam xxiv.

The prophets Jeremiah and Ezekiel, in their denunciations, speak often of these three judgments, and in a way that authorizes the opinion, that they considered them all to be closely connected. It is however remarkable that pestilence is every where mentioned as the peculiar scourge of *cities*.

In the 21st chapter of Jeremiah, the siege of Jerusalem is foretold. " I will smite the inhabitants of this *city*, both man and beast ; they shall die with a great pestilence. He that abideth in this *city*, shall die by the sword, by the famin and by the pestilence ; but he that goeth out, and falleth to the Chaldeans that besiege you, *he shall live*, and his life shall be to him for a prey "

Ezekiel v. 12. declares that a *third part* of the inhabitants of Jerusalem shall die by pestilence. This is a proportion which is not uncommon, in violent plagues. In the seventh chapter, the same prophet says, " The sword is *without*, and the pestilence and famin *within* ; he that is in the field, shall die with the sword ; and he that is in the *city*, famin and pestilence shall devour him."

Another passage in the same prophet deserves notice. Chap. xxxiii, it is said, " Thus saith the Lord, as I live, surely they that are in the wastes shall fall by the sword, and him that is in the open field will I give to the beasts to be devoured, and they that be in the *forts* and the *caves* shall die of the pestilence.".

In these passages, we have proof that in the time of these prophets, it was considered as a well known fact, that pestilential diseases are the effect of crouded propulation, raging peculiarly in *cities*, *forts* and other confined places. No evidence appears, in these early records, that the ancients, who lived in countries subject to plague, and near to Egypt, had any idea of the conveyance of the distemper from place to place by infection. It was considered as a judgment of heaven ; and piety still recognizes this idea ; to which, in a moral and religious view, there can be no objection. But philosophy endeavors to trace the hand of heaven through the medium of second causes ; and the facts re-

D

corded of pestilence in scripture, lend their aid to accomplish the object.

In 1 Samuel v. and vi. we have an account of the pestilence among the Philistines, inflicted on them as a punishment for taking the ark from the Jews, in which fifty thousand of the inhabitants of Beth shemesh perished. This plague is called *emerods* and a *deadly destruction*. This passage is noted on account of the specification of the time of the year, when the disease prevailed. It is said, the ark was in the country of the Philistines *seven months*, and was returned, during wheat-harvest, soon after which it is understood, the plague ceased. Now wheat harvest, in Syria, is in May; and it may be supposed, the pestilence was most violent in the period next preceding that time, viz. April, or during the month of May, for it was the severity of the disease which induced them to send back the ark.—This account corresponds with the modern course of pestilence in that country. It appears in February or March, increases till May or June, then gradually disappears.

See A. Russel. Hist. of Aleppo. P. Russel on the plague at Aleppo.

In this case, modern facts confirm the accuracy of the scripture-history; at the same time, they establish the identity of the disease with modern plague, and the uniformity in the operations of the laws of nature. They prove further that the climate of that country has suffered no material alteration.

In the eleventh chapter of Numbers, we have an account of a plague among the Israelites, occasioned by their eating great quantities of the flesh of quails, after being some time destitute of animal food—an obvious effect in the hot climates of Egypt and Arabia.

The scripture-history also furnishes us with ample proof that Egypt was, in early times, the nursery of plague—known and considered as such, centuries before the foundation of Smyrna, Constantinople, or other large cities in Greece or Asia Minor.

In Deuteronomy xxviii. the Israelites are warned against disobedience to the laws of Moses, and in case of disregarding them, are threatened with the *diseases of Egypt*, the botch, the emerods and the scab. These are still prevailing disorders in that country under the names of leprosy, elephantiasis, plague, &c. In verse 60 of the same chapter, it is denounced, "Moreover he shall bring upon thee *all the diseases of Egypt*, of which thou wast afraid."

Amos iv. 10. "I have sent among you the *pestilence*, after the manner of *Egypt*."

These authorities of high antiquity leave no room for doubt or controversy, on the question, whether Egypt originates the plague. The evidence is decisive against those modern superficial philosophers, who hold in contempt the most authentic ancient history, because it has claims to inspiration. Yet infidels, if they were not too wise to read, examin and be informed, might be convinced of the authenticity of the scripture history, by comparing the facts related, with the present state of the world. The present endemical and other diseases which often occur in Egypt, answer so exactly to the description given of them in the books of Moses, as to leave no room to question the genuineness of those books. It was the peculiar climate of Egypt, and the usual prevalence of scorbutic and malignant complaints, in that country, which occasioned all the minute injunctions of Moses, in regard to washing, cleansing and purifications. The same or similar regulations were enjoined by the laws of Egypt *

---

* It has been controverted whether Moses borrowed his system of purification from the institutions which he found in Egypt, or whether the Egyptians borrowed the idea from the laws of Moses. Nothing can be more idle than such a dispute. The experience of men would very readily suggest the necessity and utility of great cleanliness, to preserve health in the climate of Egypt. The custom of circumcision was established among the Egyptians, as well as among the Israelites; and Herodotus, who visited Egypt to collect facts, expressly declares that the "Egyptians circumcised their children for the sake of cleanliness."—There is not the least reason to suppose that the Egyptians borrowed this custom, or others respecting cleanliness, from the Israelites. Nor does it vary the question, that the laws of Moses were the commands of God. Divine commands have rarely introduced a new principle of right and wrong. Most of them are injunctions on man to conform to principles of moral fitness or utility, which existed *anterior to the commands*. They *unfold* to human view, and *enforce* the practice of those principles; but do not *create* them. They add the strong authority of *positive*, to the feebler authority of *implied* divine will, and are thus of the highest importance to mankind.

In the Bible alfo we find evidence of the prevalence of peftilent epidemics among cattle. A murrain is among the ten plagues mentioned in Exodus, and Ezekiel xiv. 21 fays, " If I fend a peftilence into that land, to cut off from it man and beaft."

We find the fame fact in Homer; where alfo we obferve peftilence afcribed to extreme heat, under the allegorical name of Apollo, or the fuppofed influence of the dog-ftar.

" On mules and dogs, the infection firft began,
And laft the vengeful arrows fixed in man."

" But let fome prophet, or fome facred fage,
Explore the caufe of great Apollo's rage."

" If broken vows this heavy curfe have laid,
Let altars fmoke, and hecatombs be paid;
So heaven atoned fhall dying Greece reftore,
And Phœbus dart his burning fhafts no more."

Pope's Verfion. Iliad 1 69, 83, 87.

In the following paffage, peftilence is afcribed to heat and fouth winds, according to the opinion of Hippocrates.

As vapors blown by Aufter's fultry breath,
Pregnant with plagues, and fhedding feeds of death;
Beneath the rage of burning Syrius rife—
Book 5. 1058.

" Like the red Star, that from his flaming hair,
Shakes down difeafes, peftilence and war."
Book 19. 412 *

* This evidently alludes to the received opinion among the ancients, that comets have an influence in producing peftilence In the courfe of this work, we fhall have fome grounds to determin which is moft correct, this opinion of antiquity, or that of the moderns who hold it in contempt

It is to be obferved that the idea of comets producing difeafes, is not in Homer, in the paffage from which thefe lines are taken, but is a licence of the tranflator, Mr. Pope, and the fenfe and almoft the words, are borrowed from Milton Book 2. l 710.

" ———— And like a comet burn'd
In th' arctic fky, and from his horrid hair,
Shakes peftilence and war."

" Not half so dreadful rises to the sight,
Through the thick gloom of some tempestuous night,
Orion's dog (the year when autumn sways)
And o'er the feebler stars exerts his rays :
Terrific glory ! for his burning breath,
Taints the red air, with fevers, plagues and death."

Book 22. 37.

The circumstances to be noted in the foregoing extracts, are, first that the pestilence among cattle *preceded* that among men. This is a common fact, but not always the case. Secondly, that heat and moisture, with a south wind were productive of pestilential diseases. Thirdly, that such diseases raged in Greece during the autumnal season, and were ascribed to the influence of Syrius, or the dog-star.

We read of a terrible pestilence in the island of Ægina, to the southward of Athens, in the reign of Æacus, grandfather of Achilles, about sixty years before the Trojan war ; a plague which depopulated the island. Of this calamity, Ovid has given a most affecting account Metam. lib. 7. 523. He represents the earth as covered with clouds, darkness and suffocating heat, the south wind blowing for four months, the lakes and fountains being infected, and the earth overspread with poisonous serpents. The disease first invaded dogs, birds, sheep and oxen ; then mankind. Death was sudden ; and the streets loaded with dead carcases. The symptoms began with heat in the bowels, flushings of the face, difficulty of breathing, &c. How far the poet was authorized by history in this description, I do not know ; but the whole passage is worth the attention of the learned reader.

It is certain however that the ancients believed comets to be the cause of pestilential diseases.

It is further remarkable that, in the pestilential period to which Homer here alludes, which happened during the siege of Troy, Etna was in a state of eruption, or rather at the close of the period. For Eneas, when driven from Troy, sailed with his fellow citizens to Sicily, but was frightened away by a violent explosion of Etna. See a forcible description of this eruption in Virgil lib. 3.

Dyonisius Hallicarnaffus informs us that the Pelasgi, who settled in Sicily, soon after the Trojan war, were affected with pestilence. Book 1.

Our next accounts of the plague are in the hiftories of Rome; for altho Greece contained the older ftates, and had large cities, before the foundation of Rome; yet the moft populous parts of Greece, Attica and Lacedemon, are dry, rocky countries; not calculated to generate peftilence nor to favor its propagation.

Rome, on the other hand, is fituated in a level country, on the banks of a river, and not far from extenfive marfhes. Under the influence of powerful local caufes, this city felt every derangement of the atmofphere, by intemperate feafons, or other caufes.

The firft plague in Rome happened about the 16th year from its foundation, foon after the murder of Tatius, and in time of peace. "It killed inftantly without any previous ficknefs. Even trees and cattle were not exempt from the malignity of its influence; but all nature lay one defolate and abandoned wafte. It was even faid to rain blood." This was 738 years before the Chriftian era.

Plutarch's life of Romulus

Zonaras fays that Rome was laid wafte by difeafe, and the earth and cattle were barren. "Sterilitas agrorum et pecudum."

Lib 7.

This peftilence muft have been of the moft malignant kind, and by the effect on cattle and trees, it was obvioufly during a peftilential ftate of the atmofphere, when there was a defect in the powers of vegetable as well as animal life—many fimilar inftances will occur in the courfe of this hiftory. It is to be remarked that Rome was then in its infant ftate, containing few people, and few of the artificial caufes of difeafe. Of courfe the ficknefs muft have been caufed by general contagion, or that ftate of air which is unfavorable to the prefervation of healthy life.

In the reign of Numa Pompilius A. R. 46, Italy was afflicted with fevere peftilence; on which occafion Numa inftituted the Salii, twelve dancers who had the care of the brazen target, which was fuppofed to defcend from heaven into the hands of

Numa, and to check the pestilence. See the institution and annual ceremonies of the Salii, described in

Plutarch's life of Numa, and
Kennet's Antiquities, part 2 b 2.

Another plague attacked Rome in the reign of Tullius Hostilius, about the year 110 or 112, and B. C. about 640. No important particulars are related, except that the sickness relaxed the martial spirit of the citizens. To prevent this effect, that warlike prince gave the soldiers no rest, judging " salubriora militiæ, quam domi, juvenum corpora esse," that the young men would be more healthy in the army abroad, than at home.

Livy b 1. 32.

In this opinion, the King of Rome was probably well founded; for it appears from facts hereafter to be related, that Rome was most subject to pestilence in time of peace, when the soldiers were at Rome, augmenting the population of the city, and indulging in ease and luxury.

In the reign of Tarquin, the last King of Rome, about the year 240 and B. C. 514 a violent plague infested the city. Zosimus however places this event, after the expulsion of Tarquin.

Hook, vol 1. 109   Zosimus lib 2.

In the year of Rome 261, there was a famin and pestilence in the city, and the plague depopulated Velitræ, a city of the Volsci, who applied to the Romans for inhabitants to re-people the place.

Muratori. Tom 1. 5. Hook, vol. 1. 196   Functius Chronol.

Soon after this, we read of a contagious distemper among cattle, but not very fatal.

Dion Hal lib. 7.

In the year of Rome 281 and B. C. 473, a plague raged in the city and country, but was most fatal in the city, sparing no age nor sex, and yielding to no remedies. It came suddenly and suddenly disappeared.*

Dion Hal lib 1.

---

* This account seems to contradict the doctrin of a *progression* in the pestilential principle   Thucydides remarks also that the plague invaded Athens suddenly. Such is the effect of superficial observation. So in 1794, the people of New-York alledged the city to be very healthy; when in fact the bill of mortality was higher by one fourth than

There was an eruption of Etna, according to common chronology, in the year of Rome 277, and B. C. 477. This circumstance is strong evidence that the chronology is not quite correct. The eruption took place unquestionably during the pestilential period, to which this plague in Rome belonged. It might not have been the very year of the plague in Rome, but probably was not so distant as four years. To which event, the plague or the eruption, a wrong era is assigned, I shall not determin. The early history of Rome, from the destruction of the ancient records, by the burning of the city, when taken by the Gauls under Brennus, in the year 365, is subject to great uncertainty, and authors do not agree on the chronology of that part of the Roman story.

☞ Since writing the foregoing remarks, I have discovered a fact which may serve to aid us in fixing the period of the events abovementioned. In the course of this work it will be proved beyond doubt, that the approach of comets to our system, has a prodigious influence on the elements of this globe. At present I shall assume the fact, that the eruption of Etna abovementioned, was nearly cotemporary with the appearance of a comet, during this period of pestilence. In looking into Pliny's Natural History, lib. 2. ca. 25, I find that a comet was visible, at the time of the battle of Salamis. Speaking of the different species of comets he says " Ceratias Cornus speciem habet, qualis fecit cum Græcia apud Salamina depugnavit " " A comet in the figure of a javelin, like that which appeared when Greece fought at Salamis " This battle is fixed by authors in the year B. C. 480, and consequently in the year of Rome, by common chronology 274. It appears to be a general law of nature that the approach of comets to this earth, calls into action the subterranean fire, and volcanoes discharge their contents, during or within a few months of the appearance of comets. We may safely conclude therefore that the eruption was within a year

---

usual. So the invasion of New-London by the fever in 1798 appeared to be *sudn*, altho in fact the bills of mortality show a most sensible increase in the force of the destructive principle, two years previous to the attack.

or two of the battle of Salamis. This is not certain, but probable, and I am inclined therefore to believe that Hook and others have placed the plague in Rome three or four years too late, or that the eruption is placed too early.†

The army of Xerxes, retreating into Asia, after the loss of the engagement near Salamis, suffered extremely by pestilential diseases. And it will hereafter appear that during periods when the pestilential state of air is evidenced by the existence of plague in *cities*, armies in the field and seamen on the ocean are much more subject to epidemic complaints, than at other times.

The land forces which Xerxes left behind him under Mardonius, fell a prey to famin and pestilence. The highways were strewed with dead bodies, and wild fowls and beasts devoured them.

The same period was distinguished by tempests and inundations—the constant attendants on comets. A violent storm had destroyed the famous bridge built by the great monarch over the Hellespont, before he returned from Greece; and while the troops under Mardonius were besieging Potidea, an inundation of the sea broke into their trenches, drowned some soldiers, and compelled them to raise the siege.

Herodotus lib. 8. 115, 129. Justin lib. 2. cap. 13.

These great phenomena, without any historical account, would make it nearly certain that a comet appeared at that time, and the pestilence undoubtedly happened within a short period of its approach.

A more terrible pestilence invaded the Roman city and territory, in the year 290, and B. C. 464. Several facts in regard to it, deserve particular notice. " Grave tempus et forte annus pestilens erat urbi, agrisque, nec hominibus magis, quam pecori; et auxere vim morbi, tenore pupulationis, pecoribus agrestibusque, in urbem acceptis. Ea colluvio mixtorum omnis generis animantium, et odore insolito urbanos, et agrestem confertum in arcta tec-

† Brydone mentions an eruption in the 77th Olympiad, comprehending the years of Rome from 282 to 285 inclusive, which is doubtless the same abovementioned

ta, æstu ac vigiliis angebat, ministeriaque in vicem ac contagio ipsa vulgabant morbos."

Livy. lib. 3 6 Dion Hal lib. 10.

" This was an unhealthy time and a pestilent year in town and country, affecting equally men and cattle ; and the disease was augmented by crouds of countrymen and herds of cattle, which were received within the walls of the city, for fear of being plundered or destroyed [by the Latins and Hernici, who then ravaged the country.] That collection of all kinds of animals in the city, and the unusual stench occasioned by them, severely affected both the citizens and the country people, crouded into close buildings, depressed by heat and watching ; and their fatigue and the contagion spread the sickness into every quarter."

This is Livy's representation. Dionysius Hallicarnassus mentions that the disease seized *studs* of mares, *herds* of oxen, and *flocks* of goats and sheep ; by which expressions we are perhaps to understand, that the distemper either did not seize those animals, except in collections, or was remarkably fatal to them in numerous bodies—an idea warranted by modern facts. It is generally true of cattle as of men, that pestilential diseases are most destructive, where many are collected together ; not only by reason of infection from the diseased, but by the diminution of the vital principle of the air by respiration and perspiration.

Orosius lib. 2. 12. adds other circumstances. He says there was a short suspension of war, when a grievous pestilence, which never failed to compel the Romans to a truce, or to interrupt it, if made, raged violently through all the city. Many of the patricians were victims, but it was most fatal to the poor.

It is stated that this pestilence began about the calends of September and raged in city and country. By country, *agris*, the Roman writers meant the ancient Latium, the modern Compagna di Roma, which was naturally unhealthy ; tho, in the flourishing ages of Rome, extremely populous.

That the Roman territory should be subject to autumnal complaints, is not at all surprising. At the port of the Tyber there were unwholesome marshes, called by Tacitus, Annals 15. 43. " Ostienses paludes." The shore to the southward, bordering Campania, is called by the same historian, " squalente littore." To the southward of Campania were and still are the extensive marshes, called " paludes pomptinæ," which are so noxious as to create disease in a single night, and which have caused the Appian way in modern times to be neglected, and the road to Naples to be carried round the marshes on the east.*

The territory next to the city of Rome is described by Livy, b. 7. 38. in these words " in pestilente atque arido circa urbem solo"—a dry plain, but indented with lakes, bordered with marshes, and subject to be overflowed by every uncommon rise of the Tyber, or by streams from the distant hills. Many epidemic diseases have been distinctly traced to stagnant waters on this plain, after an inundation.

Avernus, a lake of Campania, near Baiæ, emitted such a poisonous vapor, that no birds would frequent its banks, and the ancients, in their flights of fancy called it, the road to Hell.

It was this situation of Rome which gave rise to the Cloacæ, immense sewers or drains, which penetrated the city and neighborhood—Vast works intended to drain off the stagnant waters; and while these were preserved in good repair, the city was obviously more healthy.

This plague in the year 290 proved fatal to both of the Consuls Servilius and Æbutius, to many illustrious Romans, and to a countless number of the Plebeians. The Senate and people, in des-

---

* In the epitome of the 46th book of Livy, which book is among those which are lost, I find it related that the Pontine Marshes were drained or dyked [ficcatæ] and converted into cultivable land, by the Consul Cornelius Cethegus, about the year of Rome 572. The Romans were convinced that the marshes were very unwholesome, and they took incredible pains to render their city and territory healthful, by draining off all stagnant waters.

It is much to be regretted that we have not this book of Livy, to give us further information in what manner the draining of the marshes was effected It is considered by the moderns as impracticable.

The opinion of the ancients as to the unhealthfulness of Rome may be understood from the following Tetrastichon, which is preserved by Baronius.

" Roma vorax hominum, domat ardua colla virorum ;
Roma ferax febrium, necis est uberrima frugum ;
Romanæ febres stabili sunt jure fideles ;
Quem semel invadunt, vix a viventi recedent "

The brief translation of which is " Rome subdues men by the sword, and kills them with fevers "

Horace book 2. ode 29. gives to the Tyber, the epithet *udus*, wet or marshy.

pair had recourfe to prayers and fupplications, the temples were filled with men, women and children, afking forgivenefs and favor of heaven.

This violent plague was followed, anno Urb Con. 292 by a violent earthquake. "Terra ingenti concuffa motu eft," fays Livy, lib. 3. ca. 10. He exprefsly mentions this to have been in the confulate of P. Volumnius and Serv. Sulpicius, which was the fecond Confulate after the peftilence. An eruption of Etna is mentioned in the tables under the year of Rome 288, two years before the peftilence and four years before the earthquake. But there is probably a fmall variation in the chronology. The earthquake was probably at the time of the eruption, efpecially as Livy mentions, that in the fame year, "Cœlum ardere vifum," the heavens appeared to be in a flame.

Functius places thefe events one year later.

By this earthquake Locris, on the gulf of Corinth, was rent from the main land and turned into an ifland. Afterwards Locris was deftroyed by another earthquake.

Severe drouth marked this period.

In the year of Rome 300 according to Livy and the common chronology and B. C. 454, another terrible peftilence invaded Rome. The country was defolated, and the citizens were exhaufted with continual burials. "Urbs affiduis exhaufta funeribus." Famin accompanied this calamity, and cattle were victims, as well as men. This plague took place in time of peace —"ab hofte otium fuit," and in the abfence of the ambaffadors who were fent to Athens to collect the laws of Solon and the Grecian inftitutions.

Livy b 3 32.

With this period correfponds an eruption of Etna, which authors place in the year of Rome 304; of courfe, it was at the clofe of the peftilential period.

In the year 315 of Rome and B. C. 439, according to Paulus Diaconus, tremendous earthquakes fhook Italy at intervals for a whole year, fo that "affiduis Roma, nuntiis fatagaretei," Rome was fatigued with meffengers who were continually arriving with news of towns and villages demolifhed.

The chronology of P. Diaconus rarely agrees with that commonly received. The earthquakes here mentioned probably ushered in the long and formidable calamity which was to follow—and were probably cotemporary with the beginning of the plague next to be mentioned.

In the year of Rome 317, and B. C. 437 commenced a pestilential state that afflicted Rome for five years, or five seasons successively. The historian relates that the first year " a pestilence invaded the people," and as the disease increased, prodigies alarmed them and frequent earthquakes overturned houses in the country. The next year the disease was more mortal: " pestilentior inde annus." In 320, the disease was so fatal as to suspend all ordinary concerns. The people resorted to their prayers, and the Sybilline books were consulted and obeyed, to appease the Gods and avert the plague from the people. For fear of famin, corn was purchased in Etruria, the Pontine territory and in Sicily. The mortality extended also to cattle. In 321, the disease was mitigated and afterwards subsided.

Livy b 4 21, 25.

This is the first instance, in which I am able to trace distinctly a *progression* in the malignancy of the plague. That this is an important fact, in all plagues, will hereafter appear. But on this point, ancient history affords very scanty materials. This was a period of universal pestilence for many years, and was marked with all the great phenomena of nature. The last year of the plague in Rome 321, corresponds with the year B. C. 433, two years before the plague of Athens. In the year of Rome 325, according to Hook, there was a most grievous famin, occasioned by a severe drouth in all the Roman territory. " Siccitas eo anno plurimum laboratum est; nec cælestes modo defuerunt aquæ, sed terra quoque, ingenito humore egens, vix ad perrennes subfecit amnes." By this, we are led to believe, that the drouth was not solely caused by a want of rain, but by an unusual defect of subterranean springs and moisture. The expression, " ingenito humore egens," contrasted with the usual source of water, rain, evidently carries with it an idea that the evaporation from the earth was *unusual;* and this may easily be accounted for, by the violent action of internal heat or electricity which diftinguifhed this peftilential period, and was evidenced by tremendous and univerfal earthquakes, and a great eruption of Etna.

The drouth in Rome was extreme—multitudes of cattle thronged round the arid fountains, and perifhed with thirft. Difeafes followed, firft invading cattle, and the lower claffes of people and the countrymen, then extending to the city.

Livy b 4 30

Thucydides relates b 1 and 3, that earthquakes affected the largeft part of the globe, and fhook it with the utmoft violence. In many places, there was fevere drouth and a fubfequent famin. In fome places, the earthquakes produced alarming inundations of the fea, as in Euboea and Atalanta—the Prytaneum, or town-houfe in Athens, the fortifications and fome dwelling-houfes were demolifhed. Thefe events were in the fifth and fixth years of the Peloponnefian war, anfwering to 427 and 426 B. C. and confequently were at the clofe, or fubfequent to the peftilence. About the fame time there was a violent eruption of Etna; fuch as had not been known for fifty years preceding. This period was alfo marked by the approach of a comet, but I am not clear that it was in the year B. C. 431, as ftated by Dr. Prieftley in his Lectures on Hiftory. The drouth was probably within a few months of the appearance of the comet, according to numerous obfervations in late periods of the world: By which it would feem to be a law of the phyfical fyftem, that *preceeding*, *during* and *following* the approach of thofe erratic bodies, this earth is affected alternately with great rains and fnows, drouth, violent tempefts, high tides and earthquakes: Many inftances will hereafter occur.*

* We are fometimes embarraffed with the differences in the chronology of different authors. But we have, in this place, data that will fix certain points.

From the uniform operations of nature, there can be very little doubt, that all the great events of the phyfical world, in this period, happened within twelve or eighteen months of each other. The extreme drouth in Italy and Greece, mentioned by Livy and Thucydides, unqueftionably occurred, at both places, in the fame year. Livy places this under the confulfhip of A. Cornelius Coffus and T Quinctius Pennus, which Hook arranges under the 325th year of Rome, and Lempriere, under the 327th

Now Thucydides exprefsly relates, that the great earthquake which injured Athens, and produced the inundations in the Corinthian Gulf

The plague in Athens broke out in the second year of the Peloponnesian war, when all the inhabitants of the Athenian territory, were crouded into the city, to avoid the destructive ravages of the Lacedemonians. This circumstance alone would account for the production of pestilential diseases in the city. But it is probable that had the same event happened in a period of general health, the sickness in Athens would have been limited to the dysentery, the more violent camp fevers or common typhus.

But unfortunately this war broke out at a time of universal pestilence, when the diseases of the healthiest countries assume new and more malignant symptoms, and hence we account for the duration and the violence of the malady. This idea seems to be important, and the only material one to be added to the excellent philosophical account of the plague at Athens by Dr. Elihu H. Smith, late of New-York. Medical Repository, vol. 1, art. 1. The origin of this pestilence is stated by the historian to have been in that part of Ethiopia which borders on Egypt; thence extending to Egypt, Lybia, the King's dominions or Persia, and to Greece. Some of the more violent of modern plagues have first appeared in the same region. But we are not to conclude from this description that the disease is propagated by infection from person to person. It appears first where

and the Sea of Euboea, rending Atalanta from the main land, and swallowing up a town in Euboea, happened in the spring or summer of the sixth year of the Peloponnesian war. This war commenced in the second or third year of the eighty-seventh Olympiad, corresponding with the years of Rome 323 or 324. The sixth year then will be the 328th or 329th year of Rome. These data bring the drouth in Rome to one of those years, at least they will not admit of its being placed earlier than the year 327, the year preceding the earthquake. It is probable therefore that Lempriere is right, in the arrangement of the consuls. This is rendered more probable, by the eruption of Etna, in the spring of the same year; as it is a known and common fact, that earthquakes and eruptions of volcanoes are preceded by excessive drouth, owing probably to a gradual increase of subterranean heat, or unusual electrical discharges and evaporation, some weeks, or months, before the explosion.

The comet undoubtedly appeared either in the year, preceding, during or following the drouth, that is, in the year of Rome, 327, 328, or 329, corresponding with year before the Christian era, 427, 426, or 425. It was most probably in the year of the drouth, and in the fifth year of the war, A U C. 327, and B. C. 427; the earthquakes and volcanoe followed in the spring of the next year.

the original or secondary causes, that is, general and local contagion, are the most powerful. If the state of the atmosphere over the world, at any one time, is equally vitiated by some unknown cause, its effects will first appear in places where that state of air is most powerfully aided by *local* vitiation, as in cities or marshy grounds. Of this we have numerous proofs. But, in modern times, whenever the general contagion, united with local causes, produces plague in Egypt or Constantinople, it produces some milder epidemic in the neighboring countries, and often, its effects are visible, at the same time, in most parts of the world.

The Abbe Barthelemy, in his elegant Travels of Anacharsis, speaking of the plague in Athens, says, " it was doubtless bro't into Greece by a vessel from Egypt." It is to be regretted that such an accurate and judicious writer should have indulged *conjecture* on this interesting subject. He quotes no authority for his opinion, and the words of Thucydides oppose the supposition. The disease first appeared in the Piræus, the harbor; and so ignorant were the people of the cause, that they ascribed it to the poisoning of the wells by the Lacedemonians. Besides Thucydides impliedly acknowledges that he and others knew nothing of its origin; for he calls on " every one, physician or not, to assign any credible account of its rise, or the causes powerful enough to produce it."

Plutarch, in his life of Pericles, says " the enemies of Pericles, attributed this disaster to the multitude of people he had collected into the city, during the heat of summer"—a charge in which there was much truth.

But when we attend to the violent concussions of nature, that accompanied and followed the pestilence, and its general prevalence in the world for a series of ten or twelve years, all attempts to trace its origin to infection, dwindle into puerilities, and the occasional causes of sickness, crouded population, heat and bad diet, tho powerful as auxiliaries, could not be adequate to the violent and continued effects in Athens, and the neighboring cities.

The symptoms of that disease in Athens, as described by Thucydides, are known to every medical man. They correspond in all the essential particulars, with those of the Yellow Fever in its worst forms, and the disease was probably what I call the bilious plague. There is the more reason to believe this supposition, as Thucydides has not mentioned, among the symptoms, the buboes and other swellings of the glands, which distinguish the inguinal plague. The critical days were the seventh or ninth, as they have most frequently been in the bilious plague in America.

The disease extended to other towns in Attica, especially to those which were most populous, but Lacedemon escaped. It raged in Persia at the same time, and it is said, the King of Persia sent for Hippocrates to lend his aid in arresting the progress of the pestilence, but the latter declined leaving his own country.

It has been supposed that Hippocrates was in Athens during this plague; but this must be a mistake. He was probably at Thasus, an island, near the coast of Macedonia. The four epidemic years, which he has described, were cotemporary with the pestilence in Athens; and this proves what will hereafter appear more fully, that in all great plagues, the epidemic or pestilential principle extends to different countries, and often over the whole earth.

In this pestilence, as we shall have occasion to observe in many subsequent instances, the birds abandoned the infected atmosphere.

In the year of Rome 341, and B. C. 413, a pestilence arose which the historian represents as more alarming than fatal, " minacior tamen quam perniciosior." This circumstance affords ground to believe the pestilence to have been a violent autumnal bilious fever, and not rising to the utmost malignity of the plague.

The pestilence of that year was *follow'd* by famin in the next; owing to a neglect of agriculture; the people having been principally occupied with sedition, under their ambitious demagogues. It will be remarked that the famin was not the cause of the epidemic, for it succeeded it.

Livy, lib. 4. 52.

It is proper to remark here that all the preceding deadly plagues which had at times almost defolated Rome, were certainly the produce of the country. The Romans were not a commercial people, nor had they any commercial intercourfe with Egypt, till the conqueft of Carthage, two centuries and a half after this period. It was not till one hundred and forty feven years after the time now under confideration, that the Romans owned a fingle fhip When they tranfported troops into Sicily, they hired or borrowed veffels for the purpofe Egypt was a granary of corn, but until after the conqueft of Carthage, the Romans drew their fupplies wholly from Italy and Sicily. There is no pretence therefore for fuppofing the plague ever imported into Rome; nor is there a fuggeftion in hiftory, that its origin was ever afcribed to that fource.

In the year of Rome 353, and B. C. 401, happened a moft fevere winter. The Tyber was frozen over, and the high-ways rendered impaffible by deep fnow. Thefe were unufual phenomena and deemed prodigies in that city. On the opening of fpring, the weather changed fuddenly from fevere cold to great heat and drouth, and a mortal peftilence enfued among men and cattle. The hiftorian fays nothing more of the caufe of the mortality, than "Sive ex intemperie cœli, raptim ex mutatione in contrarium facta, five alia qua de caufa, gravis peftilenfque omnibus animalibus æftas excepit, cujus infanabili pernicie quando nec caufa nec finis inveniebatur, libri Sibillini ex fenatus confulto aditi funt." On this melancholy occafion was inftituted the ceremony of the Lectifternium to appeafe the Gods and folicit the reftoration of health.

Livy b 5 13 14 15 Plut Life of Camillu.. Zofimus lib 2

With this period of peftilence correfponds the dreadful plague which about 404 B C. almoft depopulated Carthage. The difeafe on the coaft of Africa preceded its appearance in Rome, as it ufually does in modern times.

Soon after, the Carthaginians under Imilco, who were fent to reduce Sicily which had revolted, were feized with the plague and the army was fo weakened, that Imilco was compelled to abandon the ifland. Juft before Imilco's arrival, an eruption of

Etna laid waste the neighboring country. By an expression of Justin, we have ground to believe a comet appeared about the same time. " Imilco, qui multas civitates cepisset, repente *pestilentis sideris vi*, exercitum amisit."

Justin lib 19 c 2 Diod Sc lib 13 14 Rol An Hist b 2 and 11.

This plague was remarkable for its symptoms, such as violent dysenteries, raging fevers, burning entrails, acute pains in every part of the body; and many were seized with madness, so that they sallied forth into the streets, and tore to pieces those who fell in their way.

It was during the dry season above mentioned that the Lake of Alba rose suddenly, without apparent cause, and overflowed its banks—an event that caused great consternation in Rome, but one that might well happen by a subterranean discharge of some water-fountains in the high adjoining hills.

This is one of the instances which will often occur, of a hard winter, followed by a dry hot summer, and therefore deserves particular notice, for such excesses in the temperature of the seasons are among the causes of pestilential diseases.

A pestilence broke out in the armies of the Romans and Gauls, while the latter, under Brennus, were besieging Rome, Anno Romæ 361, B. C. 393. The Gauls, unaccustomed to such heat, and placed between hills, where they were exposed to a burning sun, vapor and smoke, perished in such multitudes, that, weary with burying dead bodies, the survivors burnt them in piles.

Livy b 5 48

Pliny, lib. 2. 26, mentions the appearance of a comet, or light in the heavens, called by the Greeks *docus* or *doces*, and by the Romans *trabs*, from its resemblance to a beam, at the time of the defeat of the Lacedemonian fleet—" Cum Lacedemonii, classe victu, imperium Greciæ amisere," By the last expression, "the loss of the empire of Greece," I suppose he refers to the defeat of the fleet by Conon and the Persians in the year of Rome 360, and B. C. 394. If so, the appearance of this comet, corresponds in time with the period of pestilence last named.

A plague, occasioned by dearth, is mentioned to have happened in the year of Rome 371, B. C. 383, but no particulars, worthy of notice.

A great earthquake in Peloponnesus is mentioned under the year B. C. 373.

Encyclopedia, art. Chronology.

In the year of Rome 388, B. C. 366, commenced a most desolating plague of three years duration. This was a time of profound peace, " ab seditione et a bello quietis rebus, ne quando a metre ac periculis vacarent, pestilentia ingens orta." It seemed to be the destiny of Rome never to be exempt from fear and dangers; for when war and sedition ceased, pestilence arose.

Livy b 7 1

In this horrible plague, perished the great Camillus, and it is related that, in the height of the disease, 10,000 citizens died in a day.

On this occasion, recourse was had to the ceremony of the Lectisternium,* and to the institution of new games to appease the wrath of the Gods, but without success. Some old citizens mentioned an ancient practice, in such calamities, of driving a nail into the wall of a temple. This law was now revived, and a nail driven into the wall of Jupiter's temple. The time of the year, in which the law directed this ceremony to be performed, the *ides of September*, indicates the period when pestilence began in Rome to be alarming and violent.

Functius, in his chronology, assigns the absorption of Helice and Bura, two towns on the Gulf of Corinth, to the year of Rome 373, the year of the great earthquake in Lacedemon—in which case that catastrophe would make a part of the events of the pestilential period of 371, just mentioned.

Muratori and Paulus Diaconus seem not to differ essentially in arranging that event under the same period. " Sævissimo

---

* This ceremony consisted in placing the statues of Apollo, Latona, Diana, Hercules, Mercury, and Neptune, on three beds, and serving them with magnificent repasts for eight days—a mode of checking the pestilence, about as rational as the modern scheme of confining it to the infected place by bodies of armed men, which is much praised by Montesquieu!

terræmotu Achaia univerfa commota eft, et duæ tunc civitates, Bura et Helice, abruptis locorum devoratæ."

Muratori, Gen. Hift. vol. 1. 7.

Other authors refer this cataftrophe to the period of peftilence laft mentioned, which fome writers place in the year of Rome 388, and others, in 384; but all agree that it was during the approximation of a comet. This laft peftilence was dreadful in the extreme, fparing no age or fex. The year after it, the earth opened and exhibited a vaft chafm in the midft of Rome, into which M. Curtius precipitated himfelf for the falvation and profperity of the city.

Livy, b 7. 7.

P. Orofius and P Diaconus, followed by Muratori, place the commencement of this plague in the year of Rome 384. Orofius fays that " in the 103d and 105th Olympiad, Italy was fhaken a whole year, by tremendous earthquakes. The hundred and third Olympiad, according to our common chronology, comprehends the years of Rome from 386 to 389, inclufive. It is probable that in one of the fhocks of this feries of earthquakes, the chafm was made in Rome as already related. It will be obferved that this event *followed* the peftilence.

The comet that appeared, during this calamity, was probably that mentioned by Ariftotle, Meteorol. lib. 1. ca. 6, of which he was an eye-witnefs.

But I muft not omit what authors relate concerning the peculiar character of this plague. Orofius fays, it was not fuch a peftilence, as ufually proceeded from irregular feafons, extreme drouth, fudden heat of the fpring, unfeafonable moifture of fummer and autumn, or the impure air blown from the Calabrian groves; but fevere and continued, attacking all defcriptions of people, and either deftroying their lives, or leaving them in a weak and miferable condition.

The winter when the comet appeared Ariftotle relates to have been cold; but the feverity and duration of the plague cannot be accounted for on the principle of changes or irregularities in the feafons. It was one of thofe violent epidemics which never afflict mankind, without fome effential alteration in the invifible properties of the atmosphere, or a peculiar effect of the atmosphere on living bodies.

Seneca, on the authority of Aristotle and Calisthenes expressly ascribes the inundation to the approximation of a comet. "Cometes ingentis rei traxit eventus, cum Helicen et Burin orto suo merfit."

Nat Quest lib 7 16

The symptoms of this approaching calamity are described to have been these. "For several months the waters of heaven deluge the earth or withhold their beneficial effects; a dimness obscures the splendor of the sun; or his disk appears like a burning brazier; impetuous winds ravage the country; and streams of fire are seen to shoot in the air." See Travels of Anacharsis, vol. 3. 404, cited from Pausanius, lib. 7. ca. 24.

Some of these phenomena, excessive rains and drouth, tempests, celestial lights, and singular appearances of the sun, always attend the approach of comets; and it is surprising that the moderns have taken little or no notice of the fact.

The catastrophe of Helice and Bura was occasioned by violent shocks of earthquakes, with contrary and conflicting winds, which swelled the water in the Corinthian gulf, above the tops of trees on the shore. This was in the winter, during the night, and just before the battle of Leuctra. It is fortunate for us that we have a correct account of this inundation; for it perfectly unfolds the true history of the deluges in the time of Ogyges and Deucalion.

In the year of Rome 391, there was an extraordinary darkness in Italy, during the greatest part of the day; "dilata nox usque ad plurimam partem diei," and a singular hail storm.

Muratori, vol 1 11.

In the year of Rome 405 and B C. 349, a pestilence is mentioned, but with no circumstances that deserve notice, except that it was in time of peace and internal tranquillity. "Quum et foris pax et domi concordia ordinum otium esset, ne nimis lætæ res essent, pestilentia adorta"—and recourse was had to the Sybilline books and the Lectisturnium. The circumstance of the prevalence of plague in time of peace, will be often noted, to refute the idle notion, that pestilential difeafes are generated and propagated principally by armies in time of war.

☞ After writing the foregoing, I found in Pliny, Nat. Hift. lib 2. 25, an account of a comet in " the hundred and eighth Olympiad, and year of Rome 398." It refembled at firft a creft, but changed into the form of a fpear. Now, the firft year of the 108th Olympiad, according to common chronology, correfponds with the year of Rome 406. There is therefore a difference between the common mode of reckoning by the Olympiads, and Pliny's mode, of at leaft eight years or two Olympiads.—By following the common mode, and placing the firft year of the 108th Olympiad, againft the 406th year of Rome, the appearance of this comet will coincide with the general tenor of facts, hereafter to be related, and correfpond nearly in time with the plague in Rome, mentioned above.

Nearly at the fame time, there was an eruption of Etna, placed by authors in the year B. C. 350, correfponding with the year of Rome 404. It is probable this eruption was within a year or two of the appearance of the comet; according to many modern facts of the fame kind.

In the year of Rome 422, a violent plague arofe, which, fays P. Diaconus, was fuppofed to proceed from corrupt air, until the confpiracy of the Roman women to poifon their hufbands was detected, after which it was afcribed to that caufe. Livy does not appear to credit popular opinion on this occafion. He fays, " Fœdus infequens annus; feu intemperie Cæli, feu humana fraude fuit"—Recourfe was had to the ufual remedies, driving the nail, and the Lectifternium.

Livy b 8 18. Auguft Hift P Diac.

A peftilence again appeared in Rome in the year 440, but no particulars are ftated.

Livy 9 28.

In the year preceding, there was an inundation at Rhodes.

In the year of Rome 458, B. C. 296, commenced a moft fevere peftilence which continued for three or four years. In the third year, a hard winter appears to be related by Livy, who fays, " the fnow filled all places, nor was it poffible to endure the weather abroad." This was however in the mountainous country of the Samnites. The Roman confuls celebrated their triumphs over the Samnites, during this mortal epidemic, and it was a curious fpectacle to behold at the fame time, triumphal and funeral proceffions, and lamentations for the dead, mingled with acclamations of joy.

Orofius, b. 3 21 Livy, b 10 31 et feq

This plague commenced with many alarming prodigies, and violent tempefts. A remarkable cloud and extreme darknefs, for the greater part of a day, is mentioned by Livy, under favor of which the Samnites attacked the Roman lines. This darknefs is mentioned, on account of the frequency of the phenomenon, during peftilential periods.—Perhaps this appearance may be connected with the caufe of peftilence.

The violence and duration of this plague induced the Romans to fend to Epidaurus for Efculapius, which they imported in form of a ferpent, and in the ifland of the Tyber, where it was firft landed, they confecrated a temple to the God of Phyfic.

Livy, Epit 11.

It is not improbable, that the firft eruption of Lipari, recorded in hiftory, happened during this period; as it was in the reign of Agathocles, who died a few years after the time of this peftilence. The eruption is mentioned by the hiftorian Callias whofe works are loft; but the authors who cited them, have mentioned thefe particulars, that the eruption continued for feveral days, throwing great ftones to the diftance of a mile; and the fea boiling all round the ifland.

In the year of Rome 477, and B. C. 277, happened that remarkable plague which is often mentioned, as particularly fatal to pregnant women and breeding cattle. " Gravis peftilentia urbem ac fines ejus invafit; quæ, cum omnes, præcipue mulieres pecudefque corripiens, necatis in utero fœtibus, futura prole vacuabat."

Orofius, lib 4.

This alfo happened in time of peace. The words of the hiftorian are remarkable. " Sed Romanorum miferia nullis ceffat induciis. Confumitur morborum malis intercapedo bellorum; et cum foris ceſſatur a prœliis, agitur introrſum ira de cœlo." The miſeries of the Romans have no truce. The intervals between their wars are waſted with the calamities of ſickneſs ; and when they are exempt from war abroad, they are afflicted by the wrath of heaven at home.

Short on air has placed this diſeaſe in the year of the world 3712, correſponding with the year of Rome 462, but his chronology is often inaccurate.

In the year of Rome 482, a peſtilence broke out in Rome, and raged two or three years, carrying off countleſs multitudes of people. This was preceded by an eruption of fire at Calenum, which continued for three days and nights, deſtroying the ſoil for a conſiderable extent. This period alſo was diſtinguiſhed by earthquakes, in the third year of the peſtilence

Oroſius b. 4 P. Diaconus.

This period was memorable for a ſevere winter. The ſnow, to a prodigious depth, lay in the forum for forty days.

It will be found as we proceed with this hiſtory, that moſt of ſuch extraordinary ſeaſons and unuſual concurrence of great agitations in nature, happen during volcanic eruptions and the approach of comets to the ſolar ſyſtem of which this globe is a part. That comets were viſible, during the calamitous periods mentioned in the Roman hiſtory is probable ; but unfortunately few inſtances are recorded, until after the Chriſtian era.—Not an eruption of Veſuvius is mentioned, and I cannot find more than fourteen inſtances of eruptions from Etna, anterior to the ſame era. This defect of hiſtory is of no ſmall concern in a treatiſe of this kind.

In the year of Rome 529 and B. C. 225, the Roman armies which were marching into Gaul, were retarded by violent rains, and the plague which infected the ſoldiers. The Romans were, as uſual on ſuch occaſions, frightened at numerous prodigies. In Hetruria, uncommon lights were ſeen in the ſky. Meteors were ſeen at Ariminum, and the waters of a river in Picenum appeared like blood. A violent earthquake overturned the famous Colossus of Rhodes, and the shock was felt in Italy.*

Plut. Life of Marcellus. Orosius b 4 P. Diac. nus Muratori vol 1 16.

Some of the prodigies, mentioned by Roman historians, and which have been ridiculed by moderns who are too wise to study the operations of nature, and too proud to believe in extraordinary occurrences, will be hereafter explained.

During the battle near the Lake Thrasamene, a severe earthquake was experienced, which, it is said, the armies did not perceive. Pliny Nat. Hist. lib. 2. 84. This was in the year of Rome 536, and B. C. 218; in which year, Livy relates, b. 21. 61, there was a severe winter. Scipio was besieging a town in Spain, near the present Barcelona, and for thirty days, the snow was four feet deep. This is mentioned as a circumstance very unfavorable for the besiegers. I cannot help remarking how closely connected in time are great frosts and violent earthquakes. This was the winter in which Hannibal crossed the Alps and entered Italy. He reached the Alps early in November and was nine days in arriving to the summit. His army suffered incredible hardships and losses from deep snow, bad roads, and the natives who killed many of the troops. At the end of fifteen days, he gave his troops rest, on the hills near the foot of the Alps, and altho the snow was deep on the mountains, he found in the vales, pasturage for his horses and elephants. He prosecuted his route in the winter, suffering great hardships from snow, and more from rains, which swelled the rivers. Early in the spring he crossed the Appenine, and here his troops again suffered from a snow storm.

See Livy. lib. 21 Polybius, lib. 3

At the siege of Syracuse by Marcellus in the year of Rome 541 and B. C. 213, happened a remarkable mortality, among the troops, but especially among the Carthaginians, who all perished with their Generals, Hippocrates and Himilco. Of this pesti-

* The compilers of the Encyclopedia, Dufresnoy and Functius, place this event in the year B C. 224, and Rollin and Universal History in 222
Rome was overflowed, according to Universal History in 231 B C. This event may belong to the same period, but the compilers of that history differ in chronology from Hook and the common chronology which I have followed.

lence, Livy gives the following account, b. 25. 26. "A pestilence broke out in both armies, which diverted their minds from the concerns of the war; for it was in autumn, and in a situation naturally unhealthy. The heat, which was more severe without the city than within, affected almost every person in both the camps. At first, persons sickened and died, by reason of the unwholesomeness of the place; afterwards the diseases spread by infection, so that those who were seized, were neglected, or abandoned and died, or their attendants contracted the same disease. Daily burials and death were before their eyes, and day and night their ears were assailed with lamentations. At length the survivors became hardened; they neither grieved at the death of others, nor took pains to bury the dead; and the bodies of the deceased lay scattered along the streets, in sight of those who were expecting the same fate. The dead infected the sick, and the sick, those in health, with terror and pestiferous stench; and some, preferring death by the sword, rushed on the posts of the enemy.

But the disease was much more severe and fatal to the Carthaginians, than to the Romans, who, in this long siege, had become accustomed to the air and water. The Sicilian troops, on the first breaking out of the disease, abandoned their allies, and returned to their homes. The Carthaginians, who had no means of shelter, all perished. Marcellus, to avoid the evil, drew his troops into the city, where their enfeebled bodies were refreshed by the shades of the houses. Many however of the Roman army, died of the same disease."

It is observable that heat and position augmented the disease among the Carthaginians. They were encamped near a marsh or low ground; and exposed to the direct rays of a burning sun. The Romans had possession of one part of Syracuse, and had shelter under the buildings. These circumstances, and their not being accustomed to the air of the place, proved fatal to the whole Carthaginian army. Mr. Brydone learnt in Sicily from the historiographer of Etna, Recupero, that there was a great eruption of Etna, during this siege of Syracuse. I have not met with an account of it in the original histories I have consulted.

In the same year, that this pestilence raged in Syracuse, a severe pestilential epidemic prevailed in Rome. "Eo anno pestilentia gravis incidit in urbem, agrosque; quæ tamen magis in longos morbos, quam in perniciales, evasit."

Livy, 27 23.

This fact is evidence of what will be fully proved in later periods of the world, that a pestilential state of air extends, at the same time, over many parts of the world; and that if a violent plague is raging in one place, malignant diseases, if not plague, prevail in other places.

Another important fact related in the last quotation, is that the pestilence in Rome was the bilious plague, as it was not so mortal, as it was troublesome, by running out into long diseases.

It is a known fact and not unfrequent, that the Yellow Fever, in our climate, is reduceable to a bilious remittent and even to an intermittent, the pestilence on board the ships at Bulama often ran out into long and obstinate intermittents. The fever in Baltimore in 1797 began in the form of a bilious remittent, and continued in that form for many weeks, before it assumed the symptoms of a malignant Yellow Fever.

The Roman and Carthaginian armies in Bruttium, a town in the southern part of the Kingdom of Naples, suffered greatly by a pestilential disease, in the year of Rome 548; but no particulars worthy of notice are recorded.

Livy, b. 28 46.

It is however to be remarked that this period of pestilence was distinguished by the appearance of immense swarms of locusts, which overspread the whole country about Capua. Their appearance was subsequent to the plague mentioned in the armies. We shall have frequent occasion to mention the same phenomenon in the natural world as cotemporary with pestilence. But clouds of these animals rarely or never appear at any other time, than during or near the time of the prevalence of plagues; and by comparing the dates of their appearance, it will be found, that they are not, unless by accident, the cause of plague, nor the effect; but, like other animals which are generated in myriads, during pestilence, the produce of some general cause, and probably of that state of the elements, which occasions the diseases of the human race.

Livy, 30 2.

During the war between the Romans and Antiochus, king of Syria, in 563, an event took place, similar to many instances related by Dr. Lind. The Roman fleet, with that of the Rhodians, in search of the Syrian fleet, put into the gulph of Pamphylia and anchored at Phaselis. But it was in the midst of summer, and the place unwholesome; and the men, unaccustomed to the air, were seized with a pestilential disease, especially the rowers. Why the rowers? evidently because they were more exposed to a hot sun, to the air and to fatigue, than the troops on board. This sickness induced the commander to quit that station, and we hear no more of the epidemic.

Livy, b 37 23.

In the year of Rome 571 and B. C. 182 commenced a violent plague, which lasted several years, and ravaged Rome and all Italy so that the Romans could not enlist 8000 soldiers to quell a revolt. In the next year, Livy mentions a drouth of six months, and a consequent dearth of corn.

It will be remarked by any man who reads history with attention, that during pestilential periods, all the ordinary operations of nature acquire unusual strength and magnitude. Earthquakes and tempests are vastly more violent, than at other times. The ancient historians, evidently without design, have left proofs of this fact. Thus Livy mentions, that during the period under consideration, the operations of the war in Spain were retarded by continual rains, which swelled the rivers, and Flaccus, the Prætor, was compelled, *tempestatibus fœdis*, terrible storms, to order his whole army into a city in the neighborhood.

Livy, b 40. 33 and ſec 29 36.

The spring of the year 571 was remarkably tempestuous, and Livy gives a frightful account of a storm in Rome which did no small injury to the public buildings.

B. 40. 2

Short has placed this pestilence in the year of the world 3763, corresponding according to Usher with the year of Rome 507. But Short's chronology is wretched. He mentions a large comet six years after this period, of the size of the sun and of a fiery color. Of the appearance of a comet at the period under consideration, there can be no doubt, tho I have not found the original writer who mentions it and Short quotes no authority but Pozel. He however has made an egregious blunder in the time, as he has in many other instances of facts which he relates, of high antiquity.

The order of the great phenomena of nature seems to be that violent storms, rain and a cold winter, are followed the next year with excessive heat and drouth and vice versa. Violent storms however occur at all times during these periods. It will be noted, that the pestilence above mentioned could not be occasioned by the drouth and dearth of corn, for it broke out in the year preceding. The same fact often occurs, and proves that great pestilence is not solely the effect of intemperate seasons, but that both are the effects of another cause.

The present instance is one, in which a most severe winter followed the other unusual seasons. In the year 574, according to Hook, and the consulship of Q. Fulvius and L. Manlius, the winter was remarkable for deep snow and every kind of tempest. It continued longer than usual, and trees, exposed to the weather, were blasted. An earthquake happened, in the following year.

Livy, b 40 45 59

This then fixes the year of the appearance of the comet, mentioned by Short. That he refers to the same period is certain from his mentioning the circumstance of the inability of the Roman senate to raise a body of 8000 men; a fact assigned by Hook to the year 571, and which can belong to no other period. But from his description of this star, I am inclined to believe he refers to that which is hereafter mentioned, under the great pestilence of 610, and which Pliny has well described.

This uncommon season was succeeded in 576 by pestilence among cattle, and the next year, followed the plague, which made dreadful havoc in Rome. Some facts stated by the historian deserve particular notice. "Pestilentia, quæ priore anno in boves ingruerat, eo verteret in hominum morbos. Qui inciderant, haud facile septimum diem superabant: qui superaverant, longinquo, maxime quartanæ, implicabantur morbo. Servitia maxime moriebantur; eorum strages per omnes vias insepultorum erat. Ne liberorum quidem funeribus sufficiebat. Cadavera, intacta a canibus ac vulturibus, tabes abfumebat : fatisque conftabat nec illo, nec priore anno, in tanta ftrage boum hominumque vulturium ufquam vifum."

Livy b 41. 21.

It is not eafy to do juftice to this energetic defcription of the hiftorian, but the following is the fenfe of the paffage. "The peftilence which had affected cattle in the former year, now turned into difeafes of men. Thofe who were feized fcarcely lived beyond the feventh day; thofe who furvived that day, were afflicted with tedious diftempers, efpecially the quartan ague. The difeafe made its moft fatal ravages among the flaves, whofe dead bodies lay unburied along the highways. It was not poffible to bury the bodies of the free citizens. Their corpfes lay unburied, untouched by dogs and vultures, and wafted away by corruption. It was evident that in this and the former year, during the great mortality among men and cattle, no vulture was feen."

In this account, the following particulars are noticeable.

1ft. That the peftilential air firft produced its effects on cattle.

2d. That the *feventh* was the critical day—as it ufually is, in modern bilious plague.

3d. That if the difeafe had a favorable crifis on the feventh day, the patient furvived, but the diftemper changed into an autumnal bilious fever of the quartan type, and long duration—a ftrong evidence of what I have before remarked that, if peftis and peftilentia are difeafes of a diftinct fpecies, the Roman peftilence was the bilious plague.

4th. This peftilence was, as ufual, moft mortal among the lower orders of people.

5th. Carnivorous animals would not touch the dead bodies, and vultures deferted the atmofphere of Rome.

The laft fact is common in *great* plagues; but in plagues of a lefs malignancy, animals do not quit the infected places. Thefe facts feem to indicate that birds perceive the peftilential ftate of air, before it becomes fenfible to the human fpecies. It feems that the vultures difappeared, the firft year, while the peftilence was confined to cattle; and there can be little doubt, that the delicate organs of fowls perceive the derangement of the air, whether the cause may be, the infusion into it of a pestiferous vapor, or the abstraction from it of a portion of the vital principle, before its effects are visible in larger animals, and before the air is rendered offensive by the carcases of diseased and dead animals.

This was one of those violent and long continued plagues of which history has recorded many instances: and the Romans on this occasion, saw many prodigies. It is difficult, in some cases, to distinguish, in the relations of historians, truth from vulgar report; and philosophy must guard against the illusions of credulity and terrified imaginations. I take no notice of the monsters born, and an ox's speaking, on these occasions. At the beginning of the late American war, many similar prodigies were announced and believed by the ignorant and credulous. But some of the phenomena, enumerated by Livy among prodigies, in all probability, had a real existence, for it will be related hereafter that similar appearances have been observed, in modern times, during pestilence, and appear evidently to have a connection with its causes.

During the plague above mentioned, a bow was seen in the sky, in a serene day, extended over the temple of Saturn in the Roman forum; three suns or haloes appeared, and at night many torches, or meteors descended in Lanuvium. There is strong evidence for believing these phenomena to be occasioned by a vapor emitted from the earth, in superabundant quantities, and which there is reason to think, may be the cause of pestilential diseases; or there may be some changes in the combination of substances composing the atmosphere.

At the close of this pestilential period, in 581, Apulia was deluged by swarms of locusts; as the Pontine territory had been the year before. So destructive were their ravages, that the Prætor Sicinius was sent with an army to drive them away.

Livy, b 42, 2 & 10.

Orosius b. 4 relates, that a most violent plague desolated Rome in the year 610 and B. C. 144. The dead bodies lay putrefying in the houses and streets, and rendered it impossible to approach the city. In the preceding year appeared a remarkable comet. As we come down to the more authentic periods of history, this phenomenon will more frequently occur.

It is again neceffary to remaik a difference in the chronology of different authors. Seneca places the appearance of this comet, which he defcribes to have been as large and luminous as the fun, " Poft mortem Demetrii Syriæ Regis, paulo ante Achaicum Bellum"—after the death of Demetrius, king of Syria, and a little before the Achean war.

Nat Queft lib 7. 15.

Demetrius was flain, B. C. 151, according to common chronology, and the Achean war was in the year when Carthage was taken and deftroyed by Scipio, B C. 146. The appearance of the comet therefore fhould be placed in the year preceding, or 147, correfponding with the year of Rome, 607. And this is probably correct, for it is agreeable to general obfervation, that a comet appears early in the peftilential period, and often *precedes* its moft calamitous years.—The Encyclopedia affigns it to the year 146.

Seneca remarks that at firft it appeared fiery and red, emitting a bright light, fo as to overcome the darknefs of the night. Gradually its magnitude leffened and its brightnefs vanifhed.

This plague was ftill more deadly than that in which Camillus died.

Muratori, vol 1.

In the year of Rome 628, and B. C. 126, hiftorians relate, that a moft dreadful peftilence arofe in Africa, from dead locufts. Thefe animals were biought towards Numidia and Utica, by a ftrong eaft wind, in fuch innumerable multitudes, that they devoured every green thing—not fparing even the bark of trees. They weie driven by the fouth wind into the Mediterranean, and being wafhed on fhore, in the hot feafon, they putrefied, and caufed a moft deadly plague. It is related that 800,000 perfons perifhed in Numidia alone ; 200,000 on the fea coaft of Carthage and Utica, and 30,000 of the Roman troops. No lefs than 1500 dead bodies were carried out of one gate of U- tica, in a fingle day.

Livy. Epit. 60   Orofius, lib 5.   P Diac Auguft. Hift. 813.

Authors afcribe this plague to the dead locufts ; and doubtlefs that caufe had its influence. At the fame time, there is no

H

necessity of resorting to the locusts, for this was a time of general pestilence. The same state of air or other elements which favored the generation of disease, first existed, and produced this unusual number of locusts. This will appear in subsequent parts of this history.

Orosius gives a most hideous account of the pestiferous state of air from the locusts. He avers that birds, cattle and wild beasts perished by means of the corruption of the air, and thus increased the evil. He remarks further that, altho locusts had often appeared in his days, in great numbers, yet they never before had done more mischief when dead, than when living, so as to cause mankind to wish they had not perished.

We must accede to the opinion of the ancients that the stench of the locusts was one cause of the pestilence; it is possible that no epidemic disease would have been excited without that cause; but it is equally true, that in a healthy state of the atmosphere, no putrefaction of dead bodies has ever been known to produce an epidemic pestilence. It may be powerful enough to excite disease within a small extent of its own atmosphere; but if no other cause of disease exists, it will not extend beyond that infected atmosphere.

The appearance of immense multitudes of locusts, during pestilence, is a curious fact in natural history, and well deserves investigation; but these animals do not always *precede* the appearance of the diseases of the same period, nor do they often perish in such collections as to be the *cause* of those diseases. The common idea in Arabia, is, that they are generated by heat and drouth. Cold and rains are supposed to destroy their eggs.

About the beginning of this destructive period, appeared a comet. The Encyclopedia mentions *two*, in the year of Rome 629, and B. C. 125. But it is probable this is a mistake of the compilers. The universal history places one under the year 630, and a second under the following year, quoting Justin, for authority. But Justin mentions two comets, one at the birth of Mithridates, another in the year he began to reign. Now Mithridates was about eleven or twelve years old when he came to the throne, in the year of Rome 631, and B. C. 123. Of courfe the firft comet muft have been about the year 620, and B. C. 134

It is no inconfiderable proof of the truth of Juftin's account, and of the accuracy of our chronology in this particular, that there was an eruption of the great volcano of Sicily, in both the periods when thefe comets are faid to have appeared. In the year 620, and B. C. 134, there was an eruption of Etna, tho not mentioned by Juftin; and this was the year of the firft great comet, and of the birth of Mithridates. Nine years after, in 629, there was a fecond eruption of Etna. The laft year correfponds nearly with the period in which Mithridates began to reign, allowing him to be eleven years old, and with the approach of the fecond comet.

This laft comet produced moft tremendous effects, as we might expect from its magnitude, and proximity to the earth. The following is Juftin's defcription of it. " Nam et eo quo genitus eft anno, et eo quo regnare primum cœpit, ftella cometes, per utrumque tempus, 70 diebus ita luxit, ut cœlum omne flagrare videreter." For 70 days the heavens appeared to be in a flame.

Lib 37. 2.

The eruptions of the volcano were equally remarkable.

The lava from Etna laid wafte the city and fuburbs of Catana. " Ætna ultra folitum exarfit, fays the hiftorian; Catanam urbem finefque oppreffit."

Orofius, lib. 5.

In Paulus Diaconus we have a relation of fingular facts in regard to the eruption of Etna. Globes of fire were thrown from the Crater. Lipari, a fmall volcanic ifland on the north of Sicily, became fo heated, during the eruption, that the rocks were diffolved, tho it is not faid that this ifland difcharged any fire. The water of the neighboring fea was fo heated as to kill the fifh, and melt the pitch on the decks of veffels. Dead fifh appeared on the furface of the water, and many perfons, who were near the ifland, were fuffocated with heat.

This author places the appearance of the locufts which caufed the plague in Africa, in the year *after* the eruption of Etna.

Others place this event, a year *before* the eruption. It is much to be regretted that authors have been so careless of the chronology of important phenomena, on the *order* of which may depend important principles. This however is certain, that all the great agitations of nature here related belong to the same period, and it is not surprising that they were attended with most mortal pestilence.

For authorities see Livy, Epit 60 Orosius, lib. 5
P Diaconus, in August Hist 813   Juſt n, lib 37.
2, 3 Uſl er's Annals, 498 Muratori, vol 1, p. 26.

The foregoing period of pestilence was one of the most dreadful on record.

It will be found invariably true, in every period of the world, that the violence and extent of the plague has been nearly proportioned to the number and violence of the following phenomena—earthquakes, eruptions of volcanoes, meteors, tempests, inundations

During the civil wars excited by Sylla and Marius, the armies lost ten thousand men by the plague, in the year of Rome 665, and B. C. 89.

Universal Hist vol. 13. 59   Vel. Paterc. lib 2 21.

It must have been during this period that the comet appeared which is mentioned by Pliny. Nat. Hist. lib. 2. cap 25. "Civili motu, Octavio Consule," for this was the year, in which Octavius was Consul. This period was preceded by an extraordinary collision and disrupture of two mountains, and the bursting of fire from the chasm, in the territory of Modena. Pliny assures us, this was seen from the Emilian way, by an immense number of Roman knights and others.

Pliny Nat. Hist. lib. 2 83.

With this period corresponds the eruption of a volcano in Hiera, one of the Æolian isles, north of Sicily, now called Lipari, which burnt for several days, and the very sea around it appeared to be fire. Pliny says this was during the Social War.

Lib. 2 106

The year B. C. 44 was distinguished by the death of Julius Cesar, by the hands of conspirators; soon after which appeared a comet, supposed to be the same which appeared in

1680, whose period is calculated to be 575 years. If this is its period, it must have been seen in the year B. C. 1767, in the reign of Ogyges, when Attica was inundated and rendered barren for a number of years; and when the planet Venus is said to have changed her figure, color and course. When we survey the uniform effects of comets in tempests and floods, and compare the traditional account of that event with the terrible inundations which have happened in Greece at other times, and especially with that in the time of Thucydides, which rent Atalanta from the main land; which events all took place during the approach of comets; we are constrained to believe the fact of the Ogygean deluge, and fable rises to the dignity of authentic history. This inundation might have happened during the approach of some other comet, but the probability is, that it was during that of the comet under confideration, which fixes the time of the Ogygean flood, in the year B. C. 1767. This circumstance may serve to correct the chronology of the early events in Greece.

See Jackfon's chronology vol. 3 312.

Its next appearance must have been in the year A. C. 1193, when Electra, one of the pleiads, abandoned her fifter orbs, and fled from the Zodiac to the north pole.

Its third appearance correfponds with the year A. C. 618, the year of the terrible comet of the Sybill, fays Gibbon; and its fourth, is the one under confideration. Its fubfequent appearances A. D. 531, 1106 and 1680 will be hereafter mentioned. All the periods here named, which come within the limits of authentic history, have been remarkable for peftilence, earthquakes, inundations or other great phenomena. Such was the fact in 44 and 43. There was a terrible inundation of the Tyber, a violent earthquake, many unufual phenomena in the fky, and in the year 43, a violent eruption of Etna.—Peftilence, as ufual, accompanied thefe events.

But another phenomenon, the palenefs or defect of light, in the fun, deferves more particular attention. Pliny afferts that this pale color lafted almoft a year. His words are, " Fiunt prodigiofi et longiores folis defectus, qualis occifo dictatore Cæ-

fare et Antoniano bello, totius pene anni pallore continuo."
Nat. Hift. lib. 2. 30.—Virgil and Ovid, who were eye witneſſes of this phenomenon, have both deſcribed it, with the other prodigies of this period.

" Ille (fol) etiam extincto miſeratus Cæſare Romam,
Cum Caput obſcura nitidum ferrugine texit."—
Georg lib 1 466

" Phœbi quoque triſtis imago
Lurida follicitis præbebat lumina terris."
Metamorph. lib 15 785.

The words *ferrugo* and *luridus* give us an exact idea of the color—a paleneſs tinctured with the color of ruſt. A ſimilar defect of light in the ſun occurred at the time of the next appearance of this comet, A. D. 531, as will be hereafter related. The fact is curious. It is well known that this comet approaches very near to the ſun ; but whether the defect of ſplendor in the ſun was the effect of the attractive powers of the comet, or of an alteration in the electrical atmoſphere of theſe bodies ; or whether it was occaſioned by an alteration in the terreſtrial atmoſphere, is a queſtion not eaſily ſolved. It might have been owing to a vapor, like that which overſpread Europe in 1783.

This period was marked with famin alſo, with ſhooting ſtars, and numerous prodigies.

See Virgil and Ovid in the paſſages quoted.
See alſo, Zonoras' Annals, lib 10 Uſher's An p. 680.

The comet appeared in 44 and alſo the peſtilence—the eruption of Etna in 43 B. C. and therefore ſubſequent to the other events. Indeed it is more generally the caſe, that the volcano does not emit fire until ſome time *after* the appearance of the plague. To this however there are exceptions. Moſt of the great plagues appear two or three years, with different degrees of violence ; and during this period, volcanoes diſcharge immenſe quantities of lava.

By a paragraph in Uſher's Annals, p. 684, it appears the winter following the appearance of this comet, was ſevere.

The next peftilential period commenced in the year 30 B. C. An eruption of Etna, which laid all the neighboring towns in ruins, marked the commencement of this period, which however was preceded in 31 by an earthquake in Judea, in which thoufands of people perifhed in the ruins of their houfes. About the fame time appeared, fays Dion Caffius, " thofe meteors which the Greeks call comets." Thefe phenomena were followed by a peftilence in Jerufalem, which deftroyed a great part of the nobles and people of the Jews. The fame period was marked by a great inundation of the Tyber, which fpread over the low grounds of Rome, and was confidered as an omen of the future power of Auguftus.

Dion Caffius' Univ. Hift. 10. 415. Ufher's Annals, 766.

By a curious circumftance, we learn that a hard winter and peftilence afflicted Rome at this period. The Emperor Octavius Auguftus, in his 5th Confulfhip, B. C. 29, had formed the defign of refigning the empire. Horace, the Poet, his friend and flatterer, endeavored to diffuade him from this purpofe, on account of the prodigies which happened at the beginning of the year, which was the winter of the year 30 B. C. and correfponds exactly with the appearance of the comet. Among thefe prodigies, the poet enumerates an abundance of fnow, terrible hail, thunder and lightning, and a deftructive inundation of the Tyber.

> " Jam fatis terris nivis, atque diræ
> Grandinis mifit Pater—&c."

See the 2d Ode of the firft book, which is worth the notice of the philofophic reader, on account of the defcription of the inundation, which proceeded from a *fwell of the fea*.

> " Vidimus flavum Tiberim, retortis
> Littore Etrufco violenter undis."

It is a fact of which there is full evidence, that during the approach of comets, not only tempefts are more violent, than at other times, but the ocean fwells without winds—the tides are much higher and high tides are more numerous. The ancients took notice of this fact, and it came under my own obfervation, during the approach of the comet in 1797.

In the 21ft ode of the fame book, Horace addreffes Apollo who " drives war, famin and peftilence from the Roman people and the Emperor, to the Perfians and Britons."

This paffage is proof that the Romans found peftilence in Britain; but the Britons, at that time, had no trade, except with the coaft of France. How or from what quarter, they *imported the infection*, is left for the folution of Dr. Mead's followers.

In the year B. C. 25, according to the Univerfal Hiftory, a violent peftilence raged in Rome, an inundation laid a great part of the city under water, lands were left untilled and a famin enfued.

The fame year, the plague raged in Paleftine, which was *preceded* by a fevere drouth and a dearth of corn. A hard winter is mentioned about the fame time, but the order of this event is not recorded.

Univerfal Hift. vol 13 502 Ufher's Annals, 772. Dufrefnoy's Chro.

This peftilence was preceded the year before, by " epidemic diftempers which proved fatal to many." This fact is important, and will hereafter be found very material in determining the caufes of epidemic peftilential difeafes. It goes to prove a *progreffivenefs* in the peftilential ftate of air, or general contagion. And this inftance, among many to be hereafter fpecified, demonftrates that the plague was *not* produced by the famin, according to vulgar opinion in almoft all cafes of this kind. Had no malignant difeafe preceded the plague, and had the plague followed clofe on the heels of famin, we fhould have ftrong ground to believe *famin* to be the *caufe of the plague;* and a feries of fimilar facts might eftablifh that as a principle or law of nature. But it appears, that the malignant diftempers, which are found to be the conftant precurfors of peftilence, were epidemic, in the year *preceding* the famin—a demonftration that the *general* caufe, in the ftate of air, exifted anterior to the dearth.

SECTION III.

Historical view of pestilential epidemics from the Christian era, to the year 1347.

AT the close of the reign of Augustus, about the year 14 or according to some authors 16 of the Christian era, there was a great famin in Rome, and a comet is mentioned, near the same time, by Dion Cassius. This was followed by a most terrible pestilence in the east, during which twelve cities of Asia Minor were overthrown by earthquakes. Of these calamitous events, the following is the account recorded by Tacitus, An. lib. 2. 47. " Eodem anno, duodecem celebres Asiæ urbes conlapsæ nocturno motu terræ, quo improvisior graviorque pestis fuit. Neque solitum in tali casu effugium subveniebat in aperta prorumpendi, quia diductis terris hauriebantur: Sedisse immensos montes, visa in arduo quæ plana fuerint, effulsisse inter ruinam ignis memorant."

It is a circumstance not to be overlooked that the plague was prevalent, anterior to this dreadful earthquake, as the historian remarks that this catastrophe rendered the sickness more severe and less tolerable. Such is the usual course of these calamities; the pestilence appears, *before* the most destructive shocks of the earth, which rarely fail to occur, during its prevalence. It is to be observed also that men obtained no security, in this instance, by flying to open places, for the earth opened and swallowed them up—fire also issued from the earth. Large mountains subsided to plains, and plains were thrown into mountains.

Tacitus An lib 2 47 Plin lib. 2 84. Euseb. Chron. 201. Usher's Annals, 811

In the year 40 of the Christian era, there was an eruption of Etna, which frightened Caligula out of Sicily and which was followed by univerfal famin in Rome and the eaft.* This was the famin foretold by Agabus in Acts xi. 28, in the reign of Claudius Cefar. A peftilence, at the fame time raged in Babylonia, and multitudes of Jews, on account of it, withdrew to Seleucia.

Suetonius in Calig. Univ Hift vol 14 Ufher's An 864, 868.

During this famin and peftilence, a comet was vifible in the year 42.

Short on Air, vol 2 170

The clofe of the reign of Claudius and the beginning of the reign of Nero, A. D. 53 and 4, were marked by a fimilar train of phenomena and calamities. A comet is noted by Suetonius and Pliny about the year 54, the year in which Claudius was poifoned. Tacitus relates that people were alarmed by frequent fhocks of earthquakes, which demolifhed many buildings, and great dearth of corn prevailed in Rome and Greece. Pliny records that three funs, by which are doubtlefs intended, halos or mock funs, appeared the fame year. Thefe were confidered by the ancients as prodigies, but tho common phenomena, they are remarkably luminous, and frequent in the periods of peftilence.

Tacitus Annals, l.b 12 43 Plin Nat Hift lib 2 31.
Suet in Claud Functius Chronol

This period was fickly, tho not recorded as peftilential. Suetonius remarks, " Ex omnium Magiftratum generi, plerique mortem obierant." Many of all kinds of public officers died ; by which we infer that the year was fickly.

In the reign of Nero occurred the next peftilential period. Two comets are noted, one A. D. 62 and a fecond in 66. In the year 62, Laodicea was overwhelmed by an earthquake. In the year 68, occurred a moft violent tempeft in Campania which deftroyed villages, trees and grain ; and a violent earthquake. At the fame time, raged a mortal plague in Rome, which is faid to have carried off 30,000 people, but by the defcription of its

* Short places this in the 49th year of the Chriftian era, altho Caligula was killed in the year 41. No dependence can be placed on the *dates* of events, found in Short on Air, and I cannot vouch for their correctnefs, where I have not other authority

ravages, it is probable the number was much greater. Tacitus remarks that the " houses were filled with dead bodies and the streets with funerals; neither age nor sex was exempt; slaves and ingenuous plebeians were suddenly taken off, amidst the lamentations of their wives and children, who, while they assisted the sick, or mourned over the dead, were seized with the disease, and perishing, were burnt on the same funeral pile. To the knights and senators, the disease was less mortal, tho these also suffered in the common calamity."

As Rome, at the time under consideration, contained more than a million of inhabitants, so mortal a plague must have extinguished a much larger number than 30,000 people—it is not improbable, a numeral or figure has been omitted by the transcribers of the original history.

The earthquakes of this period were experienced in Asia Minor, at Laodicea and Hierapolis.

Seneca mentions that a flock of 600 sheep were killed by the pestiferous vapor, discharged during the earthquake in Italy.

Dion Cassius relates, that at this period, a most formidable inundation laid waste the Egyptian coast.

It must not be omitted that the violent tempest in which St. Paul was shipwrecked on the island of Melita, now Malta, was in the year 61 or 62, during the approach of the first comet.

Tacitus remarks, that no visible cause could be assigned for the pestilence of this period; " Nulla Cœli intemperie quæ occurreret occulis." No remarkable season had occurred, to which this distemper could be ascribed. We shall find, in subsequent periods, distinguished writers making similar remarks. The reason is, these authors did not take a view sufficiently comprehensive of the operations of nature; and if the cause of plague could not be found, *very near in time and place*, they did not observe it. It is true, that an extraordinary season does not always precede or attend pestilence, in a particular place; but by extending our view of the subject, to general causes, operating over whole quarters of the globe, and perhaps over the whole globe; and considering the causes, as invisible, and acting for a series of years, the whole myftery is unfolded.—Such may be the refult of this inveftigation.

> For authorities refpecting the laft period of peftilence here noticed, fee Tacitus, An lib 15. 47 lib 16 13 Suet in Nero. Seneca, Nat. Queft. 6 and 7 Baronius, vol 1. 620. Plin. Nat. Hift lib 2 83. Ufher's Annals, 892 Funct Chron Orof lib 7 Univerfal Hift vol 14 439 Magd Ec. Hift. lib 2 13.

Seneca places the great earthquake in Campania under the Confulfhip of Regulus and Virginius, which, according to common chronology, was in the 65th year of the Chriftian era.

The next peftilential period is one of the moft remarkable in all the circumftances, that is recorded in Hiftory.

In the year 79 [fome authors fay a year later, but the difference is of no moment, as they agree in the *order* of the events related] juft before the death of Vefpafian, appeared a comet with a long coma in the month of June. On the firft of November following, a moft tremendous ebullition of fire and lava iffued from Vefuvius and laid wafte the neighboring country. At the fame time, happened a violent earthquake, which buried the cities of Herculaneum and Pompeium; and fo fudden was the fhock, that the people, who were attending a play, had not time to quit the theater, and were all buried in a mafs.

This dreadful cataftrophe was preceded by rumbling noifes in the earth, and the earth was heated to a great degree. Violent agitations of the fea, thunder and lightning alfo announced the approach of fome dreadful event.

The eruption lafted three days, during which time fuch immenfe quantities of afhes and fmoke were difcharged, that day was turned into night, and the afhes were driven by different winds to Rome, Syria and Africa.

The agitations of the earth and the elements were tremendous and frightful. Baronius remarks, that fome perfons fuppofed the world would be reduced to chaos, or confumed with fire. The fifh in the neighboring feas were deftroyed.

This explofion of fubterranean fire was *preceded* by a fevere drouth in Italy. The next year, 80, was remarkable for a terrible inundation in England; the Severn overflowing a large tract of country, and deftroying multitudes of cattle.

These violent effects of subterranean fire were attended by one of the most fatal plagues recorded in history. A remark of Dion is here very important. He says that the " Ashes from Vesuvius caused, at the time, only slight indispositions or diseases; but afterwards produced an Epidemic distemper." The remark is incorrect, in ascribing even slight diseases to ashes; but it leads to a conclusion, which is of moment. The slight complaints which prevailed in the autumn of the year of the eruption, compared with modern observations, appear to have been the *precursors* of the plague, which broke out the next year, and as authors assert, destroyed, for some time, 10,000 citizens of Rome in a day.—The same year, while the Emperor Titus was viewing the ruins in Campania, a fire broke out in the city, which laid in ashes a great number of buildings.

The order of the events in this period was, a comet, drouth, slight diseases, and an eruption of Vesuvius, with the earthquakes, the first year.—In the second, appeared the pestilence with its most malignant effects.

In this eruption of Vesuvius, the first recorded in history, perished the elder Pliny; and the Emperor Titus fell a victim to his paternal care of his subjects.

Suetonius, 23 Aurel Victor Epit Dion Cassius Pliny Epis. Baronius An vol 1 713. Magd lib 2 14

In the year 90 appeared a comet. The plague is said to have appeared in the north of England in 88, and in 92, to have destroyed 150,000 lives in Scotland.

Short, vol 2 207.

In 102 a plague is said to have arisen from dead fish driven on shore, but I have no other particulars.

In the year 107 four cities of Asia, two in Greece and three in Galatia, were overwhelmed by an earthquake. A comet is mentioned by Short in 109, but as I have not found the original authority, I cannot depend on the accuracy of the chronology. It is probable that these phenomena occurred within the same year; and there is the more reason to believe this, as different and respectable authors differ two or three years in the chronology of Roman history. The next event to be related, is a remarkable instance of the truth of this observation.

Short mentions a plague in Wales in 114 which deftroyed 45,000 lives; but I have not the hiftory of the facts.

In the reign of Trajan, the city of Antioch was almoft totally demolifhed by an earthquake. This emperor was in the city at the time, and narrowly efcaped with his life. Some authors place this event in the year 114; others in 115; but Baronius has proved by an ancient infcription, that it happened under the confulate of P. Vipftanus Meffala and M. Virgilianus Pedo; which brings the event to the year 117. A comet was vifible the fame year.

The earthquakes of this period were extremely violent—many cities were overthrown, mountains funk, rivers were dried up and new fountains appeared.

Aurelius Victor adds to thefe calamities a great inundation of the Tyber, violent peftilence and famin; but to which of the periods, the year 107 or 117, he alludes, is not quite certain, tho probably to the latter. " Terræ motus gravis per provincias multas, atioxque peftilentia, famefque et inundia facta funt."

To remedy the danger from fire and earthquakes, Trajan limited the height of houfes in Rome to 60 feet; and for that regulation obtained the title of " Father of the Country."

The great earthquake at Antioch was accompanied with fierce winds, a circumftance not very common; it being more ufual that fhocks of the earth happen during a perfect ferenity and tranquillity of the atmofphere, unlefs in the vicinity of volcanoes.

Aurel Victor Epit Trajan. Dion Caffius
Baronius vol 2 55   Echard's Rom. Hift vol. 2, 276.

During the time that Trajan was making war on the Agarini, a people of Arabia, which had revolted from the Roman government, flies in myriads appeared and covered every veffel and utenfil, fo that the Emperor was compelled to abandon the expedition. This was near the time of the earthquake which deftroyed Antioch.

Baron 2. 54   Magd Cent 2 13.

This fact ought not to be omitted; as the generation of innumerable infects is one of the phenomena which generally attend a great peftilence.—The fame feafon was marked by terrible ftorms of wind, rain and hail-ftones of unufual fize. The winter succeeding that in which Antioch was destroyed, was so tempestuous, and the Tigris so swelled by deluges of rain, that Trajan's army suffered extreme hardships and great losses, in his expedition into Assyria.

Under the year 115, I find mentioned a sudden and violent inundation of the Severn in England, which drowned people in their beds, and destroyed 5000 head of cattle. Perhaps philosophy will place this event, under the year of the earthquake at Antioch; whichever may be the true year, 115 or 117.

In the chronological tables, a great earthquake in China is mentioned under the year 114—the year of the plague in Wales.

Under the Emperor Adrian, say the compilers of the Magdeburgh history, from Eusebius, the greatest part of Nicomedia and Nicea was overthrown by earthquakes; and not long after, Nicopolis and Cesarea were totally overwhelmed. Functius assigns the fate of Nicomedia to the year 121, and that of Nicopolis to 129. By another writer is noted a comet in 127, and a plague in Scotland.

Short, vol. 2. 207.

In 137 appeared a comet, followed by the plague.—In this year or the subsequent one, the Thames was almost dry.

The plague again made great havoc in Scotland in 146.—An eruption of fire from Lipari happened in 144.

In the year 153 happened a severe winter of three months, which covered the Thames and all rivers with ice.

In the reign of Antoninus Pius, A. D. 154, occurred an earthquake which prostrated some towns in Asia and Rhodes. A comet appeared nearly at the same time, and a pestilence in Arabia, together with an inundation of the Tyber.

Julius Capitolinus Magdeb Cent. 2 13 Baronius vol. 2 130.

Of the general and fatal pestilence in the reign of Marcus Aurelius Antoninus and Lucius Verus, we have many accounts. It appeared in Rome in 167, but its origin was in Asia, a year or two earlier. Ammianus Marcellinus, the philosophic soldier, relates that this plague originated from the foul air of a small box or chest, which a Roman soldier had opened, in search of plunder, after the taking of Seleucia. Julius Capitolinus mentions the same fact on the authority of mere vulgar report or tradition. " Et nata *fertur* pestilentia in Babylonia, ubi de templo Apollonis ex arcula aurea, quam milis forte inciderat, spiritus pestilens evasit, atque inde Parthos orbemque complesse."

A. Marcellinus gives a more particular account of this event. " Milites fanum scrutantes, invenere foramen angustum, quo referato, ut pretiosum aliquid invenirent, ex adyto quodam conclufo a Chaldœorum arcanis, labes primordialis exsilivit, quæ insanabilium vi concepta morborum, ejusdem Veri et Marci Antonini temporibus, ab ipsis Persarum finibus, adusque Rhenum, et Gallias Cuneta contagiis polluebat et mortibus."

That a close box or other confined place, which might have been shut for ages, should contain a pestiferous vapor which might destroy the life of the man that first opened it, is not only possible, but very probable. But that this trifling quantity of noxious air should be sufficient to generate a universal pestilence from the confines of Persia to Gaul, is a vulgar notion, precisely resembling the modern opinion that the plague is conveyed from country to country, in bales of goods.

The historian adds, that the Emperor returned to Rome, and " luem secum deferre videreter," seemed to carry the plague with him. But the Romans passed only from Seleucia to Rome; whereas the plague raged over the whole earth; so that the disease must have originated in other countries, through which the Emperor did *not* pass, and from other causes than the noxious air of a little box. It raged in Gaul and in Scotland.

By attending to the phenomena of the physical world, during this period, we shall find causes fully adequate to the effect, without resorting to the temple of Apollo in Seleucia. The state of the elements was deranged, and nature was every where agitated. An inundation of the Tyber at Rome laid all the low grounds, and a part of the city under water, sweeping away people, buildings and cattle, and desolating the fields. Famin and earthquakes marked the same period. The air became insalubrious, and myriads of caterpillars and other insects overran the earth and devoured vegetation.

The peſtilence was violent and mortal, correſponding with theſe ſymptoms of derangement in the elements. In Rome, at one time, it is related, that the mortality extended to ten thouſand perſons in a day. Its precife duration, I do not find to be ſpecified by the hiſtorians; but it continued for a number of years, in the midſt of which appeared a comet, about the year 169.

<blockquote>See Am Marcellinus, lib 23, and Julius Capitolinus, in Vero. Aug Hiſt 580. Hiſt of Emperors by Pedro Mexiæ, p 172. Echards Rom Hiſt vol 2. 315 to 322, who is more correct than Gibbon.</blockquote>

Of the ſymptoms of this deſolating plague, I find no account, except that the patients had a light fever, and a gangrene appeared on the extremities of the feet.

It is proper here to notice a paſſage in Gibbon's Hiſt. vol. 1. chap. 3, which deſcribes, as halcyon days, the period of the world in which this calamity occurred. The following are his words. "If a man were called upon to fix the period in the hiſtory of the world, during which the condition of the human race was *moſt happy* and *proſperous*, he would, without heſitation, name that which elapſed from the death of Domitian to the acceſſion of Commodus;" that is, from the year 96 to 180.

It is certain that, at this time, the Roman Empire was in its glory, and governed by a ſeries of able and virtuous princes, who made the happineſs of their ſubjects their principal object. But the coloring given to the happineſs of this period, is far too brilliant. The ſucceſs of armies and the extent of empire do not conſtitute excluſively the happineſs of nations; and no hiſtorian has a title to the character of fidelity, who does not comprehend, in his general deſcriptions of the ſtate of mankind, moral and phyſical, as well as political, evils.

During the period mentioned by Gibbon, not only Antioch, with the loſs of moſt of its inhabitants, amounting probably to more than 100,000, but thirteen other cities were demoliſhed by earthquakes. In the famous revolt of the Jews under Trajan, hiſtorians relate that 450,000 Romans were maſſacred in Syria, Cyprus and other countries; and in the wars undertaken by Adrian to ſubdue them, it is eſtimated that 50 cities and 985 towns were destroyed, and 580,000 men lost their lives by famine, disease and the sword. The reign of the Antonines was distinguished for multifarious and severe calamities. The description of them, by Aurelius Victor, ought to be given in his own words. Speaking of the Emperor M. Antonine, he says, "Nisi ad illa tempora natus esset, profecto quasi uno lapsu ruissent omnia status Romani. Quippe ab armis nusquam quies erat: perque omnem orientem, Illyricum, Italiam, Galliamque bella fervebant. Terræ motus non sine interitu civitatum, inundationes fluminum, lues crebræ, locustarum species agris infestæ, prorfus ut prope nihil, quo summis angoribus atteri mortales folent, dici feu cogitari queat, quod non illo imperante sævierit."

Epit. of the lives of the Emperors.

"Unless he, M. Antonine, had been born at that juncture, the affairs of the empire would have fallen into speedy ruin: for there was no respite from military operations. War raged in the east, in Illyricum, in Italy and in Gaul. Earthquakes, with the destruction of cities, inundations of rivers, frequent plagues, a species of locusts ravaging the fields; in short every calamity that can be conceived to afflict and torment men, scourged the human race, during his administration."

How can that be a "happy and prosperous condition of men," in which they were subject to continual wars, to massacres, to the ravages of insects, and to a series of plagues, which destroyed probably one fourth of the inhabitants of the globe; and when the Roman empire was upon the brink of ruin? And how can a writer be esteemed as a historian, who substitutes the flowers of rhetoric for sober truth, and sacrifices fact to embellishment?

In the year 173 a pestilence raged in the Roman armies, which threatened them with extermination.—This appears to have been a continuation of the plague before described. It prevailed in Rome in 175 and 178.

Funct Chronol Short, vol. 2

A severe winter in 173 produced famine in England, where the snow covered the earth for 13 weeks.

In 181 a comet was visible, and in 182 Smyrna was almost ruined by an earthquake. The plague prevailed in Rome in 183.

Ibid.

In the reign of Commodus, about the year 187, Rome was again afflicted with a severe plague, which was felt also in all parts of Italy, tho with less mortality than in the city. Herodian, lib. 1, gives the following account of it. " A great pestilence raged throughout Italy at that time, but with most violence in the city, by reason of the great concourse of people assembled from all parts of the earth. The mortality among men and cattle was great. The Emperor, by advice of certain physicians retired to Laurentum, on account of the coolness of the place which was shaded with laurels, from which circumstance it derived its name. It was supposed also the effluvia from the laurels acted as an antidote against the contagion of the distemper. The people in the city also, by advice of physicians, filled their noses and ears with sweet ointments, and constantly used perfumes, for in popular opinion, they occupy the passages of the senses, with these odors, and shut out the corrupt air; or if they do not wholly exclude it, they overpower its influence by superior force. But these things did not check the progress of the disease, and men and cattle continued to perish."

The deaths amounted, in Rome, to 5000 in a day, for a considerable time. A famin prevailed at the same time, and historians ascribe it to Cleander, the minister of Commodus, who had monopolized the corn, to compel people to purchase of him at an advanced price. Dion Cassius however says, the year had been unfruitful. The pestilence continued three years. Indeed we may here remark once for all, that when we read of a plague of great extent and violence in any part of the world, under the date of a particular year, we may always consider that or other pestilential diseases, as prevailing at least three years. Rarely are great plagues of less duration, but often of greater. Historians seldom mention the pestilence, except in the year of its greatest violence, but no plague, I will assert, ever yet infested a particular city or country, without precursors of a very malignant type. When therefore we speak of pestilence, as prevailing in a particular year, we are to consider the epidemic as extending to a period of three, four or five years, perhaps to a much longer period, either in the form of plague, a deadly petechial fever, or other fatal disease.

In the foregoing description of the disease under Commodus, we notice the vulgar modes of guarding against contagion, by stuffing the nose and ears with aromatics—a practice that in part subsists at this day, altho constant experience proves it to be utterly ineffectual.

It appears from Herodian that a comet appeared at this period, or other singular heavenly phenomena. He says, " Ea tempestate stellæ per diem perpetuo apparuerant, quædamque ex iis in longum productæ medio quasi aere suspensæ videbantur." Comets are sometimes visible in the day time, and it is well known that many of the ancients considered them as meteors, floating in the earth's atmosphere, as we see in Aristotle, Seneca and Pliny, who have discussed and refuted those opinions. See also Sampridius who mentions the comet and unusual darkness, at this period.

Another circumstance mentioned by Herodian deserves notice. He says, that animals at this time grew out of their usual size, assuming an extraordinary figure and disproportioned in their parts. " Preterea animalia, genus omne, minime suam naturam servantia, cum figura corporis prodigiosa, tum membris haudquaquam congruentibus edebantur." This fact the writer arranges under the head of *prodigies*, but numerous modern observations confirm the veracity of the historian. In many plagues, to be hereafter mentioned, myriads of unusual animals have appeared, and many common animals and insects have grown to an unusual size. With this fact almost invariably attending pestilence, and before the eyes of every man of science in well attested accounts ; a fact that demonstrates a prodigiously pestilential state of the elements, modern philosophers, physicians and rulers have been tracing all the plagues of the earth to one or two little spots in Egypt and the Levant—This circumstance is hardly credible ; yet is true, and indicates a lamentable decline of sound philosophy.

A slight shock of an earthquake is mentioned incidentally by Herodian, after the plague. Speaking of the burning of a temple in Rome, he says "there had been no storm or clouds, but a small earthquake preceded the conflagration:" and he insinuates that the building might have been set on fire by a flash of lightning in the night, or by an eruption of fire in the earthquake.

In 193, Canterbury in England was severely shaken by an earthquake.

The plague prevailed in London in 211, and a comet appeared in the same year. In 214, there was a most dreadful inundation of the river Trent in England, which spread over 20 miles of country, and destroyed many lives. Here is probably a mistake in chronology of at least two years—or rather a difference between different authorities. Eusebius, the learned Bishop of Cæsaria, places the birth of Christ two years earlier, than the common or Dionysian Chronology. Many authors follow one mode of computing time and many the other; and without the original authors, and a close attention to their modes of reckoning time, it is not possible to reconcile these differences. The uniform influence of comets in producing violent tempests and unusual swelling of the ocean, within a year of their appearance and after their departure, may assist in correcting ancient chronology.

In the year 218 two comets appeared, and a severe frost of five months is related to have happened in England in 220.

There was a great inundation of the Tweed in 218, and a pestilence in Scotland in 222 which destroyed 100,000 lives.

In 235 a comet is noted, but I find no other phenomena mentioned about this time, except a great death of fish in 231, multitudes of which were washed ashore on Britain; and an earthquake in Wales in 232.

In the reign of the Emperor Gordian, about the year 243, the earth was agitated by most violent earthquakes; and in 245 there was a prodigious inundation of the sea in Lincolnshire, England, which laid under water many thousand acres of land, which are said not yet to be recovered. A severe winter is mentioned in 242.

We have now arrived to one of the moſt calamitous periods recorded in hiſtory—a period of mortal plagues, which commenced about the year 250, or 252 in the reign of the Emperor Decius and continued fifteen or twenty years, through the adminiſtration of Gallus and Voluſian, Valerian and Gallienus. This period was uſhered in by a comet in 250, the winter of which in England was ſo ſevere, that the Thames was frozen for nine weeks.—An eruption of Etna is noted under the year 253, and an earthquake in Cornwall in 251.

The plague appears to have been moſt fatal in Rome at two different times, during this period ; viz. in the years 252 and 262 or 3, including the year preceding and ſucceeding each of theſe periods. It reached the northern parts of Europe, and in 266, Scotland had ſcarcely living people enough to bury the dead.

It firſt appeared in Ethiopia, on the confines of Egypt, and ſpread over all the provinces of the Roman Empire, which, ſays Zonoras, were exceſſively exhauſted by its deſtructive ravages. Zoſimus, after deſcribing the devaſtation occaſioned by the irruption of the Scythians, ſays " Lues etiam peſtilens in *oppidis* atque *vicis* ſubſecuta, quicquid erat humani generis reliquum, abſumpſit." The plague in *towns* and *villages* followed the Scythians and devoured that part of the human race which the barbarians had ſpared.

Jornandes ſays, the peſtilence " faciem totius orbis fœdavit" —deſolated or disfigured the face of the whole earth.—In the reign of Gallienus, 5000 citizens of Rome periſhed daily, in 262, or the following year, a portion of this period moſt diſtinguiſhed for convulſions of the earth.

This latter period was marked by deſtructive earthquakes in Rome, Syria and other countries. In ſome places the earth opened and ſalt water iſſued. Trebellius Pollio ſays, " Frightful earthquakes ſhook Italy, Aſia and Africa. For many days, [ſome authors ſay, *three* days] there was an unuſual or preternatural darkneſs and a hollow rumbling noiſe in the earth, which opened in many places. Many cities in Aſia were overwhelmed, and others loft in the ocean. Peftilence *followed* and defolated the Roman Empire."

In the Univerfal Hiftory, it is faid that this plague ravaged Capadocia and all Afia Minor, and was followed by famin, earthquakes and a great comet or meteor.

Orofius remarks that " Nulla fere provincia Romana, nulla civitas, nulla domus fuit, quæ non illa generali peftilentia correpta atque vaftata." Scarcely was there a province of the Empire, a city or a houfe, which was not attacked and defolated.

This paffage is worthy of notice, for it will hereafter appear, that altho the plague is ufually limited to cities, where powerful artificial or local caufes aid the general contagion, yet in fome inftances, the general ftate of the atmofphere has been fo peftilential, as to produce *plague* on the moft elevated hills and falubrious places, in detached villages and houfes, without the leaft communication with the fick and infected.

Gibbon chap. 10, has calculated that " a moiety of the human fpecies" fell a prey to this frightful epidemic.

Cedrenus page 211 fays this difeafe began in autumn and ended at the rifing of the dog-ftar; or beginning of Auguft.

The ftate of the air, during this peftilence, was uncommonly impure. The defcription of it by Eufebius, in a philofophical view, deferves notice. " Quando, inquit, aer ifte pravis undique evaporationibus turbatus, ferenus reddetur ? Tales enim ex terra fumigationibus, e mari venti, e fluminibus auræ, e portubus exhalationes fprant, ut veluti ros quidam tabidus e cadaveribus putridis, cunctis fubjacentibus elementis inferatur."

Magdeburgh. Cent. 3. p 31.

This is a remarkable inftance of a ftate of air fo highly corrupt, as to form on objects a mould or coat, like a turbid dew, from dead bodies ros tabidus—a ftate of air which the author afcribes to vapor from the rivers and the earth.—The account is analogous to what is related of other peftilential periods, and the fact denotes an utter derangement in the healthful qualities of air and water.—Cedrenus compares this dew to the gore of dead perfons. " Ros faniei mortuorum fimilis apparebat."

Page 211.

In the Traitè de la Peste, I find the following description of the symptoms of this malady, from St. Cyprian—dejection of mind, exhaustion of strength, incessant involuntary evacuations, as in certain paralifes, violent fever of the bowels, mouth inflamed, stomach swelled, eyes sparkling. The disease destroyed the feet, the hands, the sight, the hearing and organs of generation.

Aurelius Victor says of this plague "Simulque Romam pestilentia grassabatur, quæ sæpe curis gravioribus atque animi desperatione oritur." The plague spread, which often arises from the more distressing cares and despair. This describes the miserable state of mankind, at that period; but anxiety and despair do not produce the plague, except during the prevalence of a pestilential state of air. There must be a strong predisposition in the body, or an imbecillity in the powers of animal life previously induced; or the utmost pressure of grief will never occasion a plague. But at the time when general causes have impaired the vigor of the animal principles, slight causes will often induce fever and destroy life. The practical inferences from this fact are extremely important to mankind.

The articles in this account of pestilence which deserve particular notice, are the introduction of the period by a comet and an eruption of Etna—the agitations of the earth by subterranean fire—the preternatural darkness of three days, a phenomenon not unusual at such times and easily accounted for, on the supposition of the extrication of a great quantity of subterranean vapor—the pestiferous state of air which covered objects with mould and corruption—and which generated plague in every village and almost every house.

See Zosimus in Gall. lib 1 sec 26 37, 46. Zonoras lib. 12 Trebellius Pollio in Gall Jornandes Hist August 1098. Eusop lib 9 Baron vol 2. 496. Aurel Victor Ep.t. Magdeburgh Cent 3 31

Near the close of this period, about the year 272, there was an eruption of Vesuvius. At the same time, a severe famin raged in England. Five or six years later, a severe famin prevailed over the world. "Fames ingens per totum orbem grassata est."

Zosimus

It is proper here to notice an inaccuracy of the celebrated Newton, in his Differtations on the prophecies, on the 6th chapter of Revelations, in which he fays, " In the reign of Probus alfo there was a great famin throughout the world—an ufual *confequence* of famin is peftilence.—This peftilence according to Zonoras, arifing from Ethiopia, while Gallus and Volufian were Emperors, pervaded all the Roman provinces for fifteen years." But Probus began to reign in the year 276, whereas the peftilence broke out in Ethiopia under Decius or Gallus and Volufian, about A. D. 252 according to Zonoras, but according to other authors, two or three years earlier. Therefore the peftilence under Gallus, could not be a *confequence* of a famin under Probus, which was 25 years later than the plague afcribed to it. Thefe remarks are neceffary to correct that paffage of Newton, and they are ufeful in correcting the common notion, that the plague is ufually occafioned by famin. The idea is probably unphilofophical; but is certainly contrary to fact. Famin often *goes before* the plague, and as often *follows* it. But fome of the moft difaftrous periods of the plague, have originated during the *greateft abundance* of provifions.—Such was the fact in England, in 448, and in 1347, as will be hereafter related. The great error of hiftorians and phyficians has been, that obferving famin and peftilence often cotemporary, and the caufe of the plague not being obvious to the fenfes, they have taken famin to be the caufe. Whereas it will appear on careful inveftigation, that famin is an *effect* of the fame caufe which produces the plague among men. The dearth of provifions, during this formidable epidemic, is the effect of a *peftilence in vegetation*; that is, a failure in the principles of vegetable life, which proceeds from the fame derangement of the feafons, or defect in the properties of air and water, which caufes the plague among men.—Famin often augments peftilence, and modifies the fymptoms of the difeafe; but in a healthy ftate of the elements of life, air and water, famin will not produce the plague. This may be demonftrated by multiplied inftances of feamen, ftarving on the ocean, who often perifh by hunger, without difeafe, or if they had difeafes in confe-

I.

quence of mere hunger, nothing like the plague has ever been of the number.

I cannot help noticing alfo the obfervations of Mr. Gibbon on the calamities of this period. He fays, " Our habits of thinking fo fondly connect the order of the univerfe with the fate of man, that this gloomy period of hiftory has been *decorated* with inundations, earthquakes, uncommon meteors, preternatural darknefs, and a crowd of prodigies *fictitious* or *exaggerated*."

See vol 1. ch 10

If the original writers who have related the facts above mentioned, had been as fond of *decorations*, as this author, we might well have diftrufted their accounts of unufual occurrences. Had this *elegant* writer taken due pains to inform himfelf of the truth, before he had indulged fuch reflections on the moft credible hiftorians, he would have found fimilar phenomena to have attended the fame calamity, peftilence, in every age from that period to the prefent, and many of them if not all, during his own life, if not within his own obfervation.

He goes on to obferve that " famin is almoft always followed by epidemical difeafes." This point will be afterwards confidered.

He fays alfo that the plague at this period " raged from 250 to 265, *without interruption*, in every province, *every city* and almoft *every family* of the Roman Empire."

The words *without interruption*, were probably inferted for the fake of *decoration*. They are not authorized by the original writers, and cannot poffibly be true, for an uninterrupted plague in a city or country, would foon leave it without an inhabitant. The truth is, it feldom raged, more than fix or eight months, in the fame place, at one time. It feized this town, one year, and that, the next, as we obferve in modern times, through the whole period.*

The more I examin the original writers, from whom Gibbon derived his materials, the lefs confidence I place in his reprefentations of events. He appears to be a partial hiftorian and a fuperficial philofopher.

* The words of Zonoras, per quindecem continuos anno-, are to be underftood as above explained.

In 280 a comet, and in 282 an earthquake in England.

In the year 289 was visible a large comet, and in 290 the winter in England was very severe, all the rivers being closed for six weeks. Busiris and Coptis, two cities of Egypt, were overthrown by an earthquake. In 292 famin, pestilence and drouth prevailed—the bodies of men were covered with carbuncles and ulcers.

Cedrenus.

Worcester in England was almost ruined by an earthquake in 287.

Short, vol 2

In 298 also appeared a comet and earthquakes soon followed, which in Syria, destroyed several thousand lives.

Magdeburg'h Cent 4 p 1434

Earthquakes were experienced in Constantinople in 309 & 310.

In the year 311, the usual rains of winter failed in Italy, famin followed and then pestilence. Baronius, vol. 3. p. 69, describes it as a new disease of *foreign* origin, which, in consequence of excessive heat, produced the anthrax or carbuncle over the whole body, which exposed the patient to mortification. It fell upon the eyes with great severity, rendered many persons blind, and destroyed the lives of great multitudes of all ages. The reader will remark that this distemper was not of *domestic* origin! This is a stale custom of ascribing all evils to foreign sources.

It is related that Cyprus, about this period, suffered a drouth of thirty six years in consequence of which it was nearly dispeopled.

Under the chronological tables, I find a famin mentioned to have destroyed in England and Wales, forty thousand lives in the year 310; and in the following year a violent earthquake injured London.

A comet is noted in 321, and a universal famin in Britain in 325.

In the year 335, appeared a comet of great magnitude, and as it was about two years before the death of Constantine the Great, superstition held it to be the omen of that event.

In 336 Syria and Celicia were laid waste by pestilential dis-

cafes. There was an inundation of the Tweed, the fame year.
    Etrop lib 10. Orofius, lib 7. Magdeb Cent 4 1442

I have not found any particular account of the duration or extent of this calamity. But it appears that this period, like that in the time of Thucydides, was followed by moſt deſtructive earthquakes in 340, which overwhelmed or injured many cities of the eaſt. A comet marked this period in 339.

             Baron vol 3, p 536

A ſnow of 15 feet depth in England is recorded under the year 341.

In 358 happened a moſt tremendous ſhock of an earthquake, which buried in ruins the greateſt part of Nicomedia. The ſhock happened ſoon after day-break in the morning, 11th Kal. Sept. and was preceded by a collection of vapor or clouds, that covered the city with impenetrable darkneſs, ſo that the eye could not diſcern the neareſt objects. This was ſoon ſucceeded by flaſhes of lightning and moſt violent winds and tornadoes, which carried buildings to the adjacent hills. The ſcene was cloſed by a ſhock of the earth which demoliſhed a large portion of the city.

Authors relate that this earthquake levelled 150 cities.

Short indeed was the reſpite which Aſia Minor enjoyed. · In 362, the remains of Nicomedia were deſtroyed, part of Nice was overturned, Jeruſalem was ſhaken and other parts of the world did not eſcape. This was the year alſo in which Julian attempted to rebuild Jeruſalem, when fire burſting from the earth, deſtroyed the works and rendered the place inacceſſible. This event has been aſcribed to a preternatural influence; but is a common phenomenon in Italy, Aſia Minor, and in all countries ſubject to earthquakes; and as it happened when the neighboring countries were laid waſte by the exploſion of ſubterranean fire, there is no neceſſity for reſorting to ſupernatural cauſes, to account for the phenomenon.

During theſe agitations of the earth, the ſea receding left its bed, a highway for paſſengers. Inundations ſucceeded, and drouth, famin and peſtilence walked in the train of public calamities.

In the following years, the earthquakes were repeated and Baronius afferts that the whole world was fhaken; the fhores of the fea were in fome places changed; fome places funk, and in others the waters rofe and carried veffels over the tops of houfes. Authors place the deftruction of Nice in 367, and of other cities in 368 or 372.

The deftruction of Nicomedia was preceded by a fevere drouth—a common event, that a violent explofion of fire from the bowels of the earth, is preceded, fome weeks or months, by a total exhauftion of water by evaporation.

In the midft of thefe convulfions, appeared a comet in 363 or 4, and a meteor or globe of fire in 363.

A hard winter of 14 weeks duration in England is mentioned under the year 359, the year following the deftruction of Nicomedia, and the fevere drouth. This is a ufual event. A fingular light of great extent appeared in the heavens, in the year preceeding.

The whole reign of Conftantius was diftinguifhed for deftructive earthquakes, and the early writers of ecclefiaftical hiftory " make no doubt that God, by thefe judgments, manifefted his difpleafure at the prevalence of the Arian blafphemies." A dreadful famin clofed this period.

It was during the early part of this period, in 359, that the plague broke out in Amida, a city of Perfia, when befieged by Sapor, and from which, when taken, Am. Marcellinus very narrowly efcaped.

See Baron. vol. 4 121, 188, 209; vol. 3. 776 Am Marcel. lib 22 and 25 P Mexia Hift Emp p 339 Eutrop lib 11. Niceph lib 9 and 10 Magdeb Cent 4. c 13 Ech. Rom. Hift vol 3 116. Aurelius Victor, Epit Julian.

Juft before the death of Valentinian I. appeared a comet, in the year 375. Zofimus mentions a hard winter at that time, extending to an unufual length. Another author mentions a fevere drouth about the fame time. Crete, Peloponnefus and Greece in general were agitated by earthquakes and fome towns were demolifhed.* In Wales 43,000 died of the plague.

Echard's Rom Hift vol 3 156 Zofimus lib 4.
Magdeburgh Cent. 4 ca 13. Am Marcel.

* Gibbon chap 26 has well defcribed the earthquakes of 365, but

The following year was marked with famin, and universal pestilence among men and cattle. So severe was the famin in Phrygia that the inhabitants abandoned the country.

Baron. vol. 4 380

A comet appeared in 383, and the plague raged in Rome and in Syria in 383 and 4.—This star however is described by Nicephorus and others, as of a singular figure, resembling a burning column; its motions differed from those of other stars—it was visible 30 days.

Niceph lib 12 Magdeb Cent 4. ca 13.

About the same time, the Nile rose to such an alarming height as to threaten Alexandria and Lybia with an inundation.

Sozomen lib 7 20 Magd Ibm

Just before the death of Theodosius, about the year 394 or 5, happened dreadful earthquakes, storms, rain and unusual darkness.

The appearance of the fiery column and the inundation are placed by some authors under the year 394. The Magdeburgh History from Prosper's Chronicon, places it under the sixth year of Gratian, which is alledged to be the year of Christ 393. But Gratian was killed about the year 383. There is therefore a mistake as to the era of this phenomenon, which, as described by authors of credit, was one of the most singular that was ever exhibited to the people of this globe.

Niceph. lib 12 37. Magd vol 2 1452 and 5

About this period, swarms of locusts covered the land of Judea; and being driven by the winds into the sea and washed on the shore of Palestine, by Gaza, Ascalon and Azotus, they filled the atmosphere with a fetid effluvia, which occasioned pestilence among men and cattle.

Magdeburgh from Hieronymus, vol 2 p 1455

In 396 Constantinople sustained a violent shock of an earthquake, during which the heavens appeared to be in a flame. Functius places these events under the year 400, and he is probably correct.

Baron. vol 4. 20. P. Diac. lib 13.

by mistake quotes Zosimus lib 4 p. 221, whereas the latter author, in this passage, describes the earthquakes of 375.

We are now arrived at another singular and distressing period of the history of man. In the year 400, under the administration of Arcadius and Honorius, a comet appeared of a prodigious size and horrible aspect. Its immense coma seemed to sweep the earth, and Baronius, the pious author of Ecclesiastical Annals, remarks, that many of the Gentiles were terrified into christian baptism and conversion.

During its approach or appearance, happened one of the most severe winters on record. The Euxine Sea was covered with ice for 20 days. A drouth is mentioned under the same period, which was so severe that the heavens were like brass. Unfortunately historians have often neglected to arrange these phenomena in due order, throwing them into a general description.

The same period was marked by deluges of rain, and from the order of narration, it appears that the rains *preceded* the hard winter of the year 400. The rivers were so swelled as to prevent the imperial generals from passing into the east to attack Sardis.— Severe earthquakes occurred in the same year.

About the year 407 or 8, near the close of the reign of Arcadius, a celestial phenomenon of a singular species presented itself to the view of an astonished world. It was called a comet, but did not resemble one of the ordinary figure. It resembled a cone or pillar, but had not the appearance of a star, so much as of the flame of a lamp. Its motion was not regular—it began to move from the point of the heavens where the sun rises at the equinoxes, and passing the tail of Ursa, proceeded to the west.

It measured the heavens—its vertex, at some times, extended to a great length; at others, was contracted into the figure of a cone. After being visible for four months, it disappeared. This is the description of it, nearly in the words of Nicephorus. Meteors were observed at the same period.

Accompanying and following these phenomena, were some of the most distressing calamities. Violent earthquakes levelled cities—inundations of rivers and the sea, followed by intolerable cold storms of hail, and a drouth that blasted vegetation, by which means multitudes of people perished. Pestilence raged in every quarter, and famin so severe, that the populace demanded that human flesh should be sold in market. Palestine was devoured by locusts.

Nicephorus has employed a chapter to describe the physical evils, and the miseries of man, in this singular period. He declares that almost all Europe perished.—"pasa de ōleto ē Eurōpē." and no small part of Asia and Africa.

Niceph lib 13 ca. 6 and 36   Baron vol 5 20, 114, 176, 294.
Zosimus lib 5 Magd Cent 5 ca 13   Ech vol 3 254

In 418 appeared a comet; in 419 several cities of Asia were overturned by an earthquake, and in 420 there was an eruption of Etna. There was also an inundation of the sea in Hampshire, in England, in 419. Famin and pestilence prevailed also in this period.—A great storm of hail is mentioned under the year 418, and deep snow.

The next period of general pestilence commenced in the reign of Theodosius the younger, about the year 445—or a year or two earlier. A comet in 442, ushered in a severe winter, in 443, the snow fell to such a depth and continued so long in Illyricum, that multitudes of men, women and children perished. The year preceding, the Huns had ravaged the country and destroyed the provisions, which added to the public calamities. An irruption of the Sea in North and South Wales, 441, preceded the first comet, a second comet appeared in 444. In 445, severe famin and plague distressed Constantinople, and pestilence appeared in all parts of the world. In 446, Sept. 17, occured a tremendous earthquake, which demolished the greatest part of the walls of Constantinople, with fifty seven towers. The shocks continued unremittingly for six months, and extended to a great part of the globe. Many cities were overthrown, the earth, in some places, was thrown into large hills; in others, it opened and swallowed up whole towns. Islands disappeared and were lost in the ocean: the sea receding, left ships on dry land, springs of water were dried up and new fountains appeared, and in this violent concussion of the elements perished innumerable multitudes of fish.

The pestilence attending, and which rarely fails to attend such agitations of the earth, was universal and of several years duration. In this period, the plague in England was correspondent to the terrible operations of subterranean fire. In 448 or 9, it carried off incredible numbers of people, so that the living could scarcely bury the dead.—And it must not be omitted that the plague was preceded by the greatest abundance of provisions. This was in the reign of Vortigern, and in time of peace.

Niceph. lib 14 ca. 46. Beda Ec Hist. 51, 52. Baronius, vol 6 p. 30, 36, 37, 38. Echard. vol. 3 331. Magdeb Cent 5. ca. 13.

An important fact here occurs. In 446, the Picts and Scots had overrun and desolated England, so as to occasion a dearth of provisions. But this famin produced no pestilential disease. It is particularly noticed by the historian, that the plague did not occur, till a year of great plenty had intervened. This is one strong proof among others, that famin is not the *cause* of plague; but often accompanies, and sometimes increases the disease. It often happens that, during extraordinary agitations of the earth, the elements of vegetable life appear to be defective. The same cause which affects human health, seems to prevent the growth or vitiate the pabulum of vegetables.*

The close of this period was peculiarly distressing in Italy, Phrygia, Cappadocia and Galatia, where the famin compelled parents to devour their own children. The pestilence made great havoc, at the same time, and no remedy or alleviation could be found. The body was universally inflamed and covered with tumors. The disease destroyed the eyes. A cough succeeded the eruption, and ended life on the third day.

Niceph lib. 15 ca. 10.

This was in the beginning of the administration of the Emperor Marcian, which commenced in 450, in which year another comet was displayed in the heavens and a singular light or

---

* General descriptions are seldom correct. I have already taken notice of the mistakes committed by Newton and Gibbon, whose general descriptions lead, in the instances mentioned, to false conclusions. A similar mistake occurs in Henry's excellent History of Britain, vol 1. ch. 1 concerning the calamities of the Britons, in the period under consideration. The author says, " the neglect of agriculture naturally produced a famin, which was followed by a pestilence "—These facts are not correctly stated. The incursions of the Picts and Scots had occasioned the neglect of culture and a famin; but this famin was followed by plentiful crops, which were succeeded by pestilence.

flame, a severe drouth " ingens siccitas," afflicted the earth, and the calamities of this period continued for several years.

It must be remarked here that Functius has placed this comet and the beginning of Marcian's reign, in 454. Such differences in chronology cannot fail to embarrass an inquiry like the present, the results of which depend much on correctness of dates.

Nicephorus and Evagrius give a particular account of an earthquake which laid great part of Antioch in ruins in the second year of the Emperor Leo, which was A. D. 458. A comet is noted under the preceding year But they say further, that this event took place 347 complete years after the destruction of the city in the reign of Trajan, which was in 117. Now 347 years added to this number, give 464, for the year of the last catastrophe.

Niceph lib. 15 20. Evag. lib. 2. 12 and 14.

In the 311th Olympiad, which comprehends the years from 465 to 468 inclusive, appeared a comet. Whether the destruction of Antioch was in 458 or 464, the extent of the shock, through Thrace, Hellespont and the Grecian isles, together with the deluges of rain which are said to have swept away whole towns in Bithynia, leave no room to question the approximation of a comet at or near the time.

Byzantine Hist vol. 15. Evag lib 2. 14.

This latter period was distinguished for pestilence which raged in Rome, about the accession of Anthemius to the empire, and according to Baronius in the year 467.

Vol. 6 281

In the following year, a number of houses were overthrown by an earthquake at Vienna. Of the extent and duration of the pestilence, I have no particular description. A great eruption of Vesuvius is mentioned in 472, and a severe winter of four months duration, in 473 with deep snow.—The plague succeeded in Rome.

In the year 480 Constantinople again suffered great damage by an earthquake, which demolished a great number of buildings.

In 480 or the following year another comet was visible; or probably two years later. In 484 occurred a drouth most terrible and diftreffing—not a vine nor an olive branch retained its verdure—the earth was pale and defolate, and the fun affumed a melancholy face. Africa was almoft abandoned, in confequence of this event and an attending plague.

Baron vol 6 343, 426 and 7

Baronius places the earthquake at Conftantinople in 477, but others place it in 480, which is moft probably correct. The difference in the chronology of different authors, who relate the events of thefe early ages, is feldom lefs than two, three and four years.—The plague infefted Scotland in 480.

In 494 an earthquake overturned Laodicea, Hierapolis and Tripoli. According to Functius, this event was in 496.

Migdeb. vol 3 Cent 6 ca 13

In 499 appeared a comet, which was foon followed by an earthquake which deftroyed Neo Cefarea, in Pontus, and an eruption of Vefuvius laid wafte all the adjacent country.

Zonoras lib 3 Baron vol 6 541. Magd. Cent 6 ca 13 p 789.

A comet is noted in 502, and a fevere winter in 507, but I have no account of any public calamity, attending either of thefe phenomena, except a peftilence among men and cattle in Scotland, in 502.

In 517 is recorded a five year's drouth in Paleftine.

Encyclop Chronol.

In 518 a comet; and in Dardania, now Mæfia, a feries of earthquakes demolifhed twenty-four caftles, divided mountains and in one place opened a fiffure of thirty paces in length and twelve in breadth.

Baronius vol 6 702.

In 519 two cities in Cilicia were overthrown; Ediffa was inundated and part of its buildings and inhabitants overwhelmed.

Zonoras, Tom 3. Magd Cent 6 p 791

Evagrius places the inundation at Ediffa, in the following period, after the deftruction of Antioch; and as the hiftorians do not always fpecify the year in which a particular event took place, I am inclined to believe the account of Evagrius.

Lib 4 ca 8.

In the 7th year of the Emperor Juftin, A. D. 525, appeared a comet, and the fame year Antioch was again overwhelmed in ruin by an earthquake. Some authors relate that 300,000 persons perished in this cataftrophe, and among them Euphrafius, the bifhop.—This event happened on the 29th of May, about 12 o'clock. A conflagration followed and confumed what was left of the city. In the fame fhocks, Dyriachium, now Durazzo, the Epidaurus of high antiquity, Corinth and other cities were greatly injured.

Baronius vol 7. 109, 110, 111. Niceph lib. 7 3
Evag lib 4 Zonoras Tom 3

A fevere winter happened the fame year.

In 528 Antioch was again fhaken and fuffered confiderable injury. An inundation of the Humber in England is noted about this time.

In 531 appeared the refplendent comet, whofe revolution is fixed at 575 years, fuppofed to be the fame which was vifible in the year before Chrift 44, after the death of Julius Cefar. This was the fifth year of the reign of Juftinian. Famin and a flight plague prevailed in Wales.

At this period Gibbon commences his lively, but unphilofophical defcription of the formidable and deftructive calamities, which afflicted the whole earth in the 6th century. See his hiftory, vol. 4. ch 43.

Not long after the approach of the comet in 531, the fun affumed a pale color, and fhone with a feeble light. In a tranflation of Cedrenus, this phenomenon is thus defcribed. "Toto anno eo, fol lunæ inftar, fine radiis, lucem triftem præbuit, plerumque defectum patienti fimilis." During the whole year, the fun gave a gloomy light, like the moon, and appeared as if eclipfed.

Byzantine Hift 3. 293. Procop. de bell. Vandal lib 4

It is remarkable that tradition has preferved a faint account of a fimilar phenomenon, during the approach of the fame comet, at the time of the Ogygean inundation, before Chrift 1767. It is faid, that the planet Venus changed her color, fize and figure. An account is preferved in tradition, of a phenomenon of the fame nature, during the approach of the fame ftar, in a fubfequent revolution. Gibbon in the chapter above cited.—Pliny, as I have already remarked, mentions a fimilar phenomenon, about the time the same comet appeared, soon after the death of Julius Cesar.

The appearance, in the period under consideration, is a well authenticated fact, and witnesses a singular change in the properties, and reflecting powers of the atmosphere, or denotes an essential alteration in the face of the sun, which is improbable. In either case, it seemed a prelude to the most dreadful calamities, famin, earthquakes, and pestilence. I am not without suspicions that Europe might have been overspread with a vapor like that in 1783, during the eruption of Heckla.

In 534 is recorded one of the most distressing famins, that ever afflicted the earth ; it continued many years, and destroyed multitudes of the human race. Pompeiopolis was this year overwhelmed in ruin by an earthquake, and great numbers of its inhabitants perished.

Paul. Diac. lib. 16.

About this period, Vesuvius began to utter hollow rumbling noises, the precursors of an eruption.

Baron. vol. 7. 218. Procop de Bell. Goth Magdeb Cent. 6. p 793.

Excepting a flight plague in Wales—no pestilence is mentioned by the authors I have consulted, until the year 542. But the famin, in great severity, had raged eight or nine years before—a proof that something more than famin is necessary to generate the plague.

In 539 appeared another comet, and the famin now raged with double horror. The country of Italy had been ravaged, the year before by the Goths and Burgundians, and the lands left untilled. This might have contributed towards the dearth which followed. It is recorded that many persons fed on human flesh, some districts of Italy were deserted, 50,000 people perished in Picenum, and greater numbers in other districts. The bodies of the famished people became thin and pale ; the skin was hardened and dry like leather, and clave to the bones; the flesh assumed a dark appearance like charcoal, the countenance was senseless and stern, the bile redundant.

Procop de Bell Goth. lib 1.

Among these frightful effects of hunger, no plague yet appears—a circumstance that the philosopher should not pass unnoticed.

The account which Baronius gives of this famin, is, perhaps more philosophical and deserves notice. He says, the crops failed, corn ripened prematurely, and was thin, in some places, it was not harvested, and that which was gathered, was deficient in nourishment. Those who subsisted upon it became pale, and were afflicted with bile. The body lost its heat and vigor, the skin was dried, the countenance stupid, distorted and ghastly, the liver turned black. Many perished by hunger; many betook themselves to the fields to feed on vegetables, and being too feeble to pull them, lay down and gnawed them off with their teeth.

Baronius, lib. 7. 326

This is the most probable account of the famin. Repeated instances are on record, which evidently mark a pestilential state of the elements, as fatal to vegetable, as to animal life. In many periods of the world, there has been a universal defect in the powers of vegetation. This phenomenon in the vegetable kingdom is cotemporary, or nearly so, with pestilence among men; and superficial observers have ascribed the plague to a prior or cotemporary famin. But an accurate survey of facts, will probably convince any candid enquirer after truth, of the fallacy of this opinion. It will be made apparent that famin and pestilence are equally the *effects* of some general cause; a temporary derangement of the regular operations of nature.

In the present instance, the famin could not be exclusively and immediately the cause of the formidable plague that afterwards assailed mankind, for it was most severe in 539, and the next year the crops were good. But the plague did not break out till 542, at least I can find no account of any pestilence, during the famin.

An eruption of Vesuvius is noted under the year 532, the year after the appearance of the great comet—It is probable that the paleness of the sun was owing to a vapor from some volcanic eruption, as in 1783; and it is remarkable that both of these periods alike produced famin from defective vegetation.

During the remaining part of this century, a series of most calamitous events afflicted the earth. A mountain in Rhodes burst open, and a part of it rolled down upon the inhabitants below. Many places suffered by inundations, one of which overwhelmed the borders of Thrace for an extent of four miles.

In the year 543, the whole earth was shaken by earthquakes. This was the year in which the plague broke out in Constantinople; but it commenced in Egypt, the preceding year.—In 543 there was a dearth of corn, wine and oil. The plague again ravaged Constantinople in 547.

In 545 there was an inundation of the Thracian sea, and a severe winter. A terrible dysentery in France in 548.

See Cedrenus, and Paulus Diac. lib 16.

In 550 an earthquake convulsed Syria and Palestine; and Greece in 551. In 553 appeared a singular meteor in the north and west, which was preceded by a winter so severe that wild beasts and fowls might be taken by the hand. Inundations marked this period. Constantinople was shaken 40 days in 554.

Paul. Diac Madeburgh Cent. 6. ca. 13

In 557 Constantinople was almost laid in ruins by an earthquake. In 558 a comet appeared, a severe winter followed and universal plague, especially in Constantinople, where the living could not bury the dead. This year the Danube was covered with ice.

In 560 an earthquake destroyed Berytus and injured Cos, Tripoli, and Balbus. An excessive drouth in 562, and a plague began which spread over the whole world. There was a dark day in the same year.

The year 565 was distinguished for a calamitous plague, in France, Germany and Italy, which Baronius calls " vehemens pestis inguinaria,"

Vol 7. 547.

In 580 Antioch was again laid in ruins by an earthquake, and a shock was felt in Scotland. The plague again prevailed, from that year to 583, in Gaul and Germany and other countries. In 587 it ravaged Italy. Earthquakes attended this period.

In 590 appeared a comet; an inundation, from deluges of rain, overspread Rome, covering the walls of the city, and lodging innumerable serpents on the plains. In the next summer, happened the severest drouth ever known; it lasted from January to September; and the most deadly plague ravaged all Italy. In this pestilence, died Pope Pelagius.

This is a general sketch of the phenomena recorded of the period under consideration.

Of the universal and destructive plagues which dispeopled the world in the reign of Justinian I. and the succeeding age we have accurate accounts by cotemporary historians: From two of which, Procopius and Evagrius, I shall transcribe the particulars.

Procopius relates, " That this pestilence, which almost destroyed the human race, and for which no cause could be assigned but the will of God, did not rage in one part of the world only, nor in one season of the year. It ravaged the whole world, seizing all descriptions of people, without regard to different constitutions, habits or ages; and without regard to their places of residence, their modes of subsistence or their different pursuits. Some were seized in winter; some in summer; others in other seasons of the year.

It first appeared in Pelusium in Egypt and thence spread westward to Alexandria and all parts of Egypt; eastward towards Palestine, and extended to all parts of the world, laying waste islands, caves, mountains, and all places where men dwelt. If it passed by a particular country at first, or *slightly affected it*, it soon returned upon it with the same desolating rage which other places had experienced.—It began in maritime towns and spread to the interior country. It seized Constantinople in the spring of 543.

Most persons were seized suddenly without any premonition, nor was there any change of color or sense of heat; for until evening the fever was so slight that the patient was not ill, nor did the physician, from the pulse, apprehend danger. But in some cases, the same day; in others, the next; in others, at a later period, a bubo arose, either in the groin, the arm pits, or near the ear, or in some other part. All patients alike had these symptoms.

Some were seized with drowsiness and slumbering; others with furious distraction. The slumberers forgot all things—some would eat if desired; others were neglected and starved.

Neither physician nor attendant caught the distemper by contact of the sick or dead; and many, encouraged by their wonderful escape, applied themselves with assiduity to the care of the sick and the burial of the deceased.

Many were seized, they knew not from what cause, and suddenly died. Some who were given over by physicians unexpectedly recovered; others who appeared to be in no danger speedily expired. Many died for want of relief; others recovered without assistance. No cause of the disease could be devised by human reason—no means of prevention or cure. To some, bathing was beneficial; to others, injurious. Many leaped into water and the sea—In many the bubo, without sleep or delirium, turned into a gangrene, and these died with excruciating torture.

The physicians opened the bodies of some, and found within the sores huge carbuncles. Those whose bodies were spotted with black pimples, of the size of a lentil, lived not a day. Those who had running sores escaped, and these were the most certain signs of recovery. Some had their thighs withered; others lost the use of their tongues.

To women with child, the disease was certain death.

This disease in Constantinople lasted four months, raging three months with extreme mortality. In the beginning, few died more than usual, but the disease gradually increased, till it swept off 10,000 persons in a day."

Procopius calls it arrogance to pretend to assign the natural causes of this pestilence, declaring them to be undiscoverable.

Persic. lib 2 ca. 22.

Authors mention the early effects of this disease on the brain; the patients, on the first attack, saw phantoms of evil spirits, which made them imagine themselves smitten by some person.

Evagrius, who felt the effects of the same disease himself and lost many of his family by it, has enumerated so many singular circumstances, that I shall offer the reader a translation of his account. When I say, *the same disease*, I refer however to a subsequent epidemic. Procopius, as an eye witness, described the pestilence of 543 in Constantinople. It did not continue incessantly to rage in every place, for this would have soon left the earth without an inhabitant; but after an interval of a few years, it returned and revisited the same places. The plague described by Evagrius was many years subsequent to that mentioned by Procopius. He wrote about the year 594. His descriptions however are general.

See Hist Ecclef. lib 4 ca 29.

" I will now describe the plague, which has prevailed in these times, and already raged fifty-two years, a thing never before known, and has already depopulated the world. Two years after the taking of Antioch by the Persians,* a pestilential disease began to prevail, in some respects resembling that which Thucydides has described, in other respects different. It had its origin in Ethiopia, according to common report, and spread over the whole world, falling on different places by turns, and sparing none of the human race.

Some cities were so severely assailed by this disease, that they were left without an inhabitant. Some districts however were more slightly affected. The pestilence did not always begin its attacks at the same season of the year, nor cease to rage, in all places in the same manner. In some places it broke out in the midst of winter; in others, in the spring; in some, it began in summer; in others, in autumn; and in some cities, it attacked certain parts of the town, and left others untouched.

Very often we might observe, particular families all perished, in a city where the disease did not prevail, as an epidemic. In some places, one or two families only perished, while the rest of the city escaped. But we observed particularly that the families which escaped, the first year, experienced the same calamity in the year succeeding.

But what above all appeared singular and surprising was, that

* Under Chosroes A. D 540.

the inhabitants of infected places, removing their refidence to places, where the difeafe had not appeared, or did not prevail, were the only perfons who fell victims to the plague, in the cities which were not infected. And thefe effects were particularly obfervable, both in cities and in other places, in the cycles of the *Indictions*.* Efpecially in the fecond year of each indiction, was the plague extremely mortal Of this I am myfelf a witnefs, for it may not be improper, when the occafion feems to require it, to interweave into this hiftory what concerns myfelf. At the commencement of this calamity, I was feized with the *inguinal plague;* and in the difeafes, which have at different times prevailed, I have loft many of my children, my wife and great numbers of my kindred, of my fervants and laborers: the cycles of indiction parcelling out my calamities among themfelves.

At the time of writing this account, the difeafe had already invaded Antioch the fourth time; the fourth cycle of indiction had paffed, after the firft invafion of this difeafe, when I loft a daughter, and her fon.

This difeafe was a compound of various others. For in fome perfons, feizing the head, it rendered the eyes fanguineous and the face tumid: Then falling upon the throat, foon put an end to life in all that were thus feized. Some were afflicted by difcharges from the bowels. In others an abfcefs formed in the groin, a raging fever followed, and the fecond or third day, the patient died, with his body and his mind apparently found, as tho they had not felt difeafe. Some were feized with delirium and expired. Carbuncles alfo arifing on the body extinguifhed the lives of many. Others recovered once and again, and afterwards died of the fame difeafe.

The modes of contracting the difeafe were various and all calculation was baffled. Some perifhed by once entering infected houfes, or remaining in them—fome by only touching the fick. Some contracted the difeafe in open market. Others, who fled from the infected places, remained fafe, while they commu-

* The *cycle of indiction* was a period of 15 years, at the end of which the Romans paid a certain tax to the Emperors

nicated the difeafe to others who died. Many who remained with the fick, and freely handled them as well as dead bodies, wholly efcaped the difeafe. Others who had loft their children and dependents, and in defpair fought death, by attempting to throw themfelves in the way of infection and affiduoufly attending the fick, found all their efforts in vain; they could not contract the difeafe.

The diftemper has already prevailed fifty-two years, to this time, exceeding all preceding plagues: For Philoftratus was furprifed that, in his time, that calamity had prevailed for fifteen years. What will happen hereafter is uncertain, fince all things are at the difpofal of God who underftands the caufes of things and the events"

Thus far Evagrius. See alfo Nicephorus lib. 17. ca. 18.

The reader is defired to attend particularly to the foregoing relation of facts, as fome important conclufions will, in the fequel, be drawn from them, and other authorities hereafter to be cited.

It will be remarked that altho authors fpeak of this peftilential period, as of fifty-two years duration, as Evagrius and Gibbon have done, yet this is not accurate. Evagrius, from whom this number is copied, fays, the peftilence had then prevailed fifty-two years; but it was ftill raging, and what was to happen afterwards, he could not determin.

The truth is, plagues were uncommonly frequent during this period; but the difeafe did not prevail without intervals. On the contrary, the years remarkable for mortality are fpecified by hiftorians, viz 542 and 3, 547, 558, 562 to 565, 582 and 3, 587, and finally one of the moft deftructive periods of all was 590 and the few following years. Altho this was a long and fevere period of calamity, yet from the beft accounts I can obtain, I fee no reafon to believe the mortality, in any given term of five or ten years, from 542 to 600, to have been greater, than in fome other periods of the fame duration. More people probably died in a fhort fpace of time, in the reign of the Antonines—in that of Gallus and Volufian—and far more, in the dreadful plague of 1346 to 50.—It is even probable that in the last 50 years of the 16th century, the earth sustained as great a loss of inhabitants as in the same space of time in the 6th century. General descriptions are rarely correct, and Mr. Gibbon's unphilosophical, tho eloquent *flourishing* description of the miseries of the human race, in Justinian's reign is calculated to mislead a careless reader.

Evagrius indeed says, this plague exceeded all preceding ones. This is natural; Thucydides said the same of the disease in his time. But we are more able to form a correct comparison between the different epidemics that have prevailed, than the cotemporaries with any particular one.

Agathias relates that in the pestilence at Constantinople in 558, many died suddenly as with an apoplexy. The most robust constitutions survived only to the 5th day. The critical period in the Athenian plague was the 7th or 9th. Thucydides makes no mention of the stupor at the beginning of the distemper, nor of the volutatio humi, whirling of the earth, or dizziness, nor of baboes, nor of the effects of the disease on pregnant women.

Freind's Hist. of Medicine 416 et seq Baron. vol 7. 357, 358.

Warnefred relates of this pestilence, in Liguria, where it was particularly mortal, that there appeared suddenly certain marks "quædam signacula," upon the doors of houses, on garments, and utensils, which could not be washed out but grew brighter by washing. The next year, appeared in men's groins, or other delicate parts of the body, tumors like nuts or dates, which were soon followed by intolerable fever, which extinguished life in three days. If the patient survived the third day, he had hopes of recovery.

I should have ranked this account among the fictions of a disturbed imagination, had not more recent and well attested facts given me reason to credit it.

The description of the terrible effects of this disease in Italy by the same author, is melancholy and painful to the reader.

The dysentery which raged in France in 548 was accompanied with signs of the plague, and was nearly equal to it in mortality. The plague raged this year at Munster, in Ireland.

Short vol. x. 67. Smith's Hist. Cork 10.

The defolating plague of 590 was mortal almoſt beyond example, and preceded or attended with extraordinary phenomena. In 588 Antioch was overwhelmed by a violent earthquake, and 60,000 people buried in its ruins. The inundation of the Tyber exceeded all that had been known, as did the drouth of the ſucceeding ſummer. The intervening winter was equally remarkable for its ſeverity—" qualem vix aliquis prius recolebat fuiſſe," ſays Warnefied ; ſuch as the oldeſt perſons could ſcarcely recollect. Violent tempeſts overturned buildings. About the ſame time, ſwarms of locuſts appeared in Trente and devoured every ſpecies of vegetable. In ſome parts of Italy, they continued their ravages for five years. Cedrenus adds, that fiſh died, and this mortality he aſcribes to the freezing of the waters, page 332.—Modern obſervations prove the fallacy of the reaſon here aſſigned, fiſh do not die beneath a cover of ice ; but the death of fiſh by means of earthquakes, and of ſickneſs, is a common event.

Aguſt Hiſt. 1156, 1157. Magd Cent 6 ca 13

The order of the phenomena here related was this—the earthquake at Antioch—deluges of rain and inundations, tempeſts, a moſt rigorous winter, with a comet, exceſſive drouth, peſtilence.

See alſo Echard s Rom Hiſt vol 4. 246.

Africa was almoſt depopulated by this plague. So ſudden and rapid was the diſeaſe in its action, that during a proceſſion in Rome, inſtituted by St. Gregory, on account of that calamity, no leſs than eighty perſons fell dead in the ſtreet.

Authors relate that the ſerpents, waſhed from the mountains by the flood, and lodged on the earth, putrefied, and contributed to the ſubſequent plague.

Gregory of Tours relates, that the plague, at that time, was introduced into Gaul by a veſſel and her cargo ; but it did not ſpread regularly from houſe to houſe, but ſtarted up in diſtant and detached places, like fire in a field of ſtubble. Marſeilles and Lyons were made waſte by its mortality. It was moſt fatal to the poor.

Lib 9

The following facts are related of the peſtilence in Rome in

581, in the collection of German writers by Pistorius, page 683. Men died suddenly, at play, at table, and in conversation. Sometimes they fell dead in the act of sneezing, " dum sternutabant," so that when one heard another sneeze, he turned to him and exclaimed, " God help you"—which was the origin of a custom still observed in some countries.* Sometimes persons expired in the act of nodding or gaping; which gave rise to the practice of making the sign of the cross, on such occasions—a custom not yet obliterated.

In 599, the plague in the east, in Africa and Rome, was dreadful. The death of the Emperor Mauritius, in 602, was preceded by the appearance of a comet. A severe winter, about this time, killed the vines, and grain suffered by frost and blight. The army of barbarians, marching to besiege Constantinople, was so harrassed and weakened by the plague, as to be compelled to abandon the enterprize. Cayanus their commander lost seven sons.

Niceph lib 18 35   Magd Cent 6 13 and 7 13.
Baron vol 8 138.   Paul. Diac lib. 4.

The Magdeburgh History mentions a severe winter in 604, which was followed by excessive heat and drouth in 605. It places the first comet of 606 in April and May; the second in November and December.

Cent. 7. 13.

The year 615 was distinguished for an epidemic elephantiasis in Italy, and the shock of an earthquake. A comet appeared in 617 and pestilence in 618.

Baron. vol 8. 243.   Short vol. 2. 207.

Here is a period in which mention is made in history of comets, without all their attendant calamities—one in 625, another in 632. It is the first period of the kind I have been able to find; and whether this silence of history is to be ascribed to the carelessness of writers in that distracted period, when the world was overrun by barbarians, or whether men escaped extraordinary maladies, I am not able to decide.

An earthquake in Palestine however marked the approach of the comet in 632.

Funct. Chronol.

* This custom was of higher antiquity.

Short mentions an earthquake at Antioch in 637; and shocks in Palestine in 638 which continued for 30 days—a comet in 639, and the plague in Syria in 640. But I have not the original authorities. The Universal History relates that in 639, the plague was so severe in Syria, Arabia and in Medina, that the Arabs call that year the " Year of Destruction."

Vol 1 485.

A general pestilence in Italy is mentioned in history under the year 651, but no particulars. A surprising meteor had passed the hemisphere, in the preceding year. A violent plague in Constantinople in 654.

Functius Chron Magdeb. Cent. 7. ca. 13.

In 664 pestilence raged in Normandy, England and Ireland; and the historian remarks that the same disease which had afflicted England, afterwards invaded Italy in 665. Thus it would appear that this epidemic broke out *first* in the north of Europe.

Beda, Eccle Hist p 136 Baron vol 8. 496.

But the disease appeared in Egypt the same year it did in England and Ireland.

Paul Diac 980.

In the same year, in March, appeared a bow, iris, stretching across the heavens, and all flesh trembled, says the pious Diacon, expecting the last day.

Ibm *

In 669 or 70 appeared a singular meteor or flame in the heavens—the next year an unusual storm that destroyed men and cattle; and in 672 the plague raged in England, of which died Bishop Ceadda.

Beda, lib. 4

Short mentions a comet in 672, and a severe frost in 670, the year of the celestial flame.

In 678 according to Beda, and in 677 according to Sigebert, in the 9th or 10th year of Constantine Pogonatus, appeared a comet in August, which was visible for three months. The year preceding was marked by most calamitous tempests which cut short the fruits of the earth, except leguminous vegetables

* Livy mentions a similar bow at Rome, during a great plague.

which were replanted and come to maturity. About the same time appeared clouds of locusts in Syria and Mesopotamia. Universal pestilence *followed* these phenomena, in 679 and 680. England and Ireland were ravaged by it in 679; and in 680, during July, August and September, Rome was laid waste: " parents and children, brothers and sisters, were borne to their graves on the same bier." Multitudes of people fled to the mountains, and the streets of the city were overgrown with grass and weeds. A violent earthquake shook Mesopotamia and other countries in 680. The locusts appeared two years *before* the earthquake, and in the same year with the comet, according to Paulus Diaconus. A severe drouth followed the comet, which in England lasted three years.

See Paul Diac. lib 6 Beda, Ec. Hist. p 116 Baron. vol. 8 526, 544. Magd Cent. 7 ca 13. Muratori, vol 6.

In 681 famin, says Beda, raged in England, and in 683, pestilence " quæ ex more famien secuta est," says Paulus Diaconus. In this latter year, if this was the sixteenth of Constantine, according to Baronius, there was a violent eruption of fire from Vesuvius, which laid waste all the neighborhood.

Baronius, vol 8. 564 Magd. Cent. 7. cap 13.

In the same year Syria and Lybia were afflicted by famin and pestilence.

Other authors place this last pestilence two years later. The disease raged in Ireland in 685, in which year, there was a great inundation of the sea and the island of Inisfidda was torn into three parts. In 687, or according to others in 684, appeared a star, which was probably a comet, but without a coma.

Smith's Cork, p 11 Magd. Cent. 7.

Warnefred relates that a singular meteor appeared in 685.*

Notwithstanding some differences among authors respecting the time of the events here related, we observe all the violent agitations of the elements which introduce and attend great plagues.

In 690 happened in Italy, one of the greatest inundations

* We cannot but notice the coincidence in time between meteors and volcanic eruptions.

from rain that was ever known—a severe pestilence followed, "Pestis inquinoria."

In 696, the same disease raged in Constantinople; but no particulars are mentioned.

Magd Cent 7

A severe winter preceded this pestilence, when the Thames was covered with ice for six weeks.

In 707 a terribly severe winter is mentioned and a violent earthquake in Scotland. Short mentions pestilence in Scotland in 703 and in 713, but I have no particulars.

In 717 happened a very severe winter, so that animals died of cold; and the same year, a great overflowing of the Tyber. The Saracens, in an immense army, marching to besiege Constantinople, perished with cold, hunger and pestilence, and in the city, the plague extinguished the lives of 300,000 of its inhabitants. An earthquake in Syria in 718.

Paul. Diac lib 6 47   Baron. vol. 9. 15.
Magd Cent 8 ca 13   Cedrenus

Here is a chasm in the history of comets of 40 years—at least I can find no mention made of them from 685, to 729. The severe winter and the inundation of 717 however leave very little room to question the approximation of one at that time, and others doubtless appeared, during this period.*

There was a great plague in Constantinople in 724.

In the year 725, a vapor like smoke issued for several days, from the sea between Thera and Therasia, the two islands which, many centuries before, had arisen from the bottom of the sea. With this vapor issued dense substances, which, when exposed to the air, grew hard and formed a species of pumice, with which the neighboring sea and the countries of Asia Minor and Macedonia were covered. A small island arose at the same time

Magd Cent 8 ca. 13   Muratori, vol. 1. 151

---

* I have found no author that mentions a comet about this time, but it is worthy of remark that the splendid comet of 1401 was calculated to have a period of 343 years. This was therefore the same which appeared in 1744. If this calculation is just, the same comet must have appeared in 1058—in 715—in 372—and in 29 or 30; or near these years. Now it appears that there was one in 1058 and in 375 attended with all the usual calamities—it is therefore presumeable that it appeared in 715 or 16.

In 729 appeared two comets in January; one preceding the sun, visible in the morning; the other following it, was seen in the evening. The same year the plague prevailed in Norwich.

A plague in Syria raged in 732, but no particulars are mentioned. The following year, the heavens appeared all in a flame.

Magd Cent 8. ca 13

The next pestilential period is remarkable for the violence of the operations of nature.

In 740 a tremendous earthquake, or rather a continuation of successive shocks for twelve months, announced the commencement of a series of calamities. It began on the 7th Kal. November, and demolished buildings, statues and walls in Constantinople, with a multitude of cities in Thrace, Nicomedia and Bythinia. Sigibert places these events in 741.

In 742, or as others say in 743, a most severe drouth was followed by most terrible earthquakes. The next year appeared a comet and the year following, another; and the third year after the drouth, which was either in 745 or 6, according to different authors, a remarkable thick darkness covered the earth from August to October. At this time the plague was raging at Calabria in Naples, and it continued to spread with dreadful havock for several succeeding years, in the countries of the east. So violent was it in Constantinople in 746, that the living could not bury the dead; but the bodies were carried in cart-loads and thrown into empty cisterns, and any place that would conceal them from the sight. Fatal indeed was the disease, when " eodem die aliquis mortuum efferebat, et ipse mortuus afferebatur"—the man who buried a corpse, was sometimes carried, the same day, to his grave.

In the order of the events here related authors agree. Cedrenus mentions an extraordinary light or flame in the sky in 742, and a similar flame in the north, the year following. He mentions at the same time a famin in Constantinople; and limits the darkness to five days, from the 10th to 15th of August.

Paulus Diac Hist August 10. 19   Magd. Cent. 8 13
Baron vol. 9 144, 185.

At the close of this period and while the plague raged in Constantinople, in 749 or 50, Syria was laid waste by an earthquake

—whole cities were exterminated—others removed entire from mountains to plains, for a distance of six miles. This catastrophe corresponded with the approach of a comet. Short mentions two.

Magd Cent 8 13   Baron vol 9 Short 1 81

Such was the waste of people in Constantinople by the preceding plagues, that the emperor Constantine repaired the loss by introducing the inhabitants of neighboring countries.

In 760 or 61, for this difference occurs among good authorities, appeared a comet, or light, called *dokites*, by the Greeks, from its resemblance to a beam; which was visible 10 days in the east and 21 in the west.—In 762 appeared two other comets and the following winter was the most severe probably on record. It began about the first of October, and lasted till February. The Euxine sea was frozen to the distance of one hundred miles from the shore, and the snow and ice accumulated to the depth of thirty cubits. In this frost, the animal and vegetable kingdoms suffered great injury. On the breaking up of winter, the ice from the Danube and the Euxine was forced in huge masses, into the Bosphorus, and against the walls of Constantinople, which were greatly damaged.

In March, falling stars, or meteors were very frequent, and the succeeding summers were remarkable for most terrible drouths, in which all springs were exhausted. Myriads of venemous flies appeared, and a desolating mortality concluded this series of disordered seasons.

Paul Diac lib 22 Baron vol 9. 271 Magd. Cent. 8
ca 13 Short on Air, vol. 1 82

Short mentions a fatal pestilence in Wales in 762.

On the authority of Short, I have mentioned a *mortality* after the severe and unusual seasons of 763 and 4; but the original writers I have consulted do not mention it; tho the fact may be found in others which I have not seen. It is altogether probable that such extraordinary seasons should occasion great sickness; but it is equally probable that if any destructive and general plague had followed them, the writers I have consulted would have mentioned it.

I am led to notice this circumstance, by the consideration that no earthquake is recorded during this period. This circumstance is of no small confequence in this inquiry; and is a confirming proof of the juftnefs of my fufpicions, that peftilence has an intimate connection with fubterranean heat or the action of fire. It appears that the plague, for the moft part, is violent and extenfive, in proportion to the action of the fire that exifts in and about the globe. The preceding peftilential period, beginning in 740, is a ftriking inftance of the truth of this remark.

A great mortality happened in 766. In 767 a fevere drouth exhaufted all fprings and rivers and the year following was diftinguifhed by a comet. Peftilence prevailed in England in 771, and in Chichefter died 34,000 people.

Short vol 2 208.

Short mentions plague and famin in France in 779—a comet, an earthquake at Conftantinople, and peftilence in Scotland in 784; but I have no particulars.

In the reign of Charlemagne, about the beginning of the ninth century, commenced a period of great mortality. A comet in 799, was followed by an exceffively cold winter in 800. Thefe events were preceded by violent earthquakes in Sicily and Crete and in 798, an extraordinary darknefs in England of feventeen days. In 801 earthquakes fhook Italy, France and Germany, and thefe phenomena were repeated in 802 and 3. A prodigious tempeft in the year 800, levelled a multitude of buildings.

In 802 the plague prevailed in various places, " propter molitiem hyberni temporis," fays the annalift Bartianus, by reafon of a mild winter. This however could not be the true reafon.

In 808 a very mild winter was followed by the plague. In 810 happened the greateft mortality among horned cattle that is on record. In fome places in Germany, it deftroyed almoft all the fpecies.

Lancifius 146. Annal Fuldenfes 810.

In 811 fwarms of locufts from Africa invaded Italy and devoured every green thing.

In 812 appeared a comet, and after a chafm in the accounts of Etna of nearly four hundred years, that volcano is recorded to have difcharged fire in this year. P. Diaconus places the comet in 813, and a violent earthquake.

Magd Cent 9 ca. 13 Muratori vol. 2. 505, 507.
Piftarius' Germ Script vol 2 38

In 817 was a comet, and a peftilence foon after commenced, which authors relate to have arifen from exceffive rains and a humid air. This plague raged in almoft every part of France in 820, and crops failing from excefs of moifture, a famin enfued. Baronius mentions earthquakes in 820 in thofe places where the *Chriftians were perfecuted*. The following winter was fo fevere that the Rhine and the Danube were covered with folid ice for more than 30 days, and fuftained loaded carriages.

In 823 was another moft fevere winter, in which the fnow lay on the earth twenty nine weeks, and occafioned the death of many animals and men. An earthquake and a univerfal plague in France. The next year fell a fhower of hail, which killed men and cattle. Severe drouth the fame year.

Magd. Cent 9 ca 13. Muratori, vol. 2. 513, 516. Short, vol 2.

In 827 the Thames was covered with ice for nine weeks.

In 828 appeared a comet in Libra; and in 829, another in Aries; with many meteors. The earth in France was violently fhaken in 829; a violent tempeft followed, but no peftilence is mentioned.

Baron. vol 9 809 Magdeb. Cent 9. ca. 13.

In 839 appeared a comet and another in 842. In 840 Conftantinople was fhaken for five days, and fome parts of France felt the fhock. The rains were exceffive, the Rhine overflowed, and the ftorms of hail and wind were unufually fevere.

Magdeb. Cent 9 ca 13.

In 850 another comet is mentioned, and in the following year a moft fevere drouth, which occafioned a famin that compelled men to feed on human flefh.—There was a fevere earthquake in Gaul the preceding year.—A peftilence in many parts of Scotland in 853.

Baron vol 10. 73 Magd. Cent 9. Muratori, vol 2 531

It will be obferved that no peftilence is noted under fome of thefe laft inftances of comets and other phenomena. Hiftory, during the dark and barbarous ages under confideration, is extremely barren; and the smaller calamities of all kinds have been passed over in silence. Whether any confiderable mortality prevailed, at these periods or not, we cannot determin from the silence of the dull annals of the dark ages.

In 855 an earthquake at Conftantinople, and in other places, violent tempefts. In 856 another earthquake and a tremendous inundation of the Tyber, which was followed by an epidemic difeafe, called a plague of the fauces, in which the throat was obftructed by defluxions, and sudden death ensued.* In 858 a comet, and the fucceeding winter was fo severe that the Adriatic fea was covered with ice and people walked on it to Venice. This was followed by an earthquake in Conftantinople.

Muratori relates that in 855, two unusual stars appeared for ten days, alternately, and that the next year the winter was very severe, dry and peftilential, fo that a great portion of men perished. But I fufpect he refers to the same years mentioned in the preceding paragraph.

Baron vol 10 131   Muratori vol 2 534   Short vol 1. 85.

The plague was in Scotland in 863.

The winter of 864 is recorded as very severe. In 867 there were violent tempefts, and in the following year a general famin in Europe, severe earthquakes and a comet.

Magd. Cent 9 ca. 13.

In 872 a comet, and a moft exceffive heat and drouth, which cut short the grain.

Ibm.

In 874 appeared in France myriads of grafs-hoppers or locufts of a remarkable fize, with fix feet and two teeth harder than ftone. They are reprefented as having leaders, which went before them a days journey, meafuring a certain fpace; the fwarm followed about 9 o'clock and there waited for the rifing of the fun, obfcuring the heavens by their numbers, and with a broad mouth and large inteftines, devouring every green herb and tree. Their days journey was four or five miles.

Thefe animals were at laft driven into the Britifh channel by the winds, and being wafhed afhore, their putrefying bodies cauf-

* A fpecies of quinfy.

ed a ftench, and ficknefs, which, with a pinching famin, deftroyed a third of the people, on the neighboring French coaft.

The fucceeding winter, 875, was terribly fevere and continued from November to the vernal Equinox.

In this or the following year, for authors differ, appeared a comet of extraordinary brightnefs, and in June following, were deluges of rain, which, in Saxony, fwept away a whole village, with its inhabitants and cattle.

In the year 878 a mortal peftilence raged among the cattle, efpecially about the Rhine. Dogs and birds which at firft collected round the dead bodies, fuddenly difappeared.

Magd Cen 9. ca 13   Piftor. Germ. Hift vol 2. 570 vol 1. 63

In 879 there was an eruption of Vefuvius.

In Feb. 882 appeared a comet with a vaft coma preceded in January by an earthquake. In the next year Italy was feverely afflicted by famin. In 884 the plague was in Oxford.

Magd Cent 9 13   Short vol 2

In 887 the winter was unufually long and fevere; and a peftilence among cattle was fo mortal, that few furvived it.

Muratori, vol. 2 p. 92

A comet is noted under 896, and a famin in France and Germany, in the following year.—Italy was fhaken by earthquakes.

Dufrefroy. Baglivus.

In May 904 appeared a comet, followed by a fevere frofty winter of four months, and violent earthquakes with mortal peftilence in 905.

Univerfal Hift vol 17 87   Magd. Cent. 10 ca 13

In 912 appeared a comet of unufual fplendor and the following winter was very cold "acutiffimum fuit frigus," and meteors in the air very frequent. A famin followed in Germany, and Italy experienced earthquakes.

Magd Cent. 10   Short vol 1.   Baglivus. p 542

The plague was in Scotland in 922.

Short vol 2.

A fevere winter in which the Thames was frozen for 13 weeks in 929, followed by a dreadful famin, is mentioned by the laft cited authors. An earthquake is mentioned in 935, and a peftilence in 937, but no details.

In 940 there was a severe winter and pestilence among cattle.

In 942 and again 944 appeared a comet, the latter very large with a brilliant coma; followed by severe famin in France and Italy. Some authorities place the latter comet in 945. The winter of 946 or 7 was long and severe, continuing to the vernal equinox of the next year.

Magd Cent. 10—Pistor Germ Script. vol. 1.

The same period was marked by earthquakes in France and Germany.

In 954 pestilence invaded the north of Europe, with great destruction—Scotland lost forty thousand inhabitants. The following winter was severe.

Baron. vol. 10 739 —Magd Cent 10.

In 961 a flame or fiery column appeared in the heavens. In 962 a very severe winter and a famin. In 964 a dreadful plague in the Emperor Otho's army. In 968 a comet, an earthquake and violent winds which destroyed the grain and occasioned famin.

Baron vol 10 771 Magd. Cent. 10. Pistorius, vol 1. 134.

English authors mention a malignant fever in London in 961; at which time there was a large marsh on the south side of the Thames.

Maitland's Hist London.

In 975 appeared a very large comet in harvest, and the following winter was excessively severe. The next year England was afflicted with grievous famin. An earthquake preceded, in 974.

Magd Cent 10 ca 13. Simeon Dunelmensis.

In 981 a comet and in 983 another. In this latter year was an eruption of Vesuvius. Universal famin followed and a plague among the Lacedemonians.

Baron. vol 10. 831. Magd Cent. 10. 13.

This period was followed by desolating earthquakes in Lacedemon in 986.—In 987 the season was unfavorable and occasioned dearth—malignant fevers prevailed in England and the cattle died of fluxes.

Brompton, Angl Scrip. 878.

Meteors and a flaming sky were observed in 993, in which

year was a great eruption of Vesuvius. Then followed an excessively severe winter, which lasted from November to May. The rivers were frozen dry, fish perished and a scarcity of water ensued. In July a severe frost gave to the trees the gloomy aspect of winter.

With these singular seasons prevailed a famin and a deadly plague among men and cattle.

In 995 a comet was seen. The Saxon Chronicle places the foregoing events three years earlier.

In 996 an epidemic flux prevailed with great malignity in England.

The events here related are similar to what are common at the present day; a volcanic discharge of fire being followed by unusual cold and snow. Meteors also are common near the time of such discharges.

Magd Cent 10 13   Baron vol. 10. 877.

Hitherto our accounts of the great volcanoes have been very imperfect. The first instance of an eruption in Iceland, which is recorded, was in the year 1000; and from that period we have a regular history of volcanic discharges in that island, which is one of the principal outlets of fire on the globe, and which, we shall find, has no small connection with the extensive and powerful operations of fire, both in Europe and America. There are many volcanoes in the island of which Heckla is the principal.

In the year 1000, there was an eruption in Iceland, two globes of fire or great meteors were seen, violent earthquakes in England, and a severe winter followed. In the same year appeared a comet with a long coma.

In the year following a flux, and fevers with a burning ague, were epidemic and mortal in England.

Magdeb Cent 10 13

The next period of general pestilence was remarkable for its extent, violence and attending phenomena.

In 1004, an eruption of Heckla in Iceland, with a violent earthquake announced the approaching calamity. In 1005 appeared a comet of frightful aspect, and in the winter Italy was for three months, convulsed by earthquakes. In the same year commenced a famin, and a plague of three years duration, which desolated the whole earth. Cotemporary authors affirm that more than half the human race perished. The living were fatigued with burying the dead—" ut sepelientium tædio, vivi ad huc spiritum trahentes, obruerenter cum mortuis." Such was the weariness of those that buried the corpses, that the living before their breath had left their bodies, were tumbled into the graves with the dead.

At the close of this horrible destruction, Vesuvius discharged prodigious quantities of lava which laid waste the neighboring country.

In 1009 was seen a comet in May. The beginning of the year the earth was deluged with rain, and a plague among the Saxons followed.

The plague is also mentioned under the year 1012, with violent rains and inundations, followed by an earthquake in 1013. But the necessary materials for a detail are wanting.

Magd Cent. 11 13 Baron vol. 11 27 Muratori, Tom 5 55.

In 1015 appeared a comet, attended with violent tempests, and followed by famin in 1016. In 1017 another comet was seen, and the following year is noted as pestilential. But I have no particulars.

In 1020 was seen another comet, and the winter was excessively severe, so that men perished with cold. This was followed by pestilence, in which the bodies of the infected generated "serpents," says the historian; by which he probably means some species of worms. A similar fact will be related from Thuanus in the 16th century.

In 1021 was an earthquake, and the next year, the drouth and heat were extreme.

In 1025 the summer was wet. The plague raged in England, and in other parts of Europe, pestilence with violent earthquakes.

Magd Cent 11. 13.

In 1029 was an eruption of Heckla, and pestilence in some parts of Europe.

A comet in 1031 was accompanied, in its passage, through

the fyftem, with great ftorms of wind and rain, producing vaft inundations. In France, England and the eaft raged famin and peftilence. Locufts were added to thefe calamities, which were fo fevere in fome parts of the world, that multitudes were compelled to leave their country. Violent earthquakes marked this year, and what is ufual in the tempeftuous feafons occafioned by comets diftinguifhed by volcanic eruptions, a fplendid meteor, or globe of fire.

During an eclipfe of the fun in 1032 or 3, authors mention a fingular phenomenon—a faffron color in the air, which gave to the human countenance a cadaverous afpect. But it might be merely the effect of a partial darknefs, with a hazy atmofphere.

A fevere winter in 1035, was followed by an eruption of Vefuvius in 1036. The frequent coincidences of this kind deferve notice.

In 1037 is noted an igneous appearance in the heavens, like a beam. Thefe phenomena were followed by peftilence in England and in the Emperor's army, and with earthquakes.

Magd Cent 11. 13. Univ Hift vol. 17. 166
Echard's Rom Hift vol. 5. 146.

In 1042 commenced another diftreffing period. A comet in this year was followed by an eruption of Vefuvius in 1043 and fnow in harveft. The year 1042 was very tempeftuous and rainy; the dykes in Flanders yielded to the fwelling ocean, and the low grounds were overwhelmed, with infinite deftruction. At this time began a general famin in England, France and Germany. The year 1043 was alfo diftinguifhed for rains and ftorms; autumnal fnows were early, and an infectious difeafe carried off vaft numbers of cattle. In 1044 there was great mortality among men.

In 1047 fell a deep fnow in the weft of Europe, which overwhelmed fmall trees, and lay till March. In March 1048 was a violent earthquake, followed by a tempeftuous feafon and great ficknefs. There was an eruption of Vefuvius the fame year, and an earthquake in October. The reader will remark a very regular connection between eruptions of volcanoes and violent winds.

Magd. Cent. 11. 13

During this period the countries about the Hellespont were, for three years, ravaged by locusts.

In 1052 a tempest is noted which demolished many buildings. In 1053 a comet which was followed by a famin. But the seasons are not described.

In 1057 severe frost and great quantities of snow ruined the vines. During the following year, a comet was seen, the year after which the winter was very long and severe, and in 1060 prevailed famin, and plague among men and cattle.

In 1062 a trembling of the earth in Constantinople, attended with thunder and lightning, was succeeded by the plague. The next year was distinguished by a comet, visible 40 days, a tempest of four days, deep snow, and extreme cold, which proved fatal to vines, trees, birds and cattle.

In 1065 several hundred thousand Scythians, marching to invade the Roman empire, perished with pestilential diseases.

In 1066 a comet was seen in May, and a cold winter succeeded. Egypt and Arabia, countries not subject to earthquakes, were violently convulsed in November, and a plague speedily followed, which, authors affirm, swept away one half the inhabitants. This was attended with famin.

The north of Europe speedily felt similar calamities. Violent earthquakes in 1068, and a comet in May, of apparent diameter equal to that of the moon, visible 40 days, were succeeded by famin. The country in England from Durham to York was depopulated. Men subsisted on dogs, cats and every unclean thing; or perished and their bodies were left to putrefy on the earth. The winters were unusually severe.

Magd Cent 11 13 Murat vol 5 44. Baron. vol. 11. 370.

In 1074 another comet appeared and a hard winter. The winter of 1076 was excessively cold from Nov. to March, so that the roots of vines were killed. In April 1077 appeared a comet, and famin and plague raged in Constantinople with such mortality, that the living could not bury the dead. An earthquake was experienced in England. Shocks were also felt in 1081 and 1082.

In 1084 raged famin and pestilence; the latter cut off the

whole army of the Emperor Henry, in Rome. In 1085, Ruſſia was laid waſte by locuſts and the plague. The ſeaſons were unfavorable in England, the crops bad and a great mortality among cattle. In 1086, were great inundations in Flanders, Italy and other countries; and in 1087 the fiſh died in the rivers.

Magd Cent 11 Baron vol 11 564   Stowe's Annals
Knighton Hiſt Ang Script 2353

Authors relate that in 1086, domeſtic fowls left the houſes and fled to the woods. The two following years, the ſame calamities continued—bad ſeaſons, murrain among cattle, and a violent fever, which appeared in the former year, raged in theſe and affected one half the people of England. In 1089 a burning plague deſtroyed mankind. Earthquakes diſtinguiſhed theſe periods.

Functius Chro vol. 1 102.

In 1091 appeared a comet; another in 1094; a third in 1096, and a fourth in 1098.

In 1091, many violent tempeſts happened which levelled buildings, 600 houſes were blown down in London; ſwarms of locuſts darkened the ſun, and the next year a plague raged, which the hiſtorian relates to have ariſen from the putrefaction of their bodies. The place where the locuſts appeared is not named.

A moſt ſevere winter in 1093, occured after a very rainy ſummer in England. The ſummer of 1094 was alſo exceſſively rainy.—The plague at the ſame time raged in England, Gaul and Germany. A violent earthquake with a tempeſt in 1094. The comet in Oct. 1096 was attended with great rains, which prevented the ſowing of winter grain, and famin followed. Various fiery appearances and meteors were obſerved, during this period, and the winter of 1095 was ſevere.

In 1098 a peſtilence invaded cattle, from the bad quality of their food, which had been injured by great rains. This was the year of the laſt comet above named, and in the following year, was a hard winter and a dearth. Syracuſe was injured by an earthquake.

Magd Cent 11. 13. Matthew Paris, p 17. Muratori, Tom 5 59

To the year 1099 or the following, is to be aſſigned the terrible inundation which ſpread over the low lands in Kent, belonging to Earl Goodwin, and which, never having been recovered, now form the shoals, called Goodwin' Sands, of dangerous navigation.—A severe winter followed, and pestilence and famin in various places.

Pistorius, vol 1. Anderson, Hist. Com vol 1, 176.

It is probable that the events related in the two last paragraphs happened in the same year. The inundation is said to have drowned in Holland one hundred thousand people.

A dark day is mentioned in the year 1099.

In the year 1100 raged a pestilence in Palestine, said to have originated from the stench of dead bodies. In Syracuse, a violent earthquake demolished a tower, with the loss of many lives. In 1101 a singular meteor, and such multitudes of worms, called *papiliones*, from their resemblance to a pavilion, that they covered two or three miles of country.

Magd Cent. 12 ca 13.

In 1103 a new star shone for twenty five days, and a comet of a bright flaming color.—A great mortality happened this year.

Magd ibim Matthew Paris.

In 1105, there was a discharge of fire from Heckla, and in the same year, a great quantity of snow, a violent earthquake in Jerusalem, about Christmas, and about the same time, a light in the west almost equal to the sun, and two mock suns.

In Feb. of the following year, a comet* of unusual splendor for three weeks was visible from three to nine o'clock, and two mock suns. A violent earthquake happened the same year. Many meteors were seen and violent tempests and inundations, with myriads of insects in the air, marked the disorder of the elements.—The year was also noted for sterility of grain, and a consequent dearth—men were attacked with plague and unusual diseases—" ignotis morbis, igne, flamma, ardore invisibili homines excruciati et absque ad ustionis nota extincti,"

Magd Cent 12. ca. 13 Muratori, Tom, 5 485.

The reader cannot fail to remark how regularly the mention of comets is accompanied with a failure of crops, meteors, and tempests. We have proof in modern times that these were not the

---

* Supposed to be the same as that which appeared in 531 and in 1680.

fictions of imagination. See the years 1769-70—1783-4—1788-9.

In 1107 appeared a comet with a long coma—another was seen in Normandy in 1108.

In the year 1109 eryfipelous difeafes were epidemic in England; which afflicted and deftroyed many people, their limbs covered with black fpots, like carbuncles.

Magd Cent. 12. ca 13 Sigebert. Polydore Virgil.

In December 1109 appeared a comet, and in June 1110 another, which fpread its coma to the fouth. A fevere winter, with deep fnow and long continued cold, followed and fterility of grain. An unufual recefs of water in the Trente, fevere earthquake in Salop, and a mortality among men and cattle diftinguifhed the year 1111.—An earthquake and fevere plague are mentioned under the year 1112; but the year was remarkable for abundant crops of grain.—This year there was an extraordinary recefs of the water in the British Channel for a whole day, fifh died in the water and domeftic fowls took flight into the woods.

Magd Cent 12 ca. 13 Knighton, Hift Ang Script 2379.

Here we have an account of a progreffion in the peftilence—from the eruptive difeafes of 1109 to the plague in 1112—This is the modern order.

In 1113 or, as fome authorities have it, in May 1114, a comet appeared, and in a period of diftreffing calamities. In this year there was an eruption from Heckla in Iceland.

In May 1113 an extraordinary fnow very much injured trees and vegetables. In June a dreadful tempeft laid wafte whole countries, and the exceffive heat of the fummer produced dyfentery and other peftilential epidemics. In 1114 many cities in Syria were proftrated by an earthquake; and its effects were felt in all the oriental countries. In November 1115 many houfes in Antioch were fwallowed up in a chafm rent in the earth. In January 1116 various places fuffered by fhocks of the earth, and in 1117 all Italy was fhaken for forty days.

In 1113 Flanders was overwhelmed by an inundation, which compelled many Flemmings to abandon their country, and they fettled in England.

This event seems to fix the approach of the comet in the year 1113.

Severe drouth and a singular recess of the ocean left rivers dry in 1114. October 15th people walked over the Thames between London bridge and the tower. In December the sky appeared to be in a flame.

The winter of 1115 was most rigorous, and a terrible mortality swept away the cattle. A comet appeared this year also.

The year 1116 was rainy and fruits were destroyed. In 1117 swarms of locusts about Jerusalem devoured vegetation, and in England great damage was done by floods.

In 1118 and 1119 earthquakes were violent. In 1120 the locusts and mice overran Judea, and Trent suffered much from earthquakes. A severe winter followed in 1121, and a drouth the next year, which occasioned a scarcity of provision, and men and cattle perished.

In the foregoing period, no great pestilence is mentioned, but such diseases as were occasioned by intemperate seasons, except among cattle.

Magd Cent 12   Baron vol. 12 117.
Muratori, Tom 5. p 60.   Maitland's Hist Lond.

In 1124 happened a very severe winter, which destroyed trees and vines—succeeded by a cold spring which retarded vegetation. The following year was noted for a destructive plague among men and cattle, in France and Brabant. Terrible was the famin in Italy, and in England so many people perished with hunger, that dead bodies lay in the highways unburied. In 1125 the famin, accompanied with pestilence, continued in England, Germany and Italy. The season was excessively wet and all fruits were injured or destroyed. In 1126 appeared a comet in October, followed by a winter excessively severe, and in the following year, violent earthquakes occurred in Syria. Erysipelous distempers were fatal in England.

In the pestilence of 1125, it was computed that one third of the people perished.

Magd Cent 12.   Baron vol 12 160.   Dufresnoy.

In 1130, 31 and 32, happened the most destructive murrain

among cattle and fowls ever known in England. In 1131 an excessive drouth in France.

In October 1133 appeared a comet. The same year, England was shaken by earthquakes, and inundations continued a whole month. Authors assert that the sun exhibited singular appearances, changing its figure and dimensions, and that there was a remarkable intemperature in the air. In modern times, the face of the sun is often disfigured with spots, and it is not unphilosophical to suppose that moving vapor in the air may suddenly change its apparent diameter.

In 1134 the sea broke into Flanders, as it did in the following year. This year was rainy.

In 1135 the drouth destroyed vegetation and occasioned a dearth. The Rhine was fordable in almost any place. Terrible tempests and earthquakes and an eruption of Vesuvius marked this period, and a dreadful plague ensued.

Short, vol 1. 118.

The eruption of Vesuvius was in 1136 and a second in 1139. The summer of 1137 was as remarkable for drouth, as was that of 1135. The plague was universal. The disorders in the elements occasioned a long and desolating famin.

Magd Cent 12 Pistorius, vol 1 156. Matthew Paris

Knighton mentions the sun's changing its form in 1133, and adds that a darkness happened which rendered a candle necessary in the day time.

Chronocon

From this it is probable the sun presented appearances, like those which we observed on the 19th of May 1780, and which are usual in dark days.

The reader will remark the occurrence of such days, in years when electricity shakes the earth, or fire and lava are discharged by volcanoes. He will note also the drouth that preceded the eruption of Vesuvius in 1135 and 1138.

In 1140 was an earthquake in England. In 1141 a very severe winter. In 1143 the air, for a mile in extent, was filled with an unusual insect, with the body of a worm and the size of a fly. A general plague among men and cattle began the same year, and raged with great violence in various countries.

In 1144 or as some authors relate in May 1145 appeared a comet, illuminating the heavens, and the same year were violent earthquakes. In 1146 another comet, and the plague incredibly fatal. A famin prevailed with diftreffing feverity, for 12 years, including the years juft named.

Magd Cent 12. Muratori, Tom. 5. p. 65.
Piforius, Germ Script.

If men, at this period, had any refpite from natural evils, the intervals were very fhort. In 1150 a very fevere winter and fevere peftilence are recorded in the Saxon chronicle, together with famin and an eruption of fire in Iceland. Earthquakes, inundations and peftilence marked the fubfequent years. The years 1151 and 2 are mentioned to have been very rainy—the winter of 1153 and 4 fevere, and the fummer of 1156 exceffively dry. Thefe phenomena follow each other fo rapidly, and are related with fuch brevity and in general terms, that it leaves the mind at a lofs to what influence to afcribe the difeafes which afflicted nations for a feries of years about this period. In this gloomy and barbarous age of the world, hiftory is concife and deftitute of accurate obfervations.

In 1157 there was an eruption in Iceland, with a very cold winter. In 1158 an eruption of Vefuvius, an earthquake in England, and an inudation of the Tyber. Peftilence appeared in Scotland in 1154.

Not long after thefe events, Antioch, Tripoli, and Damafcus were convulfed by an earthquake, with the lofs of 20,000 lives.

After an interval of more than 300 years, during which I find in hiftory no account of any eruptions from Etna, this volcano is introduced to our notice by an almoft continual eruption from 1160 to 1169. Earthquakes were violent in 1161—in Sicily an inundation drowned 5000 people—in 1163 one of the greateft inundations in Friefland ever known, preceded by a very fevere winter. At this time the plague was raging in Milan, Normandy and Aquitain. Unufual darknefs is mentioned in 1164. In England, the fea overflowed twelve miles of country, deftroying men, cattle and improvements. In 1165, a comet appeared with a long coma; 12,000 people perifhed by an inundation in Sicily, and Norfolk and Suffolk in England were shaken by an earthquake. Most of Frederick Barbarossa's army perished by the plague in 1167. This period was remarkable for great wind and hail.

In 1169 the eruption of Etna was very violent; Catana was demolished by an earthquake, and 15,000 people perished—Asia Minor felt the shock. In the next year, so general and tremendous were the earthquakes, that many of the best cities in Syria, Palestine and other countries, were laid in ruins. Germany suffered by earthquakes and inundations. Pestilence marked this period, and in 1172 a malignant dysentery raged in England.

In 1174 mention is made, for the first time, of an epidemic cough or catarrh. There is however no question that influenza and measles always preceded or accompanied pestilence in the ancient and middle ages, as they do in modern times. Authors have neglected to record the prevalence of all the minor epidemics, or nearly all, until after the invention of printing.

In 1175 history mentions an eruption of Etna, pestilential diseases in England and a famin. In 1176 a long and severe winter, and an irruption of the sea into Holland with immense destruction—a severe drouth followed with a loss of seed time. The year 1177 was distinguished for violent winds.

In 1178 a comet was succeeded by a most rigorous winter, and destructive inundations. On the 11th of September, was a dark day, with singular appearances of the sun and moon. Another comet is mentioned in 1179 and a great hail storm.

In 1181 appeared a comet, and earthquakes, with an eruption of Etna, marked this period.—At this time Denmark was almost laid desolate by excessive rains, famin and pestilence, while Germany lost half of its inhabitants by the plague. Some allowance must be made for exaggeration in the accounts of the more destructive plagues. This was an age of superstition, and the imaginations of men were susceptible of strong impressions.

In 1185 is recorded a most violent earthquake, over Europe. Calabria was overturned, and thousands perished. On the Adriatic, a whole city was swallowed up, and the shock was felt to the Baltic.

In 1186 Ruffia and Poland were defolated by locufts and peftilence. The winter was fo mild, that the following harveft was in May, and vintage in Auguft. In Carinthia, the locufts devoured every green thing.

An unufual conjunction of planets happened, this year, in Libra ; and fo great was the alarm, in that ignorant and credulous age, on account of the calamities predicted by aftrologers, that a folemn faft of three days was appointed by the Archbifhop of Canterbury. Luckily no uncommon event happened in England, until the next year, when peftilential difeafes prevailed among men and cattle. In 1188 the plague was in Rome.

Magd Cent. 12 Murat vol 5 p 70—6—182.
Univ. Hift. vol 32 110 Henry Hift Brit vol 3 380.

I have no accounts of comets in this period from 1181 to 1211, altho it is probable that feveral were vifible.

How far may we fuppofe the conjunction of all the planets had any influence in producing the remarkably mild winter of 1186?

In January 1193 was a remarkable aurora borealis.

In 1193 and 4 exceffive rains injured the grain and produced a dearth. In England an acute peftilential fever was epidemic and left in health fcarcely a number of perfons fufficient to tend the fick. The ufual forms of burial were neglected, and dead bodies were thrown into graves in piles. A fevere winter put a ftop to this epidemic. Brompton, with a natural partiality for religious houfes, informs us that the only places exempted from the deftruction of this peftilence, were the monafteries—Cotemporary with this difeafe was an earthquake and a fingular fiery appearance in the fky. Short places this fever under the year 1196 and calls it a " burning ague." See the years 1001 and 1723.

Brompton's Hift. Ang Script. 1271. Magd Cent. 12.
Short, vol. 1. 130

The winter of 1200 was cold; the fummer of 1201 was very rainy ; and the winter fucceeding was fevere almoft beyond example. In 1203 was a fore famin from bad feafons. In 1205 a rigorous winter and a great hail ftorm ; in 1206 an eruption of Heckla ; but I have no account of any epidemics that prevailed.

In 1210 was an eruption of Heckla, and a cold winter. In 1211 appeared a comet, in May, visible for 18 days. Great tempests marked this period with inundations. In 1212 Venice and Damascus were violently agitated by earthquakes, and in Sicily thousands perished by an inundation. These phenomena were the heralds of a severe pestilence, which, in 1213, was so fatal in Italy, that authors affirm scarcely one tenth of the inhabitants survived. In the year following appeared two comets.

The year 1219 was distinguished for the approach of a large comet, distressing inundations, in one of which perished 36,000 inhabitants, an earthquake and a volcanic eruption in Iceland. In 1220 the plague was so fatal in Damietta, that authors relate three persons only survived out of 70,000. By this we are to understand the disease to have been extremely mortal, but we must reject the literal meaning of such relations. It is doubtless true that the pestilence of this period has rarely been exceeded in mortality.

This period was very calamitous in the north of Europe. In 1221 Poland was afflicted by excessive rains, and the floods which followed swept away whole villages. The winter succeeding was severe, so that frozen wine was sold by weight, while famin and pestilence almost desolated Europe. In most countries, the living could hardly bury the dead; and in some cities, scarcely a person survived.

In the year 1222 appeared a comet of unusual magnitude and the summer was excessively dry. A frost, with deep snow in April, destroyed the fruits. In autumn the earth was deluged with rains and swept with violent winds. An earthquake shook Germany and Lombardy; in Cyprus two cities were demolished; the shocks were frequent and continued for two months, in Brixia, Venice, England and other countries. The plague raged, for three years, with uncontrolable fury, in Germany, Hungary, France and other countries; falling on cattle as well as man.

During this dreadful period, the discharges of fire and lava, from the volcanoes in Iceland, exceeded what had been before known in the same space of time. There were two eruptions in

1222, one from Heckla; the other from Reikenefe; and the eruptions of the latter were repeated in 1223, 1225 and 1226. In 1224 was a severe drouth; in 1225 a rigorous winter, followed by a dearth, and mortal difeafes among fheep.

Let any candid man obferve the natural phenomena accompanying this defolating period, from 1219 to 1226; and decide for himfelf how far the fire or electricity of the fyftem is an agent in producing them, and the attending difeafes.

We obferve here the progrefs of peftilence to be the fame as in modern times. The plague appeared in Egypt almoft at the fame time with the comet, and firft derangement of the elements in 1219 and 1220; but was two, three, four and five years later in the high northern latitudes.

No comet is mentioned in the hiftories of this dark period, as far as I can find, from 1222 to 1240; but that there was one, in the vicinity of the earth, between 1228 and 1233, is very probable.

In 1228 an inundation in Friefland demolifhed whole towns, and it was eftimated that 100,000 people perifhed. Great rains in fummer and exceffive heat were followed by a fevere winter, with deep fnow.

In 1230 the waters of the Tyber rofe to the ftairs of St. Peter's Church, and drowned the lower city. July and Auguft were exceffively hot. An inundation of the Danube in 1232, and in 1233 fo fevere a froft, that rivers were converted into highways in Italy; and earthquakes marked the year, with a dark day.

During this period from 1230 to 1233, France, Denmark and Italy were wafted by dreadful famin and plague. Thefe calamities continued in 1234 and 5, in England and France. In London alone 20,000 people were ftarved. Worms and locufts devoured the fruits of the earth.

The winter of 1236 was rainy—the following fummer extremely dry, and in England moft diftreffing agues were epidemic. In 1237 was an eruption of a volcano in Iceland.

In 1239 peftilence again raged—a new ftar, like Lucifer, appeared. Famin was fo fevere that perfons fed on human flefh.

In 1240 a comet appeared in Feb. and was visible a month. Mortal difeafes prevailed, and authors relate that the fish, on the English coaft *had a battle*, in which eleven whales and a multitude of other fish were flain and caft afhore. The caufe to which this phenomenon is affigned is laughable enough; but the fact is important; for it ftrengthens modern obfervations, that when peftilential difeafes prevail on the furface of the earth, fish often perifh beneath the water. Of this no doubt can remain; and this alone demonftrates that the *peftilential caufe* is as powerful or nearly fo, at the bottom of rivers and the ocean, as on the earth—a fact that reduces the theory of propagating the fomes of epidemic difeafes in veffels, clothes and fimilar articles, from one country to another, to a thing of very trifling confideration.

The winter of 1240 was very fevere—the fnow was deep and cattle perifhed. An eruption of fire in Iceland is noted the fame year.

In 1242 the Thames rofe by means of exceffive rains and overwhelmed the country for fix miles about Lambeth. The years 1243 and 4 were remarkable for continued drouth, meteors and a moft fatal plague.—An eruption of fire in Iceland in 1245.

In 1247 a violent earthquake was experienced in England, and in September a fatal plague. The earthquake was in February and followed by a very rainy fummer. The winter following was fo mild, that people wore their fummer clothes; but from March to May was cold.

The fummer of 1250 was rainy and tempeftuous, followed by a hard winter. The fummer of 1251 was intolerably hot, and epidemic difeafes prevailed, with great mortality.

In 1252 late frofts in fpring, and fucceeding drouth deftroyed the fruits of the earth. At the clofe of July came great rains, vegetation ftarted, but great mortality prevailed among cattle. At Michaelmas began the plague in London, which fpread over England, and raged till Auguft following. This is one inftance of the plague's appearing in autumn, running through the winter, and ceasing about the time, in the hot season, when that disease usually begins.

The winter of 1254 was rigorously cold, a murrain among sheep was very fatal, and in England and France a mortal distemper among horses called the *evil of the tongue*, but it is not described.

In 1255 appeared a comet; tides rose to an uncommon height; rivers swelled with excessive rains and tempests levelled buildings. In 1256 the rains and tempests were equally violent, and another comet appeared. In 1257 the summer was also excessively rainy. From these rains came a dearth of corn in England and France in 1258, which was also rainy; and famin and diseases made havoc with human life. Fifteen thousand persons perished by hunger in London, but I have no account that the plague prevailed at that time.

To this series of wet seasons succeeded severe drouth in 1259 and 1260; and the mortality continued till the summer of 1259—after which plenty succeeded to want.

The year 1261 was rainy in England and Scotland, and a dearth was the consequence in the following year.

In 1262 an eruption of a volcano in Iceland.

In 1263 a severe frost in winter converted the Thames into a highway for men and horses. In 1264 a comet was visible from June 20th to September 28th and pestilential diseases swept away horses and cattle.

In 1266 swarms of Palmer worms devoured all vegetables in Scotland, and several villages on the Tay and Froth were swept away by floods. These were preceded by a remarkable halo.

In 1268 appeared a comet, and violent tempests and rain are noted, together with sterility of grain and dearth in Austria and Sicily.

In 1269 the winter was extremely severe; horses and carriages passing on the ice over the Thames. A plague raged among the Crusaders, on their march to the holy land, of which died the French king and his son. Some authors mention a comet of stupendous magnitude under this date; which is probably the same as that noted under the foregoing year.

In 1274 was a great earthquake and a comet of frightful aspect—an earthquake also in 1275.

In this year, it is related, the rot among sheep was first known in England. As this was said to be an imported disease, it is proper to state how it was introduced. Short on Air, vol. 1. 155, says, "This year, a rich Frenchman brought into Northumberland a Spanish ewe, as big as a two year old calf, which sheep being rotten, soon infected the country, so that the disease overspread the whole kingdom, and lasted 25 or 28 years, till it left very few sheep alive. This was the first rot ever known in England."

The reader will judge which is the greater calf, the man who gravely tells or the man who believes such a tale as this.

Historians fix upon the year 1277 for the formation of the Dollert Sea, between Groningen and East-Friesland, by a great inundation, which overwhelmed 33 villages irrecoverably; with many farm-houses in the open country.

In 1280 a great inundation was followed by a very cold winter. In 1281 Poland was afflicted with famin. The winter of 1282 was the severest then remembered; an earthquake shook Italy and a plague raged in Denmark. In 1283 the same malady prevailed in Scotland. In 1284 the winter was one of the mildest ever known; the year was also remarkable for great tempests, an unusual darkness and an eruption of Etna. The year 1285 was noted for a similar darkness, most parching drouth and the commencement of a famin in England.

This drouth was followed in 1286, by the approach of a comet. In this year, Prussia was infested with a new species of worms, whose sting was poisonous. Swarms of flies and pestilential fevers in Spain nearly destroyed the army of the French king, then making war on Arragon.

In 1287 fifteen islands in Zealand were overwhelmed by an inundation, with the loss of 15,000 inhabitants.

In 1288 the summer was excessively hot and dry. Grain was however abundant in this and the preceding year. The drouth was followed by great mortality and a severe winter.

In 1293 a comet was visible, and a great snow storm happened in May. Italy was shaken by earthquakes. In the following year, England was distressed by severe famin, thousands of the poor perishing with hunger. A severe drouth exhausted all the springs and rivers, grafs withered and cattle were fed on straw. The winter of 1293-4 was extremely cold, and an eruption of Heckla happened in 1294.

In 1295 and 6 many countries were afflicted with famin, and in 1297 the plague prevailed in Scotland.

A comet of great magnitude appeared in 1298, or as other authors say, in 1299, and others in 1300; whose approximation was attended with violent earthquakes in Germany, and other places in 1299, and with an eruption of Heckla in 1300. The year 1298 was noted for a great mortality among the Jews, and multitudes perished in the east with various diseases in 1299.

In 1305 appeared a comet, attended with fatal pestilence. A hard winter followed, and the Rhine was covered with ice.

In 1311 mount Heckla discharged its fiery contents, in 1312 appeared a comet, and a three years famin commenced in Bohemia and Poland, which was exceedingly distressing. Men became like wolves and preyed on human flesh.

In 1314 incessant rains destroyed the grain; a comet appeared in December following, and in 1316 raged a desolating dysentery in England, accompanied with an acute fever, which, like the true plague, left scarcely survivors to bury the dead. The famin continued to rage with all its horrors. Horse flesh was a delicious dish. Wheat sold at forty shillings the quarter; equivalent to £30 sterling in these days.

In 1318 the winter was severe, and in 1319 the plague prevailed in England. A murrain spread among cattle, at the same time, with fatal destruction.*

In 1321 the drouth was extreme, and there was an eruption of Etna. Eruptions of Etna are also mentioned in 1323, 1329 and 1333, and a severe winter, in the first of these years 1323, which covered the Baltic with ice. The plague raged in 1325.

The year 1330 was rainy and the crops indifferent. The year

* I have no account of any comets from 1315, to 1337;—which may be owing to the defect of my historical materials.

following, Ireland was diftreffed by famin, but Dublin was relieved by plenty of fifh, called Thurlheds, which had not been seen there for ages. In 1332 was an eruption in Iceland.

In 1336 grain was abundant. A violent earthquake fhook Venice, and a fucceeding plague laid wafte the city. This was preceded by numerous abortions.†

In 1337 happened a feverely cold winter, without fnow. Two comets were vifible, one four months, the other two. The plague prevailed in Nuremberg and other parts of Europe. The winter following was alfo fevere. Piftorius places thefe comets in 1336, and mentions an inundation at Florence. At this time, Europe was, for three years, ravaged with locufts.

In 1339 or 40, appeared another comet. Great floods, an eruption of Heckla, and a fevere winter followed, which covered the north fea with ice.

See Short on Air, vol. 1. Piftorius, vol. 1, and 2. Dufrefnoy's Chron. Henry's Hift. Eng. vol. 4. 500. Camden's Britannia. Fonctius' Chron. Knighton's Chron.

In travelling through the dark ages, we find but few interefting defcriptions; and nothing could have induced me to undertake the tedious detail of detached facts refpecting peftilence, but a ftrong defire to afcertain all that can be difcovered of the operations of nature, in producing epidemic difeafes. It is of infinite importance, in difcuffing this fubject, to know whether certain phenomena of feafons, of fubterranean fire, and unufual animals, uniformly attend peftilence; and to afcertain, if poffible, the *order* in which they proceed, for the purpofe of difcovering whether they are connected with each other as caufe and effect. Barren as the hiftory of the barbarous ages really is, we yet find it to contain a great number of facts, that will affift us in developing the caufes of epidemics. The fubfequent periods of the world furnifh more ample materials—we now approach the morning of fcience, when the clearer lights of more accurate hiftory will illuminate our path.

† To repair the wafte of population, the Senate paffed a decree inviting perfons to come and refide in the city, and promifing them the rights of citizenfhip, after two years refidence. Howel's Survey.

SECTION IV.

Historical View of pestilential epidemics, from the year 1340, *to* 1500.

THE pestilence next to be described was the most general and awfully distressing that the world ever experienced. The precise year when it appeared in Asia, where it began, is not ascertained; but probably about 1345, perhaps a year or two earlier.

The histories of that age relate, that it commenced in Cathay, China, and was preceded by the bursting of a huge meteor or globe of fire; or as others relate, the fire burst from the earth. These accounts were taken from Genoese seamen, and are recorded by Villani; but Dr. Mead, with that obstinacy that rejects truth when opposed to preconceived theory, thinks the report incredible, and questions not the disease originated in Egypt. Had he ever examined the subject, like an impartial man, he would have believed the account of the seamen, for there is not a more certain phenomenon in nature, than the appearance of meteors and the explosion of fire in pestilential periods.

Villani, book 1 ch 2 Mezeray, Tom 1 798

This plague appeared in 1346 in Egypt, Syria, Greece, Turkey; in 1347 in Sicily, Pisa, Genoa and other parts of Italy; in 1348 it appeared in the south of France, first in Avignon, which is not a maritime city, but at a distance from the sea, and afterwards in other parts of the kingdom and in all the southern provinces of Spain. At the close of the same year, it made its appearance in England, first in Dorsetshire, and soon travelled over the whole country. In 1349 it overrun Ireland, Holland, Scotland, and in 1350 all Germany, Hungary and the north of Europe.

This peftilence was remarkable for raging in winter as well as fummer, even in the north of Europe. In France it firft appeared at Avignon in February and prevailed there nearly a year.

Muratori, vol. 3. part 2. 588.

Short has placed its firft appearance in the fouth of England in September. But Archbifhop Parker has placed its origin juft after Chriftmas. His words are, " Ea ftatim poft nativitatis dominicæ celebratum feftum, ipfa nimirum hyeme et rerum omnium ad victum neceffarium copia, cum vix ulla contagionis fufpicio oriri mortalibus potuit, incepit." " Immediately after the feaft of our Lord's nativity, in winter and amidft the greateft abundance of provifions, when there could be no fufpicion that a contagious difeafe would arife among men, the plague commenced." It raged about five months and according to this author ceafed in May following; altho other authors relate, that it had not gone through the kingdom till late in the fummer.

Parker's Antiq. Brit. p. 360.

In the Englifh Annals by William Wyrcefter, in the black book of the Exchequer, it is faid that this plague prevailed in the parts of London and its vicinity in autumn 1349.

Thefe different accounts of the time of the firft appearance of this difeafe, are reconcileable on the principles which modern obfervations have unfolded. It is found that the plague is *always* preceded, for fome months, and in fome inftances, for two or three years, by other malignant fevers, which increafe gradually to the violence of the true plague; and often the degrees of violence are fo gradual, that phyficians themfelves can hardly determin a line of diftinction between the malignant difeafe, which is the precurfor of the plague, and the plague itfelf. That is, they are at a lofs to know where the malignant difeafe ends and the plague begins. Hence all the difputes, at the commencement of a peftilence, whether the *difeafe is the plague or not*—a circumftance which appears to have marked the origin of all great plagues, and yet phyficians and philofophers in Europe feem never to have fufpected the caufe.—Thefe facts will be hereafter demonftrated, and they annihilate at a blow the whole doctrine of the propagation of that difeafe from country to country by infection.

From the uniform operations of nature in the cafe of epidemic peſtilential difeafes of the kind under confideration, there muſt have been in England, during the fummer, previous to the appearance of the plague, malignant fevers, which might approach to the violence and fatality of the plague. This circumſtance might create a fmall difference in the accounts of the origin of the plague—inaccurate obfervers miſtaking the one difeafe for the other—or rather naming the previous putrid fever, the plague, before it put on the characteriſtic ſymptoms.

It is poſſible however that thefe authors may refer to the commencement of the difeafe in different parts of England.

This formidable calamity deferves a particular defcription, with all the phenomena attending it.

In 1347 appeared a frightful comet, in Auguſt. Preceding and during the prevalence of the difeafe, the whole earth was fhaken by moſt tremendous earthquakes. All Germany was fhaken in 1346. In 1349 on the 9th of Sept. Sicily was fhaken to its foundation, together with all Italy. In Greece many cities were overthrown, and in many places towns and caſtles were demoliſhed. Thoufands of people were fwallowed up and the courfes of rivers were obſtructed.

Over Avignon was fufpended a meteor or pillar of fire for an hour. The heavens were at times illuminated as with flame, and meteors were frequent.

I have no particular defcription of all the feafons, during the five years, in which this mortal peſtilence defolated Europe. But the year 1347, the year of the comet, was, in England, exceſſively rainy, and the air humid.* Short, from Johan Cole de Billona, mentions that a hot air, cloudy and moiſt atmofphere had continued for fome years, and that a malignant, contagious peripneumony followed in all Europe. But unfortunately the compiler leaves us in the dark as to the precife time of

---

* Mutius, in the collection of German hiſtory, fays that the whole year 1348 was foutherly, moiſt weather, but there were no heavy rains to cool the air. Fruit was abundant, but corn was not nutricious See vol. 3 241.—In England the rains continued from May to Chriſtmas.

its appearance, and whether before or after the other forms of this pestilence.

Mezeray relates that in China, the disease originated from a vapor, which burst from the earth, was horribly offensive and consumed the face of the country through an extent of 200 leagues. This account may be inaccurate, but is not to be wholly rejected. That some action of subterranean heat was instrumental in generating the disease, is very probable; or at least that some phenomena of fire accompanied it, because this supposition is consonant to the whole series of modern observations.

The pestilential state of air, in that period, is strongly marked by the appearance of myriads of unusual and loathsome insects, not only in China, but in Europe. They are described as young serpents, or as venemous insects, or as large vermin with tails and eight short legs—in which description, probably, a frightened imagination had some share of influence. But of the fact of their existence, there can be no doubt.

In the Ouse there was a great inundation just before Ascension day, and in York began this plague speedily after the flood.

The symptoms of this fatal malady were—violent affection in the head and stomach, buboes and other glandular swellings; small swellings like pimples or blisters; usually a fever, and a vomiting or spitting of blood.—The swellings in the glands were infallible signs of the disease; but the most fatal symptom was, the pimples or blisters spread over the whole body. Hemorrhages from the mouth, nose and other parts, indicated a universal and sudden disorganization of the blood. The patient usually died in three days or less—which denotes the virulence of the poison, or rather the activity of the disease, which destroyed the powers of life in half the time, which the bilious plague usually employs

The peripneumony which was epidemic about the same time, appeared in a burning fever, insatiable thirst, a black tongue, anxiety and pains about the heart, short breath, a cough, with expectoration of a mixed matter, open mouth, raging delirium, fury, red, turbid or black urine, restlessness, and watchings, black eruptions, anthraces, buboes, and in some, corroding ulcers over the whole body. The difeafe ufually terminated the 4th day, fometimes not till the 7th. The blood was black and thick; but fometimes greenifh and watery or yellowifh.—Venefection was certain death. The difeafe baffled medical fkill—the only remedies that appeared to relieve, were laxatives early adminiftered, cupping and fcarification, leeches applied to the hemorrhoids, and inwardly, infufions of mild, diaphoretic, attenuating, pectoral vegetables.

It will be hereafter proved that malignant pleurify and peripneumony ufually form a part of that feries of difeafes which always occur during a period of general contagion. When plague and yellow fever occur in *fummer*, in northern climates, pleurify and peripneumony often affume, in *winter*, great and even peftilential violence.

This plague was fo deadly that at leaft half or two thirds of the human race perifhed in about 8 years. It was moft fatal in cities, but in no place died lefs than a third of the inhabitants. In many cities perifhed nine out of ten of the people, and many places were wholly depopulated. In London 50,000 dead bodies were buried in one grave yard. In Norwich died about the fame number. In Venice died 100,000—in Lubec, 90,000—in Florence the fame number. In the eaft perifhed twenty millions in one year.—In Spain the difeafe raged three years and carried off two thirds of the people. Alfonfo 2d. died with it while befieging Gibraltar.

In this fatal period, the apprehenfion of death deftroyed the value of property. In England, and probably in other countries, cattle were neglected and they ran at large over the country. The corn perifhed in the fields for want of reapers; whole villages were depopulated; and after the malady ceafed, multitudes of houfes and buildings of all kinds were feen mouldering to ruin. A horfe which before had been worth forty fhillings, after the ficknefs, fold for half a mark.

Altho in the year preceding there had been a plenty of provifions, yet the neglect of agriculture during the general diftrefs produced a famin. Such was the lofs of laborers, that the few

S

survivors afterwards demanded exorbitant wages, and the Parliament of England was obliged to interfere, and limit their wages, and even compel men to labor.—See 23d Edward 3. A. D. 1350. The preamble states, that a great part of the people, especially workmen and servants had died of the late pestilence, and those who survived, seeing the necessity of men, demanded excessive wages.

This disease was particularly fatal in Denmark—all business was at a stand, towns were deserted, and all was terror and despair. It reached the highest northern latitudes; it broke out in Iceland, and was so fatal, that the settlements there are supposed not to have since recovered their population. It was called the *forte died*, black death.

In some places people attempted to escape infection by taking their families on board of vessels, and putting to sea; but it was in vain; they were seized in every place, without regard to age or sex.

In 1348 the malady swept away the Greenland merchants and seamen. This disease also, or some other cause destroyed the colony of Danes in that country, for it was extinguished and has never been found or heard of to this day.

This pestilence was remarkably fatal to the monks and regular clergy of all descriptions. In one society at Montpeliers, of 140 members died all but 7: About the same proportion perished in Magdalen Society. In Marseilles, of 140 not one survived. But a circumstance related in Knighton's Chronicon deserves particular notice. At Avignon where the disease first appeared in France, 66 of the Carmelites had died, before the citizens were apprized of the fact; and when it was discovered, the report circulated that the brethren had killed each other.

An important consequence results from the fact—that this plague first appeared in a monastery, which might be crouded with lazy, idle, filthy monks; in a city not commercial, nor a sea port. There was no idea of any imported infection; but there must have been strong *local* causes, which first excited into action the general contagion which, at that time, pervaded the atmosphere over the whole globe.

Such was the havoc made by this pestilence among the clergy

in England, fays Knighton, that a vicarage which before the plague, might have been fupplied for four or five marks a year, or two marks and the man's board, was raifed to the price of twenty marks or twenty pounds.

Col 2600.

This peftilential period was preceded and attended with all the ufual phenomena of fatal Epidemics.* The earthquakes and the infects have been noticed. Abortions were among the remarkable precurfors of this malady. The fame fact is noticed by Diemerbroeck, before the great plague at Nimeguen, in 1635. The fame has been mentioned by the authors he quoted, Foreftus, Sennertes, and others; and is afcribed to the tendernefs and debility of the heart and Vifcera. Hence pregnant women firft feel the effects of a ftate of air unfriendly to the fupport of life, and if they are feized with plague, are always its victims.

Another phenomenon attending this plague was the *death of fifh*. This circumftance, with the bad ftate of the water, which is often affected by the peftilential ftate of the elements, and was greatly affected in this period, gave rife to a report that the Jews had poifoned the wells and fprings. The prejudices againft the Jews, which have marked and fcandalized all chriftian countries, except America, were at their height in the reign of Edward the 3d of England, the period under confideration. Thefe prejudices drove legiflators and princes to exercife every fpecies of cruelty upon the Ifraelites, on account of their ufury; and when the report of their poifoning the water circulated, the populace in fome places and efpecially in Germany, rofe and affaffinated multitudes of thefe unfortunate men.

The death of animals, particularly of fheep, marked the fame period. In England, 5000 died in one pafture. The ftate of the air and water was fo peftilential that it is averred by hiftorians, the fowls and fifhes had blotches on them.

Authorities Short, on air. vol. 1. 165. Knighton, Chron. Pennant's Arctic Zoology p 67. Townfend's Travels in Spain, vol 2 219 Maitland's Hift of London. Muratori, Tom 3 588 and 594 Univ Hift vol 32 251 Stow's Survey, 478 Mazeray's Hift France Villani, and many others.

* Except eruptions of volcanoes, of which I have no account, at this period except in Iceland in 1340. But my accounts of volcanoes are very imperfect.

It may be remarked that this mortal pestilence raged in England and France, during peace, or rather during a truce, which had been concluded between Edward III and the King of France in 1347, and which lasted seven years.

Guido, an inhabitant of Avignon, when this malady appeared, and who escaped death by the favorable process of a bubo, relates a fact that throws light on this subject. He says that the malady was of two kinds—" the first, and *which preceded the other about two months*, was a fever, with spitting of blood," not unlike that which prevailed in the time of Fracastorius. All who were seized with these symptoms, died in three days.

The other kind, which succeeded the first, came on with continued fever, carbuncles and abscesses, in the glands.—This was as fatal as the other, except near its decline, and the patient died in five days.

Friend's Hist. Med. p. 564.

It is remarkable, that the disease which is technically called *plague*, pestis, is always preceded by a similar fever. It is in fact the *plague in its first stages*, tho it does not exhibit the glandular swellings, which modern physicians contend are characteristic of true plague, and mark a generic or at least a specific difference between that and any other kind of typhus fever. This fact of a *progressiveness* in the disease, annihilates the favorite notion of deducing all plagues from infection; a notion which is bandied about between physicians and legislators like a tennis ball, tho unhappily for mankind, infinitely less harmless.

At the close of this dreadful period, in 1350, were severe earthquakes in Italy. In 1356 a violent shock in Switzerland, and in Germany, especially on the Rhine, which did great injury. To this succeeded most violent rains, and famin and pestilence in Germany, with prodigious mortality.

Muratori, Tom. 3. part. 2. 594.

Brabant escaped this terrible pestilence and so did Milan.

In 1352 authors relate that 900,000 people in China perished by famin.

The rainy and humid seasons which introduced the great pestilence of 1347–50, were succeeded by drouth in 1350, a comet in 1351, with tremendous storms, and a meteor which burst with a heavy report. The winter following was severe, and in 1354 Africa and Cyprus were devoured by locusts.

In England prevailed epidemic madness in 1355.

In 1358 was a severe winter, followed by an eruption in Iceland, and a wasting plague in Italy in 1359. According to Baccace, Florence lost 100,000 citizens, and Petrarch says, scarcely ten of a thousand survived. There was a great mortality particularly among child-bed women, and cattle did not escape.

This pestilence also became nearly general. In 1361 Milan, which had escaped in 1348, was severely afflicted, as was all France, England and Ireland, and it was computed that Scotland lost one third of its inhabitants. This plague was called the *second* in the reign of Edward III, and it was in time of peace.

In this pestilential time, occurred a remarkable storm of hail and snow, in April 1360. The tendency of the elements in such periods to generate hail and snow, is a fact that well deserves consideration.

In January 1361, a violent tempest spread desolation over Europe. The winter was severe, and the summer dry. In March 1362 appeared a comet in the North East, with a vast coma, and an eruption in Iceland. A dearth and diseases among cattle followed.

This last pestilence differed from that in 1348, in two or three particulars. It raged with most violence, on mountainous districts, where the air was pure, and where the plague of 1348 did not prevail. It attacked the nobility and gentry with more violence than the poor; contrary to the usual fact; whereas the disease of 1348 was most fatal to persons in the humbler walks of life.

Muratori Tom 3 part 2 600   Liber Niger Saccarii vol. 2. 433.
Henry's Hist Britain vol. 4. 194

The comet and volcano of 1362 were followed in 1363 by a winter of extraordinary severity, which lasted from September to April. The Rhine was covered with ice for ten weeks.

The year 1365 was rainy, and the plague carried off 20,000 people in Cologne, and the vicinity. In 1366 an eruption in Iceland destroyed 70 farms. The same year was very sickly in England and deaths sudden.

In 1363 was visible in March a comet with a coma, and the crops failed. In this year commenced in England the third great plague in the reign of Edward III.; the reader will note that this was preceded by a sickly year in 1366. The mortality was great, and especially about Oxford. The most fatal year was 1369, and in Ireland the disease raged in 1370. I have no particulars of the progress of the disease on the continent; but it was very fatal.

Murat. vol. 3. 632. Pistorius vol. 1. lib. Niger 435.
Maitland's Hist. Lond. Van Trail's Letters on Iceland.

In 1373 raged an epidemic madness among the lower people in England; and in 1374 a similar disorder prevailed in France and Italy. During pestilential periods, some general cause seems to affect the brain in a powerful manner, even in persons who escape the plague.

In 1374 also was an eruption of a volcano in Iceland. There was also famin, a violent plague in Italy and some parts of France. In 1371 there had been a severe earthquake in the south of France.

Murat. Tom. 3. 646, 649.

In 1379 commenced a great sickness in the north of England, which almost laid waste the country; and in 1380 was seen a comet. The disease is not described, but it was the forerunner of a most dreadful plague. Provisions were good and cheap.

In 1381 and 2 considerable earthquakes were felt in England, and a severe pestilence appeared at Avignon in France, which raged for four or five years, depopulating many cities. It prevailed in Italy, France, Germany, England, Ireland, Greece, and the East.

There was an eruption of Etna in 1381, and the year closed with great rains. The year 1382 was without winds. The plague was most fatal to children, and great ravages were made also among the friars. In this pestilence Lubec lost 90,000 people.

Liber Niger Sac. 441. Short on Air.

In 1388 the drouth was so severe, that the Rhine was fordable at Cologne. In 1389 violent tempests raged in England, with great destruction; and in the year following, was an eruption of a volcano in Iceland. In modern days, we observe the same train of phenomena, evidently depending on one general cause. In 1389 appeared a singular meteor or light in the heavens.

The year 1389 was remarkable for the death of children in all parts of England. From the phenomena that attended and the diseases which followed, compared with the order of diseases in modern days, it appears very probable that this disease was a species of Angina, which almost invariably precedes the plague. In the next year, a deadly plague raged in the north of England. Swarms of gnats and flies marked this period, and some parts of the continent were overrun with locusts.

Pistor. vol. 1. Short on Air.

The reader will remark the excessive drouth preceding the eruption in Iceland and the fiery appearance in the heavens in the year of the tempest. In these phenomena, nature is nearly uniform.

It is a very common event that dysentery of a malignant type succeeds the plague. Such was the case in England, in 1391, when this disease was epidemic and very mortal. A dearth of corn might have contributed to the same event; but it is often the fact, without any scarcity of food.

An uncommon redness of the sun is mentioned in July of 1391, and for six weeks after, thick vapor or clouds. Perhaps these might have been occasioned by the eruption in Iceland, in the preceding year; as it appears to have been a phenomenon somewhat similar to that which Europe beheld with amazement and terror in 1783.—I have however my suspicions that while the central fires expel immense quantities of burning lava, from volcanoes, they may force through the earth in the adjoining continents, a subtle vapor, that is invisible, until it is collected and condensed in the higher regions of the atmosphere.

The beginning of the 15th century was marked by a severe and desolating pestilence. The disease first appeared in the last year or two of the former century. In 1399 the mortality was such in Spain, especially in Andalusia, that the king was obliged to suspend the law which restrained widows from marrying within a year after the death of their husbands. It was preceded by a severe winter.

Mod Univ Hist vol 20 353

In 1402-3 and 4 the plague in Iceland carried off multitudes of the inhabitants.

Van Troil

In 1400 epidemic and mortal sickness prevailed in England. A violent earthquake the same year in Persia. In 1401 Florence was nearly dispeopled by the plague. In 1402 in March appeared a comet of a fiery aspect, and coma, which was visible for three months.* In 1402 a frost so severe that the Baltic was passable for horses for six weeks. In 1406 the sea broke into Holland, Zealand and Flanders, with prodigious injury. A plague carried off 30,000 people in London ; and a comet the same year. The winters following were so severe that most birds died. In Sept. there were great floods from rain. In 1408 there was an eruption of Etna and deep snow.

Pistorius, Germ Script vol 1. Short on Air.
Maitland's Hist Lond.

The summer of 1406, when the plague raged in London, was close, moist and southerly weather.

In 1411 the dysentery carried off 14000 people in Bourdeaux, but I have no account of the seasons. The plague raged in Aquitain and Gascoigne with great mortality. In 1412, there were uncommon tides in the Thames. In 1414 a comet, and in 1416 an eruption of fire from a volcano in Iceland, preceded by great snow.

In 1421, according to some authors, happened the dreadful inundation in Holland, which formed the Zuyder Sea. In 1422 there was an eruption of fire in Iceland, and a severe winter followed. The same year, the plague raged in Poland. From these phenomena, I suspect the approach of a comet, but have no account of one.

In 1426 a comet, an excessively hot summer, and a violent earthquake which overturned twenty cities in Catalonia, in Spain, and was felt in most parts of Europe. In 1427 the seasons

---

* According to Liber Niger Saccarii, this was in 1401, and this is most probably correct. The period of this comet is 343 years and we shall find it under the year 1744.

were rainy, the winter mild, a dearth and famin followed, and the plague in Dantzick. Epidemics prevailed in England, and the year following, the plague.

In 1430 happened a general earthquake—in 1432 a great inundation in Germany—in 1433 a comet was visible for three months, in the south, and the winter following was terribly severe. The frost began in the last week in November and lasted till the middle of February.

Pistorius Germ. Script vol. 1. Short, vol. 1
Liber Niger Sac vol 2.

In 1436 there was an eruption of a volcano in Iceland and a severe winter. An epidemic fever prevailed in Venice, which was attributed to the use of stagnant water.

In 1438 and 9 violent storms and great rains injured the corn and a dearth ensued. A comet in 1439 and a hard winter followed. To these phenomena succeeded in 1440 a series of distressing epidemics, severe coughs, small-pox, fevers and dysentery, which proved exceedingly fatal.

Short vol 1. Pistorius vol. 1.

In 1443 Bohemia, Hungary, and Poland were terribly injured by an earthquake. In 1444 there was eruption of Etna and Lipari, and the explosion was repeated in 1446 and 7. An epidemic prevailed in 1445, which suddenly ended life, but it is not described. In January 1449 was seen a comet. This year the plague raged in Italy and in 1450 famin and plague. In Milan perished 60,000 people.

Muratori vol 13 Short vol. 1.

This plague of 1450 is said to have arisen in Asia, and afterwards spread over Italy, Germany, France and Spain, leaving alive scarcely a third of the human race.

In 1455 appeared a comet and another in 1456. In this latter year, Italy was violently shaken by an earthquake, and 40,000 people perished.—Pistorius places the earthquake in 1457, and says it demolished 40 towns, and destroyed 60,000 lives. In 1459 a plague began in July and raged six months in Italy.

Pistorius vol 1. 375. Muratori Tom. 5 p 50. Short vol 1.

It will be obferved, in this period and in many others, that the plague is not mentioned under the year of the earthquake. Modern obfervations explain the progrefs of peftilence, which is moft ufual, viz. meafles, catarrh, angina, and other malignant complaints *preceding* the crifis of the peftilential ftate of air, or plague. And we find almoft invariably fome of thefe difeafes to be epidemic, even *before* the comet, earthquakes and eruptions of volcanoes, altho the moft violent form of the peftilence does not always appear till a year or two *after* thofe phenomena. There is alfo a difference, in the times of the appearance of the plague in various countries. In Egypt, the peftilence ufually appears firft, and is cotemporary with the comet, or nearly fo; and the fame year, when the plague rages in Egypt, we find anginas and other malignant difeafes prevailing in Europe and America, in northern latitudes. This difference in time evinces the power of local caufes, in aiding the progrefs of the epidemic conftitution of air, and which produce the moft violent difeafes in Egypt, one, two or three years, previous to their appearance in cooler latitudes. But it will almoft always be found true, that the commencement of a feries of epidemics is nearly at the fame time in all parts of the world; the precurfors of the plague being nearly cotemporary in different countries; altho the peftilential conftitution or general contagion arrives to its crifis much fooner in Egypt, Smyrna and Conftantinople, than in places lefs expofed to the influence of local caufes of difeafe.

In 1465 peftilence again appeared in Italy, but I have no particulars. In 1467 a comet, and a *mild winter* is recorded; a remarkable fact, and the fecond inftance I have found in hiftory. Indeed fo uniform are hard winters during the approach of comets, that the accounts of exceptions are to be fufpected of inaccuracy in point of time.

In 1468 a moft deadly plague raged in Parma of which Short gives a particular defcription from Rolandus Capellatus.

Short, vol 1 194 Muratori, vol 13 Edit. Milan. Piftorius, Germ Script. vol 2

In 1471 the winter was rigorous and ftormy. In 1472 appeared three comets; two of them of diftinguifhed magnitude. In 1473 moft exceffive heat and drouth, and authors relate that the woods took fire by the heat of the fun. This drouth continued three years—all fmall rivers were dried up—the Danube was fordable in Hungary. In 1475 and 1476 appeared thofe enormous fwarms of locufts, which always denote a ftate of air highly peftilential, and ravaged Hungary and Poland. In 1474 earthquakes were felt in Germany. In 1475 an eruption of a volcano in Iceland.

Thefe phenomena, in this period, as ufual, introduced moft terrible peftilence, which began in 1472 and arrived to its height in 1477. It raged in Italy, Germany, France and England, and how much more extenfively, my authorities do not inform me It prevailed feveral years, with incredible mortality. In Paris perifhed 40,000; a large number for the population at that time. In England the number of deaths was not eftimated; but authors relate that fifteen years of civil war did not carry off one third of the number. This year 1477 was exceffively hot. In 1478 innumerable locufts overran Italy.

In 1478 and 9 the plague in England repeated its ravages; beginning like that of 1348, in autumn, raging through the winter until the next autumn.

Piftorius, vol 2. 754. Muratori, vol. 13.
Short, vol. 1. Maitland's Hift. London.
Fracaftorius de Contagione, 136.
Fernelius de morbis Peftilentibus.

In 1480 the winter was fevere.

In 1481 and 3, a moft deadly plague infefted Italy and Germany.

Muratori, vol 13 Piftorius, vol 2. 875.

In 1482 a fpecies of pleurify was epidemic in Italy.

Fracaftor p 182.

In 1484 the winter was fevere.

In 1483 or 5 appeared in England a new fpecies of the plague called Sudor Anglicus, or fweating ficknefs of the Englifh, becaufe it was fuppofed to attack none but Englifhmen. This however was a miftake; for the fame difeafe, at different times, appeared in Ireland, Germany, Sweden and Holland.

In the life of Erafmus, it is faid to have appeared firft in 1483, and to have returned in 1485. John Kaye, or Caius, a cotemporary phyfician, fays, it firft appeared in 1485 in the

Duke of Richmond's army, on his landing at Milford Haven, in Wales. But on all hands it is agreed to have had its origin in England, and to have been a species of plague. It is called "novum pestilentiæ genus," a new kind of pestilence; and instead of being peculiar to England or Englishmen, "a Britannis exortum, incredibili celeritate per orbem longe lateque divagatum est;" it originated in Britain, and with incredible rapidity spread far and wide over the earth.

Life of Erasmus, 347. Friend's Hist. Med. 566.

Sir Thomas More, in a letter to Erasmus, declares this disease in London, Oxford and Cambridge to have been more dangerous than a battle. "Minus periculi in acie, quam in urbe esse."

The summer of 1485 was excessively rainy, and an inundation of the Severn made great havoc with men and cattle.

This disease attacked persons suddenly, with a sensation like that of hot vapor running through the part affected. To this succeeded internal heat, unquenchable thirst, and profuse sweating, which often carried off the patient in two or three hours. The violence of the attack was past in 15 hours, and in 24 hours the patient was considered to be out of danger. It was most fatal to persons in high health and easy condition of life. It was attended with most of the symptoms which characterize the plague—anxiety, restlessness, violent pain in the head, delirium and excessive drowsiness.

See the life of John Caius, in Aikins' Biographical Memoirs of Medicine, p. 120, also Friend's Hist. Phys.

This was a pestilential period, for the plague infested Italy and Germany in 1483, and Denmark in 1484. And it will be found on examination, that when the sweating sickness raged in any part of Europe, that or some other pestilential disease, was in other countries. During the prevalence of this form of the plague in England, at this period, Denmark lost nearly one half of its inhabitants by the common plague; which raged terribly for two years.

The author of the Traitè de la Peste, page 23, remarks, "That until the 15th century the plague exhibited the same character; but then "its accidents degenerated," or rather it reigned a new malady, which, under different external appearances, committed similar destruction on the human body. It did not any longer show itself by buboes, carbuncles and pimples; nor by any of the eruptions which the heat of the viscera pushes out; nor was the skin withered by the parching dryness which accompanies the carbuncular spots; on the other hand, the skin was inundated by torrents of sweat, which seemed to be poured from the whole body, the viscera were dried, and the heat which dissipated the fluids, seemed to disorder all the laws of the animal economy.

About the middle of the 16th century, the plague resumed its former character, but the symptoms somewhat varied and lighter "

The sweating plague at first attacked none but Englishmen. Even Scotchmen escaped, in foreign countries, where Englishmen were seized. Foreigners in England escaped. This however was on its first invasion in 1485—for, in subsequent years, it spread over other countries But the fact of its seizing only Englishmen at first, is precisely analagous to what has happened on many other occasions, in other countries. It recurred in England in 1506, 1518, 1528 and 1551.

In 1491 appeared a comet, the season was very wet, an epidemic swept away cattle, and a famin afflicted Ireland. A severe winter is noted in 1493.

Short, vol. 1. Smith's Cork. page 30.

In 1495 and 6 the plague raged in Portugal.

Hist of Portugal by Osorio

In 1496 an epidemic leprosy prevailed in Germany, which covered the body with ulcers from head to foot.

Pistorius, vol. 2.

In 1498 the summer was very dry. In 1500 a tempest in Rome did great injury, a comet was visible in Capricorn, an eruption of Vesuvius, and a mortal plague raged which carried off in London 30,000 people. The king for safety retired to Calais. Maitland arranges this plague under the year 1499. This pestilence was preceded by an abundance of provisions.

Short, vol 1. Maitland's Hist London.

It is a current opinion that the venereal disease was *imported* into Europe by the firſt adventurers to America, with Columbus; and that it gradually ſpread in Spain; from whence it was carried into Italy by ſome of the ſoldiers, who were in the ſiege of Naples in 1494; thence it was propagated rapidly throughout Europe. This ſubject will be hereafter conſidered. It is however remarkable, that an epidemic leproſy ſpread over Germany, about the ſame time, which ſeems to indicate an unuſual tendency in the human body to ulcerous and ſcorbutic complaints.

SECTION V.

Historical view of pestilential epidemics, from the year 1500 to the year 1600.

THE comet of 1500 was followed by an excessively severe winter in 1501, to which succeeded a summer of great heat and drouth in 1502. In this latter year the plague carried off 500 persons daily in Brussels; the city was soon abandoned, the streets were overgrown with grass, and the roofs of houses with moss.

Skenkius' Obs. p. 748.

De Pauw vol. 1. 85, mentions a desolating plague in China in 1504. In the same year, the malady prevailed in Ireland.

In 1505 appeared a comet; and another in the following year, in which also was an eruption of Vesuvius, which was succeeded by a severe winter. Pestilential diseases were universal. A fatal spotted fever overspread Europe in this hot, moist summer. The plague raged in Lisbon and London was severely visited by the sweating disease.

Short vol 1. Smith's Cork p 34. Osorio's Hist of Portugal. Fracastor, de Contagione.

In 1508 a great earthquake convulsed Italy and Germany. In 1509 a shock demolished a part of the walls of Constantinople, with many buildings, and the loss of 13,000 lives: After which the plague almost dispeopled the city.

These events commenced a distressing period. In 1510 there was an eruption of Heckla, and universal catarrh or severe influenza in Europe. This was called in France *cocoluche*, from the practice of covering the head of the patient with a cap. It was preceded by a series of moist weather.

In 1511 appeared a comet; another in 1512 and a third in 1513. In 1511 the plague prevailed in Verona, and in 1513 a malignant fever or dysentery, which covered the body with black spots. Bleeding was pernicious; cupping and actual cautery were successful.

In 1514 cats perished by an epidemic pestilential disease, says Fernelius; and the plague was in Tournay; while a mortal distemper raged among the cattle in England.

In 1515 a malignant catarrh or throat distemper in Holland seized persons suddenly, and if not cured, in a few hours, fell on the lungs and terminated in death in one day. In this year and the next appeared comets, and Germany suffered universally by inundations.

To these disasters succeeded a severe winter in 1517, followed by a very hot summer. Corn was in great abundance, but the sweating plague made great havoc in London, and so malignant a murrain raged among cattle, that ravens and dogs which fed on their carcases, swelled and died.

This deadly sweating plague was preceded, in the spring of the year, by an epidemic inflammation of the throat, so virulent as to destroy life in a few hours. The malignity of this disease has rarely, if ever been equalled in modern times. It seems to have been merged in the sweating plague, about midsummer. Authors relate that half the people of England perished with these diseases.—The disease in the throat seems to have been of an inflammatory diathesis, as early bleeding and purging were the only successful remedies.

In 1518 the plague visited Lisbon, and the sweating disease prevailed in Brabant.

Short vol 1 206--7 Smith's Cork, 34.

In 1521 appeared a comet, followed by a cold winter. Inundations are said to have overwhelmed, in this year, 72 villages and 100,000 people. England suffered by dearth and sickness, and in 1522 the plague visited Munster in Ireland, and the continent.—The winter following was distressingly severe.

Pestilential fevers prevailed in 1524 and 5. The mortality in London alarmed the people, and the terms were on that account, adjourned. In 1527 appeared a comet, and one in each year, for six years in succession. In 1527, the wetness of summer injured the grain, a fevere famin enfued, and many of the poor were ftarved to death. This year is noted for a great hail ftorm in Italy.

In 1528 the fpotted fever, that almoft infallible precurfor or companion of the plague, broke out in all parts of Europe; the plague in Italy, and the fweating difeafe in London with dreadful mortality, terminating in death in fix or feven hours. The fame difeafe prevailed in Cork.

In 1529 the fweating difeafe feized Amfterdam, raging a few days with great mortality, and paffing rapidly to other places.

In 1530 was an eruption of Etna, and an earthquake in Lifbon demolifhed 1400 houfes. In 1531 was another eruption of Etna, the fweating plague raged in Germany, and peftilence, in fome form, was almoft univerfal.—A great hail ftorm, the fame year.

See Skenkius' Obf. Smith's Cork 35. Short vol. 1. Maitland's Hift London.

Fracaftor informs us that the petechial fever of 1528 was preceded by a mild winter and foutherly rainy weather, together with inundations in fpring, and unufual darknefs. He obferves, that appearing in many places, it muft have had a common caufe.

De Contagione, p 160.

The laft remark is verified by modern obfervations. The petechial fever is an almoft infallible forerunner of the plague in the Levant, in Italy and other countries. It may be laid down as an axiom, on this fubject, that altho the appearance of this fever is not *always* and *certainly* followed by the plague, yet that the plague, in moft parts of the eaft, is *always* preceded by a petechial fever.

In 1533 there was a volcanic eruption in South America, but I have no account of the difeafes of that year.

In 1534 the plague was in Narbonne.

In 1535 there was a terrible plague in Cork.

In 1538 appeared a comet, which was preceded by eruptions of Etna in 1536 and 7 and a hard winter. In 1539 another comet and in 1541 a third.

U

In 1538 a mortal dysentery raged all over Europe, as also in the following year. The preceding summers had been moist, and an acute fever, with violent pain about the heart, delirium, moist and black tongue, anthraces and buboes, had been epidemic. But Fernilius remarks that the unusual dysentery of 1538 and 9 could not be ascribed to any visible cause in the seasons.

In 1538 also was a violent earthquake at Puteoli, near Naples and Vesuvius, where there was an immense eruption of fire. This year the plague raged in Constantinople, and in 1539 was still more destructive.

In 1539 the drouth in Ireland was excessive——and nearly dried up the river Lee at Cork.

In 1540 there was a terrible drouth. In England a pestilential ague and a dysentery were epidemic and mortal. Another eruption of Etna happened this year, and the next year a comet.

  Short, vol. 1. Mignot's Hist. Turkish Empire, vol. 2. p. 4.

In 1541 the plague raged in Constantinople.

The year 1543 was very wet and cold, and a great mortality among cattle. In 1542 the plague was in Geneva. In 1543 it raged in London in winter. In 1545 there was an eruption of Etna. The plague again raged in Geneva, and all over Europe a pestilential epidemic, called the Troup Gallant, which seized chiefly the young and robust, with a mortality nearly equal to that of the true plague, of which it seems to have been the precursor. Patients had a violent pain in the head, heat in the kidneys, universal lassitude, continual watchings ending in frenzy, or drowziness ending in lethargy; and worms rising into the throat, with danger of suffocation. Bleeding was the only remedy; then detergents and cordials. The disease terminated on the 4th or 11th day. Charles, duke of Orleans, died of this disease at a monastery in Abbeville.

In 1547 the plague prevailed in most parts of Europe, as in Ireland and in Germany; and in 1548 in London. Here my labors begin to receive aid from that accurate and elegant historian Thuanus, who, in lib. 4, describes the disease as it prevailed in Saxony. "Such was its violence that all other distempers gave way to it or ran into it. Most of the soldiers in the

Emperor's army were seized. They experienced a moft intolerable pain from the heat of the head; the eyes were fwelled and fiery; the tongue bloody; refpiration difficult and breath fetid; vomitings of bilious matters frequent; finally the body became livid, with pimples here and there fcattered over it, which bred worms. Death took place the fecond or third day."

During this year great rains inundated Tufcany. Locufts in 1547 were unufually numerous.

Short, vol 1   Thuanus, lib 1 and 4.
Univ Hift vol. 37.   Smith's Cork p 40.

This peftilential period was long and fevere. In 1548 the plague was in London. A contagious peripneumony prevailed over Europe, with fpitting of blood and difficulty of breathing. In 1549 the plague prevailed in Pruffia and Portugal.

In 1550 a comet in March, and the fame year an eruption of Etna and Lipari. The fummer was very rainy and the winter dry. In 1551 the earth was deluged with rain, and infinite damage was done by floods The catarrh was epidemic in France. An epidemic peftilential fever raged all over Europe, and the fweating ficknefs in London. The plague followed in various parts of Europe. In 1552 it raged in Mifena, and the patient difcharged blood by the pores for three days before death. In 1553 the fame diftemper raged in Paris, with extreme mortality, and to appeafe the wrath of heaven, many heretics were burnt.

At the fame time, peftilence fpread over Hungary and Tranfylvania for two years and fufpended the operations of war. This year alfo there was an earthquake from the Elbe to Saxony.

Thuanus, lib 12   Skenkius' Obf p 766.

In 1554 there was an eruption of fire in Iceland and in the fame year appeared a comet. In 1555 the fummer was excefsively rainy, and fevers were very mortal in England and France.

In 1556 a comet and a drouth; the fevers of the laft feafon raged with augmented violence; as alfo the fpotted fever and confluent malignant fmall pox

This year there was an eruption of Etna, and in China a large diftrict of country was funk by an earthquake, with all its inhabitants, and became a Lake. Thefe phenomena indicated a great disorder in the elements and introduced most deadly epidemics.

In 1557 a comet; an inundation of the Tyber; and a violent catarrh was almost universal. The cough was severe, and pain in the side, difficulty of breathing and fever attended. In general bleeding the first or second day was successful; but in a small town near Madrid, bleeding was fatal, and 2000 patients died after venesection.

In Alemar this epidemic assumed the form of a sore throat; 2000 persons were seized almost instantly in October, of whom 200 died. Forestus ascribes it to a vapor, for it was preceded by thick clouds of an ill smell.

In 1556 the plague raged in Vienna.

In 1557 a violent plague broke out in a small inland village between Delph and the Hague in Holland—an instance of its origination at a distance from a sea-port; and it spread over the country, in June. This disease was preceded by meteors in the air, and attended with abortions. Such was the mortality, that the poor fought for coffins for their dead relations. In Delph only, died 5000 of the poor. It continued through the winter to May 1558.

In the same summer pestilential fevers raged with great mortality in France, Holland and other countries.

In de Thou's history of his own times, vol. 2. 227, we have an account of the spotted, or petechial fever, which appeared in Spain in 1557, which was nearly as mortal as the inguinal plague. He calls it a " new disease" and unknown to the ancients. The spots differed from the florid pimples of the purple fever. It was putrid, malignant and much resembling the plague, but " did not carry so pestilent a contagiousness." It was called in Spain the " puncticular disease." Innumerable people perished by it that year. The same fever in Florence " was succeeded by a violent plague," which had raged on the Tuscan coast.

In 1558 appeared a comet. The summer was excessively hot and the winter very cold. Dysenteries raged in France, and in Holland semitertians, which affected principally the rich, as the plague, the laft year, did the poor. In fome places quartan agues were fatal, and malignant fevers, in others.

Violent tempefts and inundations are mentioned, this year and the laft. In 1558 died Charles V. emperor of Germany.

Short vol 1 Van Swieten vol. 16. p 23.
Maitland's Hift Lond   Univ Hift vol 27. 373.

In 1560 a comet, and a dearth of corn in England.

In 1562 and 3 the plague fpread over Europe. It broke out in 1562 among the Englifh foldiers, who were fent to garrifon New-Haven in France. The next year it raged in London and carried off 20,000 of its inhabitants. Authors fay, the foldiers from New-Haven introduced it into London; but who introduced it into New Haven, we are not informed.

The truth is, this terrible difeafe appeared in moft parts of Europe about the fame time. In Frankfort, Nuremberg, Magdeburgh, Hamburgh, Dantzick, and in the vandalic maritime towns, Wifmar, Lubick, Roftock and others, perifhed by computation 300,000 perfons in the year 1563.—This difeafe alfo raged in winter, for Thuanus mentions the death of Caftalion, a literary character of that age, by the plague at Bafle in January.

This year was remarkable alfo for earthquakes. In Sept. was a violent one in England, efpecially in Lincoln and other northern parts In January the river Thames was agitated by preternatural fluxes of the tides, which forced back the natural tides, three times. In winter, fevere cold rendered that river paffable as a highway.

The fame year earthquakes were felt in Illyrica, and Dalmatia, and Catana fuffered a great lofs of lives.

In 1564 a comet appeared, and remarkable northern lights, or meteors, and a deftructive inundation of the Thames.

Short vol 1 Maitland's Hift Lond   Thuanus.
Strype's Life of Archbifhop Parker, 131.

In 1564 epidemic quinfies were very mortal, and in fome places, the fpotted fever or the plague.—In winter came on as fevere a froft for two months as was ever known.

This epidemic quinfy was a fpecies of angina maligna, and fatal as the plague. It fpread over Europe.

In 1565 France was afflicted by peftilential epidemics, in

which bleeding and purging were fatal. The next year appeared the plague in Lyons.—Charles IX. demanded of the physicians the best mode of treatment, and they all decided against venesection.—One fourth of the inhabitants of France perished.

In 1566 the spring was rainy and the harvest dry. The Hungarian fever broke out in the Emperor Maximilian's army, and as authors affirm, the soldiers, when disbanded, spread it all over Europe, with great mortality. This disease invaded the patient at 3 o'clock in the afternoon, with slight cold and shivering for about fifteen minutes. This was followed by intense heat, and intolerable pain in the head, mouth and stomach, so that the slightest touch of the bed clothes, made the sick utter shrieks: The pain in the mouth and stomach being the pathognomonic symptoms of the disease.—The thirst was unquenchable, and a longing for wine, which was fatal, if taken. The tongue was dry and lips chopt. Delirium came on the third day. A critical looseness and deafness were favorable—Swellings behind the ears were frequent. The most miserable crisis was, tubercles on the top of the foot, which, if neglected, ended in mortification. Many suffered amputation. Spots, like flea bites, appeared on the body, and if livid or black, they were fatal symptoms. Copious bleeding, on the first seizure, was, of all remedies, the most successful.

Skenkius' p. 770. Short vol. 1.

In the year 1567 was an eruption of Etna, and in Tercera, one of the Azores, fire burst from a lake on the top of a hill, and the water released from its bed, rushed down and swept away part of a settlement below. In 1568 a spotted fever raged in Paris, in which prostration of strength rendered bleeding fatal. The winter of 1567 was very severe, and the summer excessively dry.

In 1569 appeared a comet.—The spotted fever in this year became epidemic in Europe, raging for three years with great destruction. The plague was in London. Short remarks that this spotted fever " in several places turned to the plague, and where the plague raged, it turned to this fever."—Indeed this spotted fever was a milder form of the pestilence, raging as it ufually does, for fome time, *before* the glandular plague appears. In this period, it was the herald to announce one of the moſt general plagues that Europe ever knew. The petechial fever prevailed principally from 1569 to 1574, interſperſed with the real plague, in a few places ; and the real peſtis followed it, with mortal rage, and prevailed for three or four years.

In 1570 a moſt dreadful earthquake in Chili, S. America, deſtroyed many villages and buried the inhabitants in their ruins. This is the firſt occaſion I have of introducing America in this hiſtory.

Ulloa b. 8. ch. 7.

Thuanus, whoſe authority is very reſpectable, and who was cotemporary with this period, relates that in 1570 the dikes in Holland were broken by a ſwell of the ocean, and that 400,000 people were overwhelmed in the floods. He ſays further that ſimilar phenomena were obſerved, that year, in different places over the whole world. Reggio, Florence, Venice and Modena felt ſevere ſhocks of earthquake in 1571, and Ferara was laid in ruins.

The ſummers of 1570 and 71 were moiſt and warm ; and in general the ſeaſons were ſimilar for the two ſucceeding years. The winters were rigorous. Fluxes, meaſles, worms and ſemi-tertians were epidemic in many places. In 1572 appeared a comet or new ſtar, very bright and clear, larger than Jupiter, in the conſtellation of Caſſiopeia, behind her chair. It was ſtationary for 16 months and by degrees evaniſhed. The winter ſucceeding was remarkable for hard froſt and deep ſnow. The author of Obſervations de Phyſique et de Medicine, ſays, that all maladies in France in 1572 turned to epilepſy and palſy.

This year the plague raged in Poland , and at Baſle a malignant fever, chiefly fatal to men of robuſt conſtitution.

In 1574 the petechial fever, which had ſpread mortality over Europe, eſpecially in Italy and Spain, began to change into the uſual form of the plague. This diſeaſe made its appearance in London, in a ſmall degree, in October and November of this year.

In 1575 the plague appeared in many parts of Europe, and

raged with incredible mortality for three years. It was reported in Italy to have been *imported* into Verona and Venice, from Trent. Such was the current vulgar opinion. But men of science held the difeafe to be generated in cities from the *filthinefs of private dwellings*, and not to be produced by the pofition of the ftars or malignant conftitution of the air.

The truth was, the difeafe in Italy firft appeared in Trent, an *inland town, far from the fea*—another inftance in which the advocates of importation from Africa or the Levant are filenced. Philofophy difdains to look abroad for the caufe of an epidemic, when the ftrongeft of all caufes exift in the place. Trent is fituated in a valley, on the bank of the Adige, a river which often overflows the adjacent low lands; and after the flood recedes, the place is fometimes fo fickly that the people are compelled to retire to the neighboring hills. Strong local caufes therefore account for the *firft* appearance of the plague in that city. The general contagion of the atmofphere, which had produced fpotted fevers and other deadly difeafes all over Europe for four years preceding, was aided by the local unhealthinefs of Trent, and here appeared firft, the crifis of the peftilence, or plague. See the defcription of that country in Zimmerman on Air.

The difeafe almoft depopulated Trent in 1575, and became mortal in the neighboring Venetian territories. This mortality however was only the forerunner of greater evils. The difeafe indeed fubfided in winter, and the people fuppofed its violence to be paft. They might have known otherwife, had they attended to the *progreffivenefs* of the malady, and the certain indications of its increafe.

In 1576 the difeafe appeared in Venice; and as it carried off a few people at firft, in fcattered fituations, opinions were, as ufual in all fuch cafes, divided as to the nature of the diftemper. In this ftate of the public mind, two eminent phyficians, Mercuriale of Forli, and Capavacca of Padua, undertook to affert the difeafe not to be peftilential. The fenate, obferving the controverfy among the Venetian phyficians, as to the nature of the diftemper, liftened to the two foreigners, who declared they could cure it, and put a stop to the removal of the diseased from the city. By this means, says the historian, the distemper was obviously increased; and it raged with terrible fury, till it carried off 70,000 of the citizens, with fifty-seven valuable physicians and surgeons. The two foreign physicians were dismissed, with applauses for having preferred the good of Venice to their personal safety.

This account from Thuanus deserves particular notice. We here see the same doubts about the nature of the disease on its first appearance, which prevail in all similar cases—as in Marseilles in 1720—in London in 1665—and in America, with respect to the yellow fever, which is only another form of plague. The source of all these doubts and controversies, which have so often embarrassed the citizens and disgraced the faculty, is, the *progressiveness* of the pestilence. The malignant diseases preceding, slide into the glandular plague so gradually, that physicians themselves do not know precisely when the distemper should lose the name of *malignant fever* and take that of *plague*. Sydenham honestly confesses that, in 1665, he did not know whether the malignant disease which appeared in May and became epidemic, just before the plague, was the real plague or not. And the truth is, that the disease often assails people, in a few scattering cases, at the beginning of a plague, with a mortality equal to the true pestis, and *without* the distinctive marks of plague, the glandular tumors.

These facts will hereafter, with careful observation, obviate all controversies at the beginning of pestilential diseases; and they will decide infallibly all questions relative to the domestic or foreign origin of such maladies.

This pestilence was severely felt in Padua, Milan, Cremona and Pavia. Vicenza, which escaped this year, was visited the next, with equal severity.

Dr. Mead is puzzled to know why Vicenza, which lies between Verona and Padua, should escape the plague, in the year when both those cities were infested; and yet the next year, should suffer equally with her neighbors, when *they* were exempt from the calamity. He finds some difficulty in accounting for the conveyance of the *infection* from one to another, without communicating it to the intervening city. This subject will be considered in a subsequent section; I will only here remark, that nothing is so fatal to truth and science, as for a man of popular talents to espouse an erroneous theory, and then strive to bend facts to its support.

See Thuanus, lib. 62. Shenkius, 756. Short, vol. 1.

In 1575 multitudes of flies and beetles were found in England, and in 1576 an earthquake was experienced.

In November 1577 appeared a comet of surprising magnitude, with a long coma—and most terrible tempests accompanied its approach. In 1578 another comet, and in 1579 an eruption of Etna. In 1578 were earthquakes in England.

Short, vol. 1.

In the great pestilence of the preceding ten years, not only Europe, but Asia was laid waste. So general and severe was the disease that the operations of war, in the Turkish empire, were suspended. Messina in Sicily lost 40,000 inhabitants—and Europe must have lost in ten years, by the pestilence under the various forms it assumed, one third, or more probably one half her people.

In this period we see all the extraordinary operations of nature united. Comets, earthquakes, in Europe and S. America tempests, volcanoes, unusual animals, excessive floods from rain or an extraordinary intumescence of the ocean all mark an extreme agitation or disorder of the elements.—The vast comet of 1577, the year when the plague was at its height, was calculated to approach within 840,000 miles of the earth. Upon the Newtonian principles of the power of attraction, the influence of that body on the earth must have been prodigious.

Encyclop. art. Astronomy.

In this year appeared in Moravia a new disease, evidently distinct in its symptoms from any known malady, and which Thuanus has described.

This also was the year in which a sudden disease seized the court and attendants at the Oxford assizes in England. Early in July, while the court was sitting, " there arose, says Stowe, amidst the people such a damp that almost all were smothered—

very few efcaped, that were not taken at that inftant. The jurors died prefently—after which Robert Bell, Lord Chief Baron. There died in Oxford 300 perfons—and fickened there, but died elfewhere, more than 200 from the 6th to the 12th of July. After which died not one of that ficknefs, for one of them infected not another, nor died thereof any one woman or child."

Chronicle, p. 681.

This fudden cataftrophe is afcribed to a damp or vapor. But there is no need of reforting to fuch a caufe. The atmofphere, during the period under confideration, was not furnifhed with the power of fupporting animal life, in as ample a manner as it ufually is.—This is evident, from the univerfality of mortal epidemics. In this ftate of the atmofphere, a multitude, crouded into a court room, in the hot month of July, muft fpeedily deftroy all the refpirable air, and death muft enfue. That the principal caufe was not only local, but fudden, is demonftrated by the circumftance, that no infection accompanied the difeafed. Had the caufe of their illnefs been long in operation, it would have produced in the body that fpecies of poifon, which is noxious to perfons in health. Perfons, fuddenly deprived of life, as by damps in wells or the fumes of charcoal, communicate no infection.

It is fuggefted by fome writers, that this difeafe was occafioned by an infected prifoner, who was brought from jail into court; but Stowe does not mention this circumftance. And it is poffible the cataftrophe might have been owing to a fudden difcharge of mephitic vapor.

Scarcely had the laft period of peftilence come to a clofe, when another feries of maladies fucceeded, and nearly in the order of thofe laft defcribed.

In 1580 appeared a comet on the 10th of October which was vifible for two months. The preceding fummer was very moift and rainy, and about the rifing of the dog-ftar, came on a cold dry north wind. In June began an epidemic catarrh in Sicily, which fpread over Europe. In July, it was in Italy; in Auguft, in Venice and Conftantinople; in September, it extended over Hungary, Bohemia and Saxony; in October, on the Baltic; in November, in Norway and in December, in Sweden, Poland and Ruffia.—Its fymptoms were nearly the fame, as in this country, but the difeafe was more violent and fatal.—In Rome, died of it 4000 people—in Lubec, 8000; at Hamburgh, 3000; and multitudes in other places. It appears to have been attended with more fever than in ordinary cafes—The fever was continual for four or five days, with a pain in the head, ftraitnefs of the breaft and cough—it terminated in profufe fweating.—In general bleeding and purging were found to be prejudicial.

Riverius, lib. 17.

In this year and about the time, when the catarrh had overfpread Europe, broke out in Grand Cairo, one of the moft defolating plagues ever known. Profper Alpinus, who lived in that age, reports the number of deaths, from November 1580, to July 1581 to have been 500,000. It will be found on examination that the plague, in a feries of peftilential and epidemic difeafes, appears in Egypt, *before* it does in Europe and America, and is nearly cotemporary with the catarrh, angina or other precurfor of the peftilence in more northern latitudes. This fact deferves notice. The plague which followed the catarrh in Europe, did not appear in many places, perhaps in none except in France, in the year 1580.—In northern latitudes, the malignity of the epidemic conftitution does not appear, till the fecond or third year, after its commencement in catarrh or meafles.

In Paris however the plague raged in 1580, the fame year it appeared in Egypt, and carried off 40,000 people, moftly of the poorer fort; and at the fame time, it prevailed in many of the neighboring towns, efpecially, fays Thuanus, " at Laon in Vermandois, which city is in a pofition expofed to a hot fun, in which died 6000."

The hiftorian further remarks, that the " crops that year were plentiful, and the fky ferene; fo that it was thought the difeafe was produced rather by the influence of the ftars, ab aftrorum impreffione, than by the malignity of a corrupt air." This is another proof that a ftate of air, as defcribed by Hippocrates, is not always the caufe of peftilence.

Altho this malady broke out in France in 1580, yet it had been preceeded by the catarrh. The historian remarks, that the catarrh was not so much dreaded for its mortality, tho many died of it, as for the astonishing rapidity with which the contagion spread from place to place. It seized the lower spine of the back with a chill, *horrore ;* to this succeeded *gravedo,* a dull pain in the head ; and universal languor or debility, resolvens membra, loosening or unhinging the joints. If the crisis was not favorable in five days, the disease terminated in a fatal fever.

See Thuanus and Riverius, also lib 17.

In 1580 confiderable earthquakes were felt in Belgium, at Cologne and about the Mediterranean. The same shocks were felt in various parts of England, but Short places them under the following year. The German sea was agitated, and a great swelling of its waters was observed.

See Thuanus, lib 71, 72. Short, vol. 1. p 260

In 1580 also, the marshes in Essex, and some parts of Kent in England, were laid waste by mice, which were so numerous as to destroy the herbage, and a murrain among cattle succeeded.

In this year was issued a proclamation of Queen Elizabeth, upon the representation of the Mayor and Aldermen of London, prohibiting any new house to be built within three miles of the gates of the city, and more than one family to reside in a house. The reasons assigned for the prohibition are connected with this subject. The increase of London had long been considered as an evil, by swelling the head too large for the body, and several attempts had been made to restrain the increase. The resort of people to the city from the country was held to be prejudicial to agriculture.

But the proclamation states further, that " such great multitudes of people, brought to inhabit in small rooms, whereof a great part are very poor, yea such as must live by begging, or by worse means, and they heaped together, and in a sort, smothered with many families of children and servants, in one house or small tenement, it must needs follow, if any plague or popular sickness should, by God's permission, enter amongst those multitudes, that the same would not only spread itself, and invade the whole city and confines, but a great mortality would enfue the fame, and the infection be difperfed through all other parts of the realm."

In this paper, we obferve fome powerful caufes of peftilence in London to be explained—and events fhowed how little good was done by the interference of authority with private rights, and an attempt to check, by pofitive prohibitions, the natural growth of towns. This proclamation, like all which had preceded it, was ufelefs. The city increafed, and the plague continued to ravage it, until the good providence of God arrefted the evil, by a general conflagration, and men had become wife enough, to build large, airy houfes, and keep them clean.

Maitland's Hiftory of London.

In 1582 a remarkable tempeft is mentioned, and a comet in May. A fevere earthquake was felt in South-America, and a fmall city near Lima was deftroyed.

Ulloa's Voyage, vol. 2. b. 7.

In 1583 feveral concuffions of the earth were experienced in England, and the plague appeared in London. At the fame time it appeared in Germany or Holland; as Diemerbroeck mentions this as a peftilential year. The following winter was fevere. In Rome there was a famin.

Maitland's Hift. Lond. Short, vol. 1.

In 1585 in fpring appeared very malignant pleurifies. In 1586 Thrace was overrun with locufts, and the plague raged in Hungary, Auftria and Turkey. A comet appeared in each of thefe years, and in 1586 Lima in South America was nearly ruined by an earthquake. See Ulloa, from whom my accounts of earthquakes in Spanifh America, are all taken.

In 1587 a very cold fpring, but a plentiful year in moft countries. The plague raged in Flanders, which was almoft depopulated by difeafe, war and famin. In fome parts, the wild beafts took poffeffion of the houfes. Dogs ran mad, and did no fmall mifchief, and fields were covered with weeds and bufhes. The catarrh appeared in England, this year, but how extenfively, I am not informed. An eruption of fire in Iceland is recorded under the fame year.

In 1589 the English fleet, returned from *Portugal*, with the *Hungarian* fever, says Short, and introduced it into England. What an influence have *names*, and what mischief is done by ignorance and false philosophy! The Hungarian fever! As tho this fever had been a native of a particular soil, and transplanted from country to country, like a fruit-tree. Names are not always harmless. The name, Sudor *Anglicus*, given to the sweating plague, because it appeared first in England and was at first peculiar to Englishmen, has led the moderns to suppose, the disease to have been limited to England or to Englishmen, altho it repeatedly spread over all Europe. In the same way, the insect which injures wheat in America, was ignorantly called the Hessian fly, and altho the animal was never known in Germany, yet people believe, that, like yellow fever, it *was imported*. It is thus that ignorance gives currency to an improper name, and the name in turn assists to propagate and perpetuate an error.

The truth, in regard to diseases, is, that they often assume peculiar symptoms; such as are not usual. These are not properly *new* diseases, but modifications of common fever, proceeding from the infinite variety of that cause of sickness, which I denominate general contagion, and which Sydenham called the Epidemic Constitution of the air. This or other causes are perpetually diversifying the symptoms of diseases; so that physicians are often at a loss whether to call a disease by an old or new name. Wherever the peculiar causes *first* exist, there will the peculiar symptoms of disease first appear—and when similar causes exist in other places, the same symptoms will attend the disease.

In 1590 multitudes of people perished by famin. A comet approached the system, the winter was cold, a violent earthquake convulsed Hungary, Bohemia and Vienna; near the latter place, the earth emitted an offensive smell. The drouth was extreme. The Azores were shaken by an earthquake, and a tempest in September threatened to overwhelm them in mass.

In 1591 universal catarrh in Europe was a prelude to most destructive pestilence. It is singular also that the plague broke out in Narva and Revel, in Livonia, on the gulf of Finland, in the 59th degree of latitude, and raged through the succeeding cold winter. Six thousand persons perished in Revel. As to its origin, the great Thuanus could not decide whether it was "a belli incommoditatibus, sive cæli inclementia," from the distresses of war, or intemperature of the air. There could have been no suspicion of a foreign origin.

Thuanus, lib. 100.

Cotemporary with the catarrh was a malignant spotted fever in Trent. A distressing famin caused a great mortality in Italy.

In 1591 the plague began to show itself in Italy, but attended with peculiar symptoms. A fever, little infectious, seized the head, inducing delirium, and in many patients, was attended with fluxes and flatulent bowels. It terminated fatally on the tenth day. The remedy was bleeding "Secta vena capitis, quæ in brachio est, aliisque a capite manantibus," says Thuanus. It attacked chiefly men between the ages of 30 and 50; but was fatal to few women. It raged in Umbria, Tuscany, Romagne and Lombardy, sweeping away, in some towns, almost every man. From August to August, it was computed that 60,000 persons perished.

Thuanus, lib. 102.

In 1592 the petechial fever spread over Florence, with a malignity that entitled it to the name of plague. It was most fatal to the nobles.

In England the drouth in this and the former summer was extreme. The Thames was fordable at London. The plague appeared in Shropshire in the west, and carried off 18,000 citizens in London. Persia suffered much by an earthquake in the same year.

Short, vol. 1. Sims on Epid. Mem. Med. Soc. vol. 1. Maitland's Lond.

In the same year a furious pestilence prevailed in Candia. It appeared in spring, increased till July and then abated. On its first appearance, all infected and suspected persons were removed to a distant hospital, but without effect. The disease continued to spread—a proof that it was an epidemic. In September, it was supposed to be extinguished; but in October, it broke out with fresh violence, and the diseased were confined to their houses—a useless and pernicious regulation. The city lost 10,000 inhabitants.

In 1594 was a severe winter. The years 1594, 5 and 6 were very rainy in England and Germany. Crops failed, and in Hungary, the famin was extreme.

In 1596 appeared a comet. Violent earthquakes shook different countries, and several cities in Japan were swallowed up.

In 1596 and 7 prevailed in Cologne, Westphalia and other parts of Germany, a singular disease, which authors ascribe to the famin which had preceded. It was a malignant fever, which was attended with convulsions and raving madness, or delirium. Sometimes the convulsions were attended with little or no fever. The patient was contracted into a knot or ball by the violence of the convulsions, or extended to full length, like a dead body—sometimes the extension of the body was succeeded by a contraction in the same paroxism. The particulars respecting this disease do not fall within the plan of this history, but may be found in Short, vol. 1.

In 1597 appeared a comet, and the same year the catarrh was again epidemic. Malignant fevers, accompanied with worms in youth, were predominant also, and the plague was in Juliers and Geneva. A dearth in England. The winter of 1597 was severe, as was that of 1599.

The summers of 1598 and 99 were remarkably dry, and swarms of fleas, gnats and flies abounded. Tertians, with petechiæ, were frequent, and continual fevers which yielded to bleeding and purging, or went off with a bilious diarrhea.— Small-pox and measles were also epidemic.

These diseases, as usual, were the precursors of a very distressing plague, which, in the autumn of 1598, raged in London, Litchfield, Leicester and other places in England. It even broke out in the small towns in Wales and the northern counties, as in Kendal in Cumberland, where died 2500—in Richmond, where died 2200—at Carlisle which lost 1196 inhabitants; and at Percrith which lost 2266.

See Camden's Britannia.

In 1598 Pegu, in Asia, was depopulated by famin, and Constantinople was almost stripped of its inhabitants by the plague,

Seventeen princeffes, fifters of the Sultan, Mahomet III. died in one day. To arreft the progrefs of this mortality, cannon were fired and aromatics burnt in all parts of the city; but with what fuccefs the hiftorian does not inform us.

Hiftory of the Turkifh Empire.

In Italy an inundation of the Tyber injured Rome.

In 1599 the fpring was cold and dry; the fummer hot and rainy, with great floods. A very mortal diftemper raged among cattle in Italy. In Spain and Lifbon died 70,000 people of the plague. In fome places, a fatal dyfentery prevailed.

Short, vol. 1. Sims on Epid.

SECTION VI.

Historical view of Pestilential Epidemics from the year 1600 to the close of the year 1700.

THE year 1600 was remarkable for pestilence in almost every part of Europe. Spain, where the disease was fatal the year before, was this year almost depopulated. There raged throughout Europe, a pestilential, mortal cholic which destroyed the lives of all whom it seized, within four days. The patient, as soon as he was seized, became senseless—the hair fell from his head—a livid pustule arose on the nose, which consumed it—the extremities became cold and mortified.

In Florence a terrible earthquake destroyed many buildings.

The winter of 1600 was very cold. In the summer of 1601 there was a severe drouth of four or five months; and a violent dysentery followed, with double tertians and continual fevers. The plague raged in Portugal, attended with black round worms. At Christmas, there was an earthquake in England. The same year there was an earthquake at Arequipa, in Peru, accompanied by an eruption of a volcano.

In 1602 a cold and dry summer and winter, the catarrh was epidemic, and acute fevers prevalent. These diseases and phenomena accompanied a series of calamities in all parts of Europe.

The famin that marked this period, for a series of years, exceeded in extent and severity, what had been before recorded. Famins are usually local; but in the present instance, there was a failure of crops for several years, in almost every part of Europe; while the plague committed most desolating ravages.

In Muscovy the famin raged for three years at the beginning of the century under consideration, attended with the plague. Parents devoured their dying children; cats, rats and every unclean thing was used to sustain life. All the ties of nature and morality were disregarded; human flesh was exposed to sale in the open market. The more powerful seized their neighbors; fathers and mothers, their children; husbands, their wives, and offered them for sale. Multitudes of dead were found, with their mouths filled with straw, and the most filthy substances. Five hundred thousand persons were supposed to perish in Muscovy, by famin and pestilence.

At the same time, the famin in Livonia, and the cold winter of 1602, destroyed 30,000 lives. The dead bodies lay in the streets, for want of hands to bury them.

Thuanus, lib. 135. Encyclopedia, art. Russia.

At the same time, raged a most dreadful pestilence in Constantinople, which also followed a famin.

In England, there was also a dearth, and in 1603 perished 36,000 in London, of the plague, which was said to be imported from Ostend.

Maitland's Hist. Lond. Mignot's Hist. Turkish Empire, p. 256.

Even in this case, the report of imported infection into London was believed, altho the nation had before their eyes, a demonstration to the contrary; for the same malady broke out in every part of the kingdom, and had actually prevailed in Chester, in the north-west corner of England, the year preceding.

It is idle to ascribe the plague to infection, communicated from person to person, or from clothes to persons. The disease, in 1602 was in every part of Europe, and appeared nearly at the same time, in the most distant parts. In this case, as in those before related, of 1580 and 1591, it had been preceded by catarrh, and a course of malignant fevers. The malignity of the disease in 1602 resembled that of 1348—persons were seized with spitting of blood, and died in three days.

In August 1603 in Paris died 2000 persons weekly of the plague. This disease was attributed to the diet and filth accumulated, under a defective police.

Wraxall, vol. 3. 458.

Why the filth of Paris did not produce the plague in other seasons, writers have not informed us.

The period under confideration was remarkable for the univerfality of the action of fubterranean fire. The earthquakes of 1600 and 1601 and the burfting of a volcano in South-America have been mentioned. In 1603 there was an explofion of Etna. In 1604 a fecond eruption in Peru, and a comet.

The plague abated, in fome places, the year following; but London was not free from it for a number of years, and from 1606 to 1609 inclufive the diftemper carried off from two to four thoufand citizens in each feafon.

In 1607 commenced an unufual concurrence of great agitations in the elements, and fevere peftilence attended.

In this year appeared a comet, and another in 1609. The winter of 1607-8 was the fevereft that had been known for an age, boats were built on the Thames. And here for the firft time, I am able to introduce North-America, into this hiftory; from which will be derived fome of the moft important evidence in regard to the univerfality of the caufes of peftilential epidemics.

The feverity of the winter mentioned was equally great in America, as in Europe. George Popham, and a company of fettlers under the patent of king James, to the London merchants, attempted a fettlement at Sagadahoc in 1607; but Popham, the Prefident, died during the winter, and the extreme cold was one of the difcouragements that contributed to break up the fettlement.

Gorges Hift New-England. Purchas, vol. 4. 1637.
Hutchinfon's Hift Maff vol. 1 2.

In this fame year was an eruption of Etna.

The comet of this year produced a moft remarkable tempeft, with a fwell of the ocean, that did incredible damage in England. In the latter part of winter, the tempeft brought in a flood into the Severn, which overflowed the country, near Briftol, to the extent of ten miles, with a rapidity, that left no time for the people to fave their effects, and many lives were loft. The flood rofe above the houfes, where people had reforted for fafety, and overwhelmed them. The lofs of cattle and goods was immenfe.

In Somerfetfhire, the inundation laid wafte an extent of 20 miles by 10; overwhelming five towns. So fudden was the irruption, that laborers were caught in the fields, and were seen floating on the timbers of their houses. In Norfolk, the inundation was not less destructive.

Thuanus, lib. 138.

In 1608 a very malignant dysentery prevailed.

In 1609 the approach of the second comet produced effects equally remarkable with the last. The action of subterranean fire was extensive. There was an eruption of Etna, and a violent earthquake at Lima in Peru. The winter was so severe, as to convert the Thames into a common highway.

In this year the plague was augmented in London; and it raged in Alemar and Denmark. In the years 1607 and 8, it had been very mortal in Cork.

The pestilential state of air, at this time, was experienced at sea. The people on board the fleet under Sir Thomas Gates and Sir George Somers, bound to Virginia, were seized with the calenture, a spotted pestilent fever, which, on board of one of the ships, was so malignant as to be called the plague. Thirty-two dead bodies were thrown out of two ships. Was this disease imported? In the same passage, the fleet met with a tremendous storm of four days continuance, and Sir T. Gates was shipwrecked on Bermuda.

Purchas, vol. 4. p. 1733.

In 1610 the catarrh was again epidemic. In some parts of the continent prevailed the Hungarian fever like the plague, and severe bilious complaints. A remarkable fiery bow in the heavens was observed in Hungary; and Constantinople was infested with clouds of grass-hoppers, of great size, that devoured every green thing. The malignant sore throat was fatal in Spain, and authors relate that this was its first appearance in that country.

In 1611 the plague carried off 200,000 of the inhabitants of Constantinople. It appeared also in some other places. The summers of the three last years were very hot and dry.

In 1612 appeared a comet. A terrible tempest made great havoc with shipping—2000 dead bodies of sailors were found on the coast of England, and 1200 on that of Holland. Some towns were injured. In the following year, Provence in France was greatly injured by an inundation; and swarms of locusts succeeded, which laid waste the vegetable kingdom.

The summer of 1612 in England was excessively dry, and a malignant fever severely afflicted the nation.

In 1613 the plague appeared in detached parts of France, and in Montpelier, a malignant disease so fatal, as to want only the buboes, to prove it the true plague. It was marked with red and livid spots, swellings behind the ears and carbuncles. One third who were seized died.

Riverius, lib. 17.

The preceding summers, the earth was covered with grass-hoppers, and the air filled with clouds of flies.

In this year also Constantinople was ravaged with the plague; and as cats were supposed to spread the infection, the physicians, who were mostly Jews, advised the emperor Achmet I. and he accordingly ordered all the cats to be transported to a desert island near Scutari.

Short, vol. 1. Mignot's Hist. Turkish Empire.

In 1614 the winter was severe; there was an eruption of Etna, and an earthquake in the Azores. The heavens appeared, at one time in a flame, and afterwards very dark.

This year was remarkable for the most universal small-pox, and most fatal ever known. It laid waste Alexandria, Crete, Turkey, Calabria, Italy, Venice, Dalmatia, France, Germany, Poland, Flanders and England. The mortality equalled that of the plague. In Persia also it raged, with measles.

In 1615 the seasons were cold. In 1616 a very hot and dry summer—quartan agues epidemic—not a family in Germany escaped; but not fatal.

In 1617 the summer was hot and dry.

In 1618 appeared a remarkable comet in November, (Short mentions four) and a town in Rhetia was overwhelmed by an earthquake. Violent tempests, inundations and hurricanes are recorded of the same year, and in Bermuda, the year following, a storm tore up the strongest trees by the roots. In 1619 Heckla discharged her fiery contents.

In 1618 broke out in Naples a malignant Angina which ravaged the place for many years. The plague appeared at Bergen, in Norway, in Denmark and in Grand Cairo. This was the beginning of a very pestilential period, and here must be introduced the terrible pestilence which wasted the American Indians, just before our ancestors landed in Massachusetts. As this is one of the most remarkable facts in history, and one that demonstrates the general causes of plague to belong to other climates, besides those of Egypt and the Levant, I have taken great pains to ascertain the species of disease, and the time of its appearance.

Capt. Dermer, an English adventurer, who had arrived in America, in a fishing vessel, a year or two before, passed the winter of 1618-19 in Monhiggan, an Indian town on the northern coast. On the 19th of May 1619 he sailed along the coast, on his way to Virginia, and landed at several places, where he had been the year before, and he found many Indian towns totally depopulated—in others a few natives remained alive, but " not free of sickness;" " their disease, the plague, for we might perceive the sores of some that had escaped, who described the spots of such as usually die." These are his words. He found some villages, which, in his former visit, were populous, all deserted—the Indians " all dead."

Purchas, vol 4 1778

Richard Vines, and his companions, who had been sent by Ferdinando Gorges, to explore the country, wintered among the Indians, during the pestilence, and remained untouched, the disease attacking none of the English. Belknap's Life of Gorges, American Biography, vol. 1. p. 355, but the year is not specified.

Gookin, in his account of the Indians, Historical Collections, p. 8, places this pestilence in 1612 and 13, about seven or eight years before the English arrived at Plymouth. But this cannot be accurate, unless the disease began to rage for a number of years previous to 1618. Capt. Dermer's letter in Purchas is decisive of the time of the principal sickness, and fortunately we have another authority which is indisputable.

A sermon was preached by Elder Cushman at Plymouth, in 1620, just after the colony arrived, and sent to London to be published. In the Epistle Dedicatory which is dated December, 21, 1621, the author has these words. " They [the Indians] were very much wasted of late, by a great mortality, that fell amongst them, *three years since*, which, with their own civil diffentions and bloody wars, hath so wasted them, as I think the twentieth person is scarce left alive."

Hazard's Collection, vol 1 p 148.

This corresponds also with the accounts in Prince's Chronology from original manuscripts. This fixes the time in 1618, precisely agreeable to Capt. Dermer's account. This was the year of the principal mortality; but like other pestilential periods, this continued for a number of years; for some of the Plymouth settlers went to Massachusetts, (now Boston) in 1622, to purchase corn of the natives; and " found among the Indians, a great sickness, not unlike the plague, if not the same." It raged in winter, and affected the Indians only.

See Purchas 4 1858. Prince's Chron. 124.

The time then is fixed. The disease commenced, or raged with its principal violence in 1618 and through the winter. This was the year of the remarkable comet, when the plague was raging in many parts of the world. So fatal was the pestilence in America, that the warriors from Narraganfett to Penobscot, the distance to which the disease seems to have been limited, were reduced from 9000 to a few hundreds.* When our ancestors arrived in 1620, they found the bones of those who perished, in many places, unburied.

Magnalia, book 1. p. 7.

The kind of disease is another important question. Dermer seems to think it a species of plague, and he saw some of the sores of those who had survived. Hutchinson, vol. 1. p. 34, 35, says some have supposed it to have been the small-pox, but the Indians, who were perfectly acquainted with this disease, after the English arrived, always gave a very different account of it, and described it as a pestilential putrid fever.

Fortunately General Gookin, in the passage above cited, has left us a fact, which leaves no doubt as to the nature of the malady. His words are—" What the disease was, which so gen-

* Hutchinson says, 30,000 of the Massachusetts tribe alone were supposed to be reduced to 300.

erally and mortally swept them away, I cannot learn. Doubtless it was some pestilential disease. I have discoursed with some old Indians, that were then youths, who say, that the *bodies all over were exceeding yellow* (describing it by a yellow garment they showed me) both before they died and afterwards."

This account may be relied on for its authenticity and it decides the question, that the pestilence was the true American plague, called yellow fever. If any confirmation of this evidence were necessary, we have it in Prince's Chronology, where it is recorded that this fever produced hemorrhagy from the nose.

At the time Gookin wrote, about forty or fifty years after the settlement of New-England, the infectious fevers of autumn were called "pestilent," and they were frequent in the country, but had not then acquired the appellation of *yellow*.

Winthrop's Journal, p. 51.

This fever has been frequent among the Indians since the English settled the country. Some instances will be hereafter related.

The evidence then of the origin of the yellow fever in this country, between the 41st and 44th degrees of latitude, is complete, leaving no room for doubt or controversy. No intercourse existed, in 1618, between this continent and the West-Indies; nor did a single vessel pass between New-England and the islands, till twenty years after that pestilence. Not one of the islands was then settled, except by the Spaniards, with whom our ancestors had no commerce. Not an European was among the Indians, except a French seaman, who had escaped from a wreck a year or two before, and Mr. Vine's men, who arrived directly from England. These men escaped the disease; none being attacked but the Indians; another evidence of the origin of the malady in the country.

In Gorges' description of New-England, there is the following account of this pestilence. "The summer after the blazing star, which moved from the east to the west, even a little before the English removed from Holland to Plymouth, in New-England, there befel a great mortality among the Indians, the greatest that had ever happened in the memory of man, or been taken notice of by tradition, laying waste the east."

The author further remarks that this ſtar was much noted in Europe. In America it was ſeen in the ſouth weſt, for " thirty ſleeps," as the Indians expreſs themſelves. The deſcription of the comet here given anſwers to that of Riverius, who repreſents it as very ſplendid, larger than Venus, moving from the eaſt to the weſt, and viſible from Nov 27, 1618, till the cloſe of December. This was the time the peſtilence was raging among the Indians. Gorges indeed ſays, it was the ſummer *after* the blazing ſtar. It is true, that the diſeaſe continued not only into 1619, but occurred in autumn for ſome years ſubſequent. We hear of it among the Maſſachuſetts Indians in 1622. From this it appears that this was a long and ſevere period of peſtilence, between 1617 and 1623, or a later year; like the preſent period in the United States.

It muſt be remarked that in 1618, the ſame year when the Indians in America were falling a prey to this malady, the angina maligna broke out in the kingdom of Naples, and ſpread mortality over the country, as authors affirm, for eighteen years. This however is not underſtood, as affirming the diſeaſe to have been conſtantly epidemic; but as prevailing at certain times and ſeaſons.

The ſame deſtructive principle operated in Virginia. Capt. Dermer relates that when he arrived in the Cheſapeek on the 8th of September, " The firſt news ſtruck cold to our hearts, the ſickneſs over the land."* Three hundred of the ſettlers died in 1619.

It appears from Purchas that the emigrants to Virginia in 1619, 20 and 21, amounted to 3570, in 42 ſail of ſhips.† There were 600 ſouls in that colony before theſe arrived, making the whole number 4170. Of theſe, 349 periſhed in the Indian maſſacre of 1622, which would leave 3821 ſurvivors. But in 1624 no more than 1800 were living. Scanty means of ſubſiſtence might have contributed to this mortality; but moſt of it was in conſequence of fevers, that were probably the ef-

* Capt Dermer was probably the firſt Engliſhman that ever paſſed through the rapids between Long-Iſland and the main land, now called Hell-Gate He deſcribes this paſſage as a cataract, and mentions the difference in times of high water, from the eaſt and weſt.
† Mr Jefferſon allows only 2516 perſons to have arrived in that period.

fects of the climate, and a very unfavorable state of the atmosphere.

In 1620 a comet was followed by a cold winter. In England the year was distinguished by a violent tempest, a preternatural tide, and a very wet summer. The Hungarian fever, so called, spread along the Rhine, and in the next year became infectious. London became sickly. The year 1621 was remarkable for an epidemic malignant small-pox.

In 1622 a comet is noted, and an earthquake in Italy In New-England the spring was excessively dry, from the third week in May to the middle of July.

In 1623 the epidemic fevers in Europe became more fatal, as the period of pestilence approached. This is obvious from the London burials, which show a considerable increment. Riverius, who has written on the epidemic fevers of this period in the south of France, observes that the mortality was great, until he began to bleed and purge, when it abated. He refers to the city of Montpelier, where almost half died who were seized. The disease was a species of pestilence.

This author concurs with the ancients in ascribing pestilence to comets. Speaking of the singular star of 1618, he says, " Hunc vero Cometam, morborum malignorum et pestilentium, necnon etiam bellorum, quibus universa penè hactenus Europa devastata est, præsagium ac prenuntium fuisse, credere non alienum est."

De febre pest 533 fol

The author falls into the error, which has brought into contempt the opinions of the ancient sages, in regard to the influence of the stars on man, and the state of the elements. He ascribes *moral* as well as *physical* effects to that influence. Admitting the distant orbs to have some effect on the air or fire of our system, and through that medium to augment or diminish the stimulus which acts on the human body and of course on the passions, by the exciting powers; yet any moral effects derived from this source, must be so inconsiderable, or so blended with the effects of other causes, as interest, ambition, love, revenge and the like, that the degree of influence could not be ascertained, nor the effects of one cause distinguished from those of the other. I reject therefore all *moral* effects ascribed to comets; but the *physical* effects are, beyond question, great and extensive.

The diseases of this period continued to multiply and grow more malignant in 1624, when the epidemic assumed the form of the spotted fever. In 1625 this fever turned to the plague, and in 1626 changed back to the spotted fever, says Lotichius, cited by Short. This is not an unusual fact.

The plague in 1625 swept away 35,000 of the citizens of London. It raged at the same time in Italy, Denmark and Leyden, and how much more extensively, I am not informed.

In this year another comet was seen; several cities in Spain were overwhelmed by inundations; the winter was severe; the summer, hot and moist weather; and there was an eruption of a volcano in Iceland. It is remarkable also that, in this year, a volcano burst forth in Palma, one of the Canaries, with a violent earthquake.

The summer of 1626 was very hot, and the plague continued its ravages in many parts of Europe, as in Wittemburg and the vicinity; and in Lyons, which lost 60,000 of its inhabitants. This was the prelude to more general calamity in France; for in the following years the whole country felt the distressing effects of the malady.

In 1627 and 8 the same disease prevailed in various other countries, especially in Augsburg after a famin. In 1629 the pestilence raged in Amsterdam. In 1630 Cambridge in England was visited. It was a very sickly summer in London, so that the citizens were alarmed and many retired to the country; but finding the country very sickly, they returned.

In 1629 Pola, a town in the Venetian territories, lost 7000 inhabitants by an earthquake.

Of the pestilence in this period, there was hardly a suspension. Particular countries enjoyed short intervals of health; but Europe and America were severely annoyed by pestilential diseases between 1632 and 1637.

In 1630 happened great explosions of subterranean fire. Apulia lost 17,000 people by an earthquake; and Lima, in South-

America, was laid in ruins by the like cataſtrophe. At this time the plague prevailed in Vienna.

In 1631 happened a memorable earthquake in Naples, with a tremendous eruption of Veſuvius, which continued or was repeated in 1632. In this eruption, Baglivus aſſures us, Veſuvius loſt 240 feet of its altitude.

Cotemporary with theſe diſcharges of fire and lava, was an eryſipelous fever in Europe with inflammation in the jaws, and an increaſe of mortality, antecedent to a general plague. See the bills of mortality for London, Augſburg and Dreſden, where the progreſs of the malignity in the epidemics, is diſtinctly marked, by an augmentation of the bills, till the plague in 1636.

In 1633 appeared a comet, which was followed by a ſevere winter. The ſame winter in America was mild, ſays Winthrop, p. 61. Southerly winds prevailed till the cloſe of winter, when there were great ſnows. It is very common that ſevere cold is progreſſive, happening in Europe one year before it does in America, as will hereafter appear.

In 1633 the year of the comet, commenced an eruption of Etna, which continued for four or five years, through this whole peſtilential period. London was ſhaken by an earthquake, and at Halifax in Yorkſhire raged a very malignant fever.

In this year alſo a "peſtilent fever," invaded the little colony at Plymouth in Maſſachuſetts, and carried off twenty of their number. This was a great mortality for that ſmall ſettlement. It muſt have been occaſioned by a fever of domeſtic origin, as the colony had, at that time, no intercourſe with foreign countries, except with England. No ſuſpicion has ever been entertained that the diſeaſe was of foreign origin.

At the ſame time, the Indians were invaded by the ſmall-pox which ſwept them away in multitudes. It ſpread from Narraganſett to Piſcataqua, and weſtward to Connecticut river.

The ſummer of this year was remarkable for innumerable large flies, of the ſize of bees, which made the woods reſound with a humming noiſe.

Hubbard's M. S. p. 131.
Winthrop's Journal, 51—56—59—61.

We have then a remarkable evidence of the extent of a peſtilential principle in the elements. The same species of diseases appeared, at the same time, in Augsburg, Dresden, London, and in America. Probably the same species prevailed over most of Europe; for we hear of them in every part of Holland in the following year. The diseases predominant, previous to the plague, are of the eruptive kind. Such was the case in the present instance. In America, the epidemic among the Indians took the form of the small-pox; and altho it is the current opinion that the small-pox is communicated only by contagion, yet my investigations have satisfied me that this is a great error. The small-pox is one of the *family of eruptive diseases*, which belong to almost every pestilential period. Before its origin and progress had been affected by the art of innoculation, it used to be epidemic, in large cities, under that inflammatory condition of the atmosphere, which originated measles, influenza, anginas and plague, and *rarely or never at any other time*. This disease therefore, tho communicable at any time by infection, is generated in particular habits without any infecting cause ab extra; and is the offspring of that state of the atmosphere which generates other eruptive epidemics.

In 1634 the plague showed itself at Ratisbon. The summer in America was hotter than usual, and the following winter was very cold.

In 1635 the plague appeared in Leyden and 20,000 inhabitants perished. This year was distinguished for an eruption of Vesuvius, violent earthquakes, an inundation in Holstein which destroyed 600 people and 50,000 head of cattle, and a terrible tempest in America on the 15th of August O. S. which brot in a remarkable swell of the ocean. It will appear hereafter that most of the violent storms and hurricanes, which sweep the earth, happen during or near the time of the discharges of great quantities of fire from volcanoes. In this year, Etna and Vesuvius were both in a state of eruption. The plague appeared also in Mentz and other parts of Germany.

In 1636 there was an eruption of Heckla. The pestilence was general in proportion to this universal agitation of the central fires. In London it prevailed in 1636 after a regular increase of previous malignity in diseases.

Of the progress of the pestilence in Holland, and especially in Nimeguen, we have an accurate account in the treatise of the able Diemerbroeck, which is by far the most learned and philosophic work on the plague, that I have seen. Not that I believe his opinion of the cause of the plague; but his view of the subject is otherwise correct and worthy of universal attention.

In 1635 when the plague appeared in Leyden, the malignant diseases, its precursors, appeared in various parts of Holland. In Nimeguen, these precursors were measles, small pox, dysenteries of the worst type, but especially the spotted fever. The malignity of this fever increased, until it *changed into the real plague*—" donec in apertissimam pestem transiret," says Diemerbroeck.

The plague appeared, in a few cases, in November 1635, but made little progress, during the winter. In January appearances were more alarming; in March the malady spread rapidly and continued to increase till autumn. Scarcely a house escaped; more than half who were seized, died; and medical aid was baffled. The disease declined in the following winter, and was extinguished by a severe frost in February 1637.

The summers of 1636 and 7 were warm, the winds constantly from the south and west, " cum magnis aeris squaloribus," says Diemerbroeck.

In 1635 a dysentery prevailed in most parts of Germany. In 1636 the eruption from Etna was augmented, and Rome was severely afflicted with the plague. In 1637 the same distemper raged in some parts of Holland, in Denmark, Constantinople and Natolia; after which year the disease declined or disappeared.

This period of disease was also experienced in Virginia, where, says Winthrop, died 1800 people in the year 1635.

The summer of 1638 was very hot and dry in England, as it was in America, after a very severe winter, and cold spring.

In this year was a most tremendous earthquake in Calabria, memorable for the destruction of whole towns and the loss of 30,000 lives.

On the firſt of June, between 3 and 4 o'clock in the afternoon, in a clear warm day, with a weſterly wind, happened a great earthquake in America, which extended from the Piſcataqua to the Connecticut, and perhaps over the whole northern region. The year was alſo diſtinguiſhed for tempeſtuous weather; not for ordinary ſtorms which occur many times every year, but violent hurricanes of vaſt extent. On the third of Auguſt a tempeſt raiſed the tide, on the Narraganſett ſhore, fourteen feet above common ſpring tides. Autumn was very rainy and conſiderable ſnow fell in October, which our anceſtors aſcribed to the earthquake. On the 25th of September, another mighty tempeſt occurred and the higheſt ſwell of the ſea that had then been obſerved in America. If I miſtake not, the ſtate of the atmoſphere, during earthquakes and eruptions of volcanoes, is peculiarly diſpoſed, not only to produce high winds, but to generate ſnow and hail.

This year was very ſickly in America. In December a general faſt was obſerved, one reaſon for which was the prevalence of the " ſmall-pox and fevers."

Winthrop, p 165.

The ſpring of 1639 in America was very dry, there was no rain from April 26th, to June 4th, O. S. and from the ſouthward came ſwarms of ſmall flies, which covered the ſea, but they did not invade the land.

Winthrop, p 181—184.

The plague continued to infeſt London, without interruption, from 1636 to 1648 ; ſee the bills of mortality ; but it was not epidemic, nor very fatal.

In 1640 a hard winter, and epidemic pleuriſies were fatal in Europe. The following year, a malignant fever was epidemic, in England, and other countries.

In September 11th appeared, in the evening, a remarkable light in the heavens, about 30 or 40 feet in length ; it moved rapidly and was viſible about a minute. It was ſeen in Boſton, in Plymouth and in New-Haven, and to the ſpectators every

where, appeared to be in the same part of the heavens—of course must have been of a great altitude.
Winthrop, p. 232.

I notice this fact as it confirms the testimony of ancient writers, who, in describing the seasons and phenomena of pestilential periods, frequently mention similar appearances. This seems to have been of the figure of a beam, called by the Latin writers, *trabs*, but it differed from those meteors described by ancient writers, in the rapidity of its motion.

In November following a series of tempests took place, and the highest tide ever known at Boston.

This summer of 1641 was remarkably wet and cold, so that a great part of the corn did not come to maturity. Those who fed on it, the year following, were exceedingly troubled with worms, and some persons found a remedy in leaving bread and living on fish.
Winthrop, p. 234.

The following winter was the most severe that had been known for 40 years. The bay at Boston was frozen so that teams and loads passed to the town from the neighboring islands. The snow was deep, and Chesapeek bay was nearly frozen. At Boston, the ice extended to sea, as far as the eye could reach. The following spring 1642 was early, but wet.
Winthrop, p. 240, 243.

The oldest Indians declared they could scarcely recollect such a winter.

This severe winter was followed by a very sickly summer on the Delaware river. Such was the mortality among the settlers from New-Haven, who had not long been in that country, that it broke up their settlement. The Swedes settled there suffered much by the same disease.
Ibm. 254.

The very wet weather of the last year produced a dearth of corn in Boston, in the spring of 1643, and myriads of pigeons appeared also and did no small injury, the same season. It is an old observation, in America, that pigeons are uncommonly numerous in the spring of sickly years. The Massachusetts colony suffered also from the number of mice which devoured their grain, and the bark of the fruit-trees.

Several singular meteors were seen this year in the neighborhood of Bolton.*

One fact in the foregoing account deserves notice; the extreme winter in America was in 1641-2, one year later than in Europe. Several instances have occurred in other periods, which seem to indicate a kind of progressiveness in great cold from east to west. It often happens however that the winter is severe at the same time, in both hemispheres, as in 1607-8—1685-4—1762-3—1779-80.

In England, in 1643 a malignant fever was epidemic and few escaped. In autumn, it put on pestilential symptoms and petechiæ. The same year, an eruption of Vesuvius and of Etna.

In 1644 a malignant fever was epidemic in Denmark.

The summer of 1645 being excessively hot, there prevailed a contagious dysentery, which was fatal in England. For the great mortality in England, through a series of years at this time, see the London bills.

In this year a great sickness prevailed among the Indians on Martha's Vineyard—few escaped.

Neal's Hist. New-England, vol. 1 264.

In 1646 inundations laid a part of Holland, Friesland and Zealand under water so suddenly, as to destroy more than one hundred thousand lives and three hundred villages. Gorges relates that two mock suns, with other singular celestial phenomena, were seen this year in America.

P 41.

In 1647 May 13th, a most tremendous earthquake in Chili, South-America, sunk whole mountains into the earth and nearly ruined the large city of Santiago.

Ulloa, book 8 ch 7.

This year appeared a comet. The plague in London also was more severe, and appeared after this year to subside.

In 1646 and 7 the Ukrain was ravaged by locusts.

---

* Here ends Winthrop's Journal—a circumstance to be regretted. Hubbard's Manuscript will in part supply materials for this work, for some years subsequent But for the last 30 years of the last century, I can obtain very little information of the state of the seasons and health in America.

A. D. 1647. This year appeared an epidemic catarrh in *America*, and the first of which we have any account. It is not named either influenza or catarrh, but is clearly the same disease. It is thus described in Hubbard's Manuscript, p. 276. " In 1647 an epidemic sickness passed through the whole country, affecting the colonists and the natives, English, French and Dutch. It began with a cold and in many accompanied with a light fever. Such as bled or used cooling drinks died—such as made use of cordials and more strengthening things, recovered for the most part. It extended through the plantations in America, and in the West-Indies. There died in Barbadoes and St. Kitts, 5 or 6000 each. Whether it was a plague, or pestilential fever, in the islands, accompanied by great drouth, which cut short potatoes and fruits."

This epidemic was in the same year with the earthquake in Chili, but the date of the disease is not recorded.

In Connecticut prevailed a malignant fever, occasioned by the excessive heat of the summer.†

The year 1648 appears to have been less sickly, in London; but in the south of Europe, malignant diseases were the harbingers of the plague, which in 1649 carried off 200,000 people in the southern provinces of Spain. In Ireland and Shropshire the plague prevailed in the same year, and a fatal fever in France. The small-pox was epidemic in Boston.

Townsend's Travels, vol. 2. 219. Short, vol. 1.
Douglas' Summary, vol. 2. 395.

In 1650 was an eruption of Etna, and an earthquake in the north and west of England. In this and the following year the plague continued in Ireland.

In 1650 the influenza spread over Europe. In 1651 many desolating floods happened in Holland and France—in Italy, a quinsy or sore throat proved very fatal to children. These diseases were succeded by malignant fevers, and plague in most parts of Europe, except in England. The summer of 1651 was hot.

In 1652 appeared a comet. A dangerous synochus prevailed in France and a tertian fever in Denmark.

† Of this fever died the Rev. Thomas Hooker, and many others in Hartford. See Neal's Hist. N. E. vol. 1. 289. Magnalia, b. 3. 67.

In 1653 a flight earthquake occurred in New-England, in Oct.

The years 1652 and 3 were remarkably dry in England, and in 1654 public thanks were ordered for a supply of rain.

Mercurius Politicus.

In 1654 the plague made its appearance in Denmark. Some severe epidemic had prevailed in New-England; for in the spring of 1654 a general faft was appointed by the government of Connecticut, one reason affigned for which was, " the mortality which had been among the people of Maffachufetts." What the difeafe was, I am not informed.

Trum. Hift. Con 225.

In 1655 occurred the second epidemic catarrh, recorded in the Annals of America. The following is the account of it in Hubbard's Manufcript, p 285.

" In 1655 there was another faint cough that paffed through the whole country of New-England, occafioned by fome ftrange diftemper or infection of the air. It was fo epidemical, that few perfons efcaped. It began about the end of June. Few were able to vifit their friends or perform the laft teftimony of refpect to any of their relations at a diftance. Of this died Mr. Nathaniel Rogers, minifter of Ipfwich."

See alfo Magnalia, b 3 108.

It will be obferved that this epidemic commenced in the heat of fummer, and that its invafion was fudden and univerfal. In November 1655 occurred an earthquake in South-America.

Of the feafons in America I have no account; but in Europe the winter of 1654-5 was extremely fevere. The rivers and harbors in Holland were all made faft with ice, a feries of fnow ftorms took place in April, and as late as the 19th there was a fevere froft at Bruffels.

See Mercurius Politicus, a London paper for 1655.

In March 1655 was an eruption of Vefuvius; it was very fickly in the north of England; and there were great tempefts of wind and hail in 1654 and 5.

In 1654 the plague appeared at Chefter in England, but did not become epidemic; owing, it was fuppofed, to the precaution of confining the difeafed to their houfes.* At the fame time

* This may poffibly have been the cafe, but it is probable the opinion is not well founded See this point confidered in the 16th fection.

the difeafe was raging in Turkey, in Prefburg, Hungary and in the city of Mofcow, it is alledged, perifhed 200,000 inhabitants. We have here precife and authentic evidence, that the plague appeared in Chefter, in the north-weft of England, in Denmark, in Ruffia, Hungary and Turkey, in the *fame feafon*. To prove this to be the effect of a general principle, we have numberlefs authorities, in the Gazettes of that and the next year, that malignant difeafes prevailed over Europe. See the paper above cited. Thus when a few cafes of plague occurred in Chefter, fatal difeafes prevailed over the north of England. And it is remarkable in this inftance, that the epidemic plague appeared *in the north of Europe before it did in Italy*—an exception to the general courfe of that difeafe.

In 1655 the plague was more general in Europe. It prevailed in Sardinia, Malta, Leyden, Amfterdam, and in Riga, a Ruffian port at the mouth of the Divina. There died in Riga 9000—Amfterdam 13,200—Leyden 13,000.

In 1656 the fame difeafe invaded Naples, Rome, Genoa, Candia, Benevento, and moft parts of the Neapolitan territories. In the city of Naples, perifhed three fourths of the inhabitants, and in Benevento, a greater proportion. The numbers of deaths were eftimated as follows—

In the city of Naples died 240,000—furvived 50,000.

In the Neapolitan territories 400,000.

In Benevento died 9000—furvived 500.

In Rome about 10,000.

In Genoa in 1656, 10,000, and in 1657, 70,000, and 14,000 only furvived.

In Riga 9000.

In Thorn 8200.

I have not materials for a complete view of the difeafes of this peftilential period. But it is to be obferved, that influenza prevailed over Europe in 1650, and difeafes of the throat in Italy in 1651—difeafes which feem to precede peftilential fevers on moft occafions.

The fummer of 1656 was hot, and an earthquake in the fouth of Italy accompanied the dreadful mortality.

See Univ. Hift. vol. 28. 318. Mercurius Politicus, 1656. Encyclopedia, art. Plague.

The influenza in America was also succeeded by fatal epidemic diseases, altho I have no means of determining what they were. The account recorded is that there " was a great sickness and mortality, throughout New-England in 1658. The season was intemperate and the crops light." Trumbull, p. 244. This year was also distinguished for what is called in our annals, the " Great Earthquake." This is an instance of a violent concussion of the earth, in the same year with violent rains; but unfortunately I can find no account which phenomenon preceded the other. The summer was so rainy, that the christianized Indians observed days of fasting, on that account, apprehending that their crops would fail and the world be drowned.

Neal, vol. 1. 259.

The introduction of the plague into Naples was ascribed to a transport of soldiers from Sardinia. How the disease came to be in Sardinia, we are not informed. But this report, like nine tenths of all the stories about infection, is demonstrably a mistake. The account given in the history of the disease, is, that it was at first called by physicians a " malignant fever." One of the faculty, a man probably of more observation and firmness than the others, affirmed the distemper to be pestilential, and for his audacity, was imprisoned by the Viceroy, who apprehended the report might injure the business and reputation of the city.

We have then another instance of the uncertainty in the minds of medical gentlemen, about the nature of the disease, when it first appeared, because it was not characterized by the distinctive marks of the plague, the glandular tumors. This circumstance demonstrates that the disease was *not* imported, but an epidemic; appearing first, as *all great* plagues first appear, in the form of catarrh, inflammatory fevers, affections of the throat, and typhus fevers.

There cannot be a more clear and demonstrable truth, than that a disease of specific contagion, must communicate a disease of the same specific character. If the plague has this species of contagion, it cannot communicate another disease, a malignant fever, for instance, which has a different character or type, and is deſtitute of the diſtinctive marks of the plague. A ſingle inſtance might occur, in which the diſeaſe might not bear the character of its original; but it is abſurd to ſuppoſe, that a plague *with* glandular tumors, can communicate and render epidemic a fever *without* glandular tumors.

Yet all ſevere plagues firſt appear in the form of ſuch fever, or other diſeaſes *without tumors*. I challenge the followers of Mead to produce an exception. Hence the uncertainty that perplexes the phyſician and the magiſtrate at the commencement of the plague—an uncertainty that has originated in the errors reſpecting the ſpecific nature of the diſeaſe and its propagation by infection—errors as fatal to great cities, as to truth and philoſophy.

Had the real origin of this diſeaſe been known, the certainty of the exiſtence of it in Naples, Venice, Rome, Vienna, Amſterdam and London, would have induced the citizens to abandon the places, before the diſtemper had made much progreſs, and multitudes of lives would have been ſaved—an expedient practiſed in America, with the moſt ſalutary effects.

In Genoa, the diſeaſe manifeſted a more diſtinct progreſſion; 10,000 died the firſt year, and about 70,000 the ſecond.

When this diſtemper appeared in Malta, Candia and Sardinia, every poſſible precaution was taken to prevent its introduction into Genoa, by ſtopping intercourſe with thoſe places; but in vain.

When the report of a malignant infectious fever in Naples prevailed in May 1656, an alarm was excited in Rome; a committee of health watched over the ſafety of that city; four of the gates were ſhut and barred; the others were guarded with vigilance to prevent any perſon from entering who could be ſuſpected of infection; but all efforts were uſeleſs. The real truth was the diſeaſe was an epidemic, no more under the control of health laws, than the influenza and ſore throat which had preceded it.

The ſummer of 1657 in England was very hot, and ſucceeded by a long ſevere winter and deep ſnow.

In April 1658 commenced in Europe an epidemic catarrh, which was ſo ſudden in its attack as to ſeize a whole village in a night. It was fevere and fatal to old people—its courſe was finiſhed in about ſix weeks. The ſummer was hot and fevers with vertigo and delirium, were epidemic.

See Short, vol. 1. and Morton's Treatiſe.

It will be remarked that the year 1647 when the influenza invaded America, was a ſickly year in Europe. In 1655 when the plague was epidemic in Europe, the influenza again prevailed in America. In 1658 when the influenza invaded Europe, great ſickneſs and mortality occurred in America. Theſe alternations of epidemic diſeaſes will be obſerved in the ſubſequent ſtages of this hiſtory.

In 1659 prevailed the Cynanche Trachealis in America—the firſt inſtance mentioned in our annals. Magnalia, b. 4. 156.— This diſeaſe was alſo ſucceeded by malignant diſeaſes, for the Legiſlature of Connecticut in October 1662 appointed a day of thankſgiving, two reaſons aſſigned for which were, the " abatement of the ſickneſs in the country, and a ſupply of rain in time of drouth."

This was the commencement of a very ſickly period in Europe. In 1660 occurred an eruption of Veſuvius, and of a volcano in Iceland. The year was very tempeſtuous, and earthquakes ſhook England, France and America. In 1661 appeared a comet.

In 1662 another conſiderable earthquake happened in New-England ; and in this year was the drouth above mentioned.— In 1663 Canada was convulſed for five months by a ſeries of ſucceſſive ſhocks—ſmall rivers and ſprings were dried up—the waters of others were tinctured with the taſte of ſulphur—an immenſe ridge of mountains ſubſided to a plain. Such were the phenomena in America which marked this peſtilential period.

Mem. Royal Society, vol. 6 86. Neal's Hiſt. N England.
Mem. Amer Acad vol 1 263

In 1663 a malignant diſeaſe ſeized the inhabitants of the Venetian territories and 60,000 periſhed. The country, at the ſame time, was overrun by innumerable ſmall worms.

In the ſame year, a memorable mortality occurred in England, among the cattle and ſheep, by means of a diſeaſe in which the

A a

liver was eaten by small worms, and in some cases, the lungs. These phenomena were the precursors of the plague in many parts of Europe. In England, all diseases assumed new violence, as early as in 1661, preparatory to the great plague. See Sydenham. In Holland, the plague appeared at Heusden, in 1663.

The winter of 1663-4 was mild. In the following summer, Prussia was afflicted by a malignant purple fever, attended with tumors or inflammation in the throat, very fatal to the young. Bonnetus. Med. Septen. p. 206. A species of scarlatina.

In 1664 appeared a comet; another in 1665, and a third in 1666. In 1664 began an eruption of Etna, which lasted, with various degrees of violence, till the year 1669, when it ended with a most dreadful explosion. This period corresponds with the epidemics described by Sydenham.

In 1664 the summer in England was wet, and cattle died of diseases. In New-England commenced the mildew of wheat, which has rendered it impossible to cultivate that grain, on the Atlantic coast of the three Eastern States. The winter of 1664-5, was terribly severe in England; the Thames was a bridge of ice, and in January happened earthquakes, in Coventry and Buckinghamshire. During this winter inflammatory fevers and quinsies, says Sydenham, were more frequent in London, than were before known. These gave way in May to a malignant fever, which could hardly be distinguished from the plague, which, in June, became the controling epidemic.

Such were the phenomena of the pestilential period under consideration; and at this time, the plague appeared in Holland, and in England. English authors all agree that the disease was imported into England from Holland in some bales of cotton! O fatal bales of cotton! says Short. This tale has been recorded and repeated by every writer on the subject, without a single document in evidence to prove that any cotton was imported, or that the first persons seized had ever seen such cotton. The whole tale rests on assertion. That the seeds of the distemper were *not* imported is evident from the acknowledged facts relative to its origin; and is demonstrated by the history of the preceding diseases found in the works of Sydenham.

The origin of the pestilence, which arrived to its crisis in 1665, is to be traced back to the year 1661, when malignant diseases began to appear in different and distant parts of the world. In London, the intermitting tertian fever, says Sydenham, became epidemic, and differed from the same disease in other years, by new and unusual symptoms, which in short, amounted to this, that they were "*all more violent.*" In winter, the disease yielded, as usual, to cold, but continued fevers prevailed every winter. These fevers, with some variations, continued until the spring of 1665, and the bills show how much they augmented the mortality in London. This increased malignity in usual diseases, with an increase of the number and mortality of epidemics, is the constant precursor of the plague or other pestilential fevers.

Notwithstanding the clear evidence of these facts, authors have conjured up a tale of importation which would disgrace a schoolboy by its inconsistency.[*] The account states, "That a violent plague had raged in Holland in 1663, on which account, the importation of merchandize from that country was prohibited by the British Legislature in 1664. Notwithstanding this prohibition, *it seems the plague had actually been imported;* for in the close of 1664, two or three persons died suddenly in Westminster, *with marks of the plague on their bodies.*—Some of their neighbors, terrified at the thoughts of their danger, removed into the city; but too late; for they soon died of the plague, and communicated the infection to others. It was confined however through a hard, frosty winter, till the middle of February, when it again appeared in the Parish of St. Giles, to which it had been originally brought; and after another long rest, till April, showed its malignant force afresh, as soon as the warmth of spring gave it opportunity. *At first, it took off one here and there, without any certain proof of their having infected each other.*

Encyclopedia, art London 21

In the substance of the foregoing statement, all authors are agreed, and I want no other proof that the report of the importation of the disease is all a vulgar, childish tale, the propagation

---

[*] If this language should be thought too severe, I can sincerely say, that in my opinion, no language can be too severe for the carelessness which has originated a system of error on this important subject.

of which is a disgrace to philosophy and to the faculty of that age.

In the first place we have no authentic evidence in any author, that any bales of cotton were brought from Holland to London, at that time. The whole assertion rests on vulgar report, and is wholly unsupported by proof—had the report been well founded, the fact might have been ascertained, and in an affair of such magnitude, probably would have been. The importation of goods from Holland was prohibited by act of parliament.

In the second place, the disease first appeared in Westminster, not in the commercial city of London, but in a place where bales of cotton would be the least likely to be deposited and opened; Westminster being the residence of the nobility and gentry, rather than a place of commerce.

In the third place, no proof is stated that the persons first seized had any connection with bales of cotton.

In the fourth place, the death of two or three persons, with the plague-marks on their bodies, in December 1664, is no evidence of any imported infection at that time; for the bills of mortality show, and the reader is desired to turn to them, to be satisfied, that a smaller number died that year of the plague, than had died of it in any of the six preceding years. In the year 1659 died of that disease 36—in 1661 died 20, and every year more or less. In 1664 died but 6 of the plague, and yet this number, small as it was, must be proof of the importation of infection, *that year*, when *greater numbers*, in preceding years, are passed over in silence ! In such accounts, there must be want of knowledge, or want of honesty. The plague imported from Holland ! when the city of London had not been free from it, for 28 years preceding ! See the bills of mortality !—

Besides, why in the name of common sense, should " two or three," infected persons in 1664, spread the plague over London, and desolate the city, when twelve, fourteen, twenty and thirty-six infected persons, who died in preceding years, produced no ill effects ? To account for such effects on the principle of *infection*, is not possible ; and men of science ought to be ashamed of such absurdities.

In the fifth place, the suspension of the disease, during six weeks, is evidence, that infection had no agency in spreading the disease. It is a fact known and acknowledged, that *infection* cannot be preserved, for a tenth part of that time in the open air. Air dissolves the poison of any disease, in a very short time. Infection can only be preserved in confinement, as in close vessels or packages of goods. The walls of an infected house will be cleansed by the action of air, in a very few days, so as to be perfectly harmless. During the six weeks suspension of the plague in London, where was the infection concealed to preserve it from air and frost?

Was the fomes shut up by design for a few weeks and then set at liberty? Had the persons who were first seized in February, any access to the infected houses or clothes of those who died in December? Is this probable? There is no suggestion of this sort.

Then again another interval of several weeks elapsed from the death of those in February, before others were seized. It is not solely improbable; but I aver, that the fomes or infecting principle of no disease whatever, can be suspended in a state of inaction, in the open air, and afterwards give rise to disease. Unless therefore it can be proved that the persons who died in April had access to infection, which had been closely confined from the air, they could never have received the disease from the virus generated in February or December. Now it appears from the statement, that the persons, seized in February, lived in a different part of the city, from those who died in December, and no suggestion that they had an intercourse with any infected object.

But the last sentence of the statement disproves fully all assertions and suspicions respecting infection. It seems that when the disease showed itself in spring, it seized one here, and another there, in scattered situations, " without any certain proof of their having infected each other." This is usually the case in the plague, and in the yellow fever, in the ulcerous sore throat, the dysentery and other contagious, epidemic diseases. The whole mystery is, that any disease will *first* seize the constitutions least capable of refisting that state of air, from which the disease proceeds. One person will sustain a vitiated air, for one day only; another for two days, and a third for a week, before his constitution yields to the destructive principle. It is precisely with the access of the plague, in a city, as with a company of men going from a healthy situation, into a marshy place—one man will be seized very speedily with the ague and fever; another will sustain his health for a week or two, and some perhaps escape unaffected. This example explains the phenomena which attend the invasion of pestilence, as related by Evagrius, Diemerbroeck and others, and which will be more fully discussed in a subsequent section.

The account therefore of the origin of the plague in London in 1665, not only does not prove the disease to have proceeded from imported fomes, but actually demonstrates the impossibility of the fact.

But we have better evidence than the popular accounts afford us, that the disease was generated in the city of London. Sydenham has left facts on record, which place this point beyond controversy.

After describing the multiplied diseases of increased malignity, which prevailed in London, from 1661 to 1665, and which swelled greatly the bills of mortality in that city, he informs us that in May 1665 he was called to assist a woman of a sanguine habit, who was seized with violent fever and frequent vomitings. He was surprised at the singularity of the symptoms, and puzzled to know how to treat the disease. The woman died the 14th day. He observed her face, during the fever, to be red, and that a little before her death, a few drops of blood issued from her nose. These and other circumstances suggested to him the use of bleeding, and his next patient recovered.

This species of malignant fever soon spread and towards the close of May and beginning of June, became epidemic. Soon after appeared the true plague with its characteristic symptoms. After stating these facts, Sydenham says, " Whether the fever under consideration deserves to be entitled a plague, I dare not positively affirm; but this I know by experience, that all who were then seized with the true plague, attended with all its peculiar concomitants, and for some time afterwards, in my neighborhood, had the same train of symptoms, both in the beginning and through the course of the disease."

He then observes that he attended some persons with the true plague, and afterwards, he saw several cases of a similar fever.

See chap. 2. sect 2.

Had not the faculty been blinded to truth by their theory of *specific contagion*, it would not have been possible so long to overlook the *progressiveness* of the plague, which not only Sydenham, but many physicians of the 16th and 17th centuries observed and recorded.

The malignant diseases which prevailed from 1661 to 1664 marked a *pestilential state of air* in London. We now know what Sydenham could not know, that this unhealthy state of air extended not only over Europe, but over Persia and America. But the malignant fever which appeared in May, as described by Sydenham, was the *first stage of the plague*, or mild form of the disease, which *always* precedes that state of it which is characterized by buboes. This form of the disease appears before the season or state of the atmosphere is advanced sufficiently to give the destructive principle its full force.

The same species of fever preceded the terrible plague in Venice and in Naples, as before related; and this is always the cause of uncertainty and controversy respecting the nature of the disease, at its commencement. And it is remarkable that this milder form of the plague, often rages for many months, before the disease arrives to its crisis. Thus in London, the pestilential principle produced a few cases of real plague, in the winter of 1664-5. The cases must have occurred in constitutions more irritable, or susceptible of the cause, than bodies in general; or the persons must have been exposed to the action of powerful local causes, or to extreme debility. The severe frost doubtless suspended the operation of the pestilential principle—but on the opening of spring, the operation began, and proceeded from the malignant epidemic of May to produce the most deadly effects.

I have one obfervation further to make on this fubject. It has been alledged and generally admitted that the plague was introduced into Amfterdam, in 1663 by a veffel from the Mediterranean. It is probable that if this queftion could be fully canvaffed, the popular belief would appear to have had no better foundation, than many opinions in America, in regard to the importation of the yellow fever, which are proved to reft merely on conjectures, fuppofitions, and vague reports. But in regard to the origin of the peftilence in Holland, in this inftance, it is wholly immaterial, whether popular opinion was well founded or not; for we have the exprefs authority of Diemerbroeck, that anterior to the arrival of the fhip, with the fuppofed infection, the plague broke out in Heufden, a town on a branch of the Meufe, furrounded by a morafs, not a maritime place. Befides the fpotted fever, which precedes the plague and turns into it, had been prevailing in all parts of Holland in the preceding year. The peftilence therefore originated in Holland, *before the infection arrived;* and the tales of importation vanifh in fmoke.

According to the bills of mortality, London loft upwards of 68,000 inhabitants by the plague in 1665, and more than 28,000 by other difeafes. As the 28,000 deaths by common difeafes muft have occurred moftly in the fix firft months of the year, before the plague raged, this circumftance fhows what a great increafe of mortality preceded the plague. With fuch evidence before their eyes, how can difcerning men look abroad for the fources of the malady!

It fhould alfo be remarked that this calamity among the human race was preceded by a great mortality among cattle in 1664.

It muft not pafs unobferved that the fummer of 1665 in England was very temperate, the weather fine and the fruits good. All the writers of that day agree, that no caufe of peftilence could be obferved in the vifible qualities of the feafon.

This was the laft plague that has appeared in London, or in Great Britain. The difappearance of the plague in that and other countries, is a moft confoling fact, and one that has not a little engaged the minds of philofophic men, to difcover the cause. The causes usually assigned are, the destruction of the city by fire in 1666, the more airy, convenient construction of the modern city, the introduction of fresh water, with more cleanliness, and improved habits of living.

These reasons would have more weight in my mind, if the other large cities in England, in France, Spain, Holland and Germany, which have neither been burnt nor improved in their general structure, had not also escaped the ravages of pestilence. But as the plague has not visited Paris and Amsterdam, which retain their ancient construction, no more than London, which has been improved, we must resort to other circumstances for the causes of this exemption. The consideration of this subject will fall under another part of this work.

In 1666, appeared a comet, the summer was very hot, and a tremendous hurricane, tore up a thousand trees in Nottingham forest, and of 50 houses in one village, seven only were left standing. In this tempest fell hail-stones, as large as hens eggs. An earthquake occurred in Oxfordshire. Persia did not escape the effects of this pestilential constitution. In 1667 prevailed famin and epidemic diseases, and an earthquake demolished great part of Teflis, the capital of Georgia, and four villages, with the loss of 30,000 lives; and another city with the loss of 2,000 lives.

Chardin's travels, 86 126

In 1666 dysentery prevailed over England and many parts of Europe and in St. Domingo. This disease seems to be the successor of the plague, and other epidemics. During the inflammatory stage of an epidemic constitution, evidenced by measles, influenza, a mild small-pox, we rarely hear of destructive dysentery. But after those diseases have run their course, dysentery appears in many parts of a country, and sometimes becomes almost universal. It would be a curious question, by what means the inflammatory diathesis, so to speak, of the epidemic period, acts upon the nerves, muscles and intestines, to give to the subsequent autumnal fevers this particular direction.

During the foregoing series of epidemics in Europe, America did not escape. Slight shocks of earthquake were felt in 1660, and in 1665. Great sickness prevailed at this period also, but I am not informed of the species of disorder, except the small-pox in Boston in 1666.

In 1668, appeared a comet with a stupendous coma. This was attended by an excessively hot summer, and malignant diseases in America. In New York the epidemic was so fatal, that a fast was appointed in September, on that account. This was undoubtedly the autumnal bilious fever in its infectious form. In this same year was an earthquake in America, and a meteor in the west, in form of a spear, pointing towards the setting sun, which gradually sunk and disappeared.

Neal's Hist. vol. 1. 567. Magnal b. 4 184

This year was marked also by violent earthquakes in Europe and Asia. The winter of 1668-9 was very severe, and ice was seen in the Bosphorus; that of 1670 covered the Danube with a bridge of ice.

In winter appeared in Hungary two mock-suns of resplendent brightness—the infallible forerunner of great discharges of electrical fire, or of violent tempests.—On the 11th of March 1669, the eruption of Etna which had commenced in 1664 redoubled its fury, and by immense discharges of lava laid waste the country below. Its violence subsided in July; but tremendous hurricanes marked the year. The summer of this year also was excessively hot.

In this year, the cats in Westphalia died with an eruption on the head, accompanied with drowsiness. In England prevailed a dangerous fever, with slimy tongue and sore mouth.

In Norway prevailed measles of a malignant kind, attacking old and young. Donetus, Med. Sept. 223.—In the two following years measles was epidemic in London alternating with the small-pox—See Sydenham—In 1673 winter was cold; and catarrhs were frequent with spotted fevers—A comet appeared in the preceding year.

In 1675 a wet and cool summer, the influenza prevailed in Europe with the usual symptoms. In Italy was seen a meteor or fire ball, from the north-east; and the following winter in America was colder than usual.

The summer of 1676 in England was cold. Measles and small-pox prevailed in some places.

In 1677 was seen a comet in April and May; an earthquake was experienced in England; and in Charlestown, Massachusetts, raged the small-pox with the mortality of a plague.

Mag. b. 4. 139.

The summer of 1678 was very hot and dry. There was a comet and an earthquake in Lima. Fevers and affections of the throat were epidemic in the north of Europe. The plague raged with most desolating fury in Algiers and Morocco. Authors relate that four millions of people perished, and that the waste of population has not since been repaired.

Chenier= Morocco, vol 2. 180.

On the 12th of January occurred in England a most extraordinary darkness, at noon.

Notwithstanding the barrenness of my materials, this pestilential period may be very clearly distinguished, by the measles from 1669 to 1672 with the small pox, the catarrh of 1675, the subsequent malignant fevers and affections of the throat, and finally the pestilence of 1678.

The same deleterious principle extended to America. Our annals relate that the seasons were unfavorable and the fruits blasted, while malignant diseases prevailed among the people. The sickness and bad seasons were attributed, by our pious ancestors, to the irreligion of the times, and to their disuse of fasting. On this occasion, a synod was convened to investigate the causes of God's judgments, and to propose a plan of reformation. The small-pox prevailed at Boston in 1678, and a singular epidemic in England, France and Holland.

See Neal's Hist. N. Eng vol 2. 32. Mag. b. 5. 85. Hutch vol 1. 324. Doug vol 1. 440. Short, vol 1.

The comet of 1678 was followed by a very cold winter, after a rainy autumn, with an epidemic cough. A comet is mentioned in 1679, and the plague was in Vienna.

The year 1680 was distinguished also for a severe winter, and the noted comet that had appeared in Justinian's reign. In Dresden raged the plague. The summer was hot and sickly.

A large meteor was seen in Germany, descending to the north and leaving behind it a long luminous stream.

The summer of 1681 was excessively dry. This was the forerunner of violent earthquakes, which, in 1682 shook all Germany, Italy and Switzerland. In some places, the shocks were preceded, for four nights, by lights or flame, like ignes fatui, on the mountains. The convulsions were attended with a disagreeable sulphurous smell. In this year also was visible a comet, and an eruption took place, both of Etna and Vesuvius.

In this year 1682 a mortal disease spread among the cattle in Italy, Switzerland and Germany, that was called the angina maligna, and of which cattle died in 24 hours. Authors relate that a blue mist appeared on the herbage of pastures. The disease moved about two German miles in 24 hours, and spread over Germany and Poland. Cattle at rack and manger were affected equally with those that grazed.

At Halle in Saxony prevailed the plague, and at Dublin, a petechial in which the brain was severely affected, and bleeding pernicious.

The discharges of fire already mentioned were productive, as usual, of violent winds. In Sicily, a tempest, preceded by great darkness, almost laid waste the island.

In 1683 was an earthquake in England, in September, preceded by meteors or lights and fetid exhalations. A comet appeared in this year, and another in the following.

The winter of 1683-4 was the coldest that could be recollected by the oldest men living. Trees of large size split with the frost. The same winter was excessively severe in America, and from a passage in a letter of the Rev. John Eliot, the season appears to have been sickly

Hist. Col vol 3.

The year 1683 was also remarkable for general sickness in Connecticut, and in some places, unusual mortality. Some towns suffered by excessive rains.

Trumbull's Hist. p 383

These unusual seasons were accompanied with singular diseases. In Leyden in 1683 prevailed what was called the hungry fever, which came on with a chill, succeeded by ravenous hunger

To gratify this appetite was fatal. When the hot fit came on, the hunger subsided. In 1684 was a terrible earthquake in St. Domingo.

Description of St Domingo, vol. 1. 142.

After the severe frost in 1684, a malignant dysentery raged over Europe. This and the two succeeding summers were hot and dry. In 1685 Languedoc in France was overrun by grasshoppers, and the petechial fever was prevalent.

In September 1686 was seen a comet. At Lille in France, fell a storm of hail, the stones of which were of a pound weight. There was an eruption of Etna, in this year also, and a meteor was seen at Leipsick on the 9th of July, which was stationary for 7 minutes, at the height of 30 miles. It is curious to remark the coincidence in time between the phenomena of the electrical fluid, tempests, snow and hail.

The summer of 1687 in Europe was very rainy. In October the city of Lima in Peru, was demolished by an earthquake.

The winter of 1688 was cold, and in the summer following epidemic catarrh spread over Europe. This was preceded by a disease of the same species among horses, attended with a defluxion of rheum from their noses. Swarms of insects in some countries announced a pestilential period. In the interior of Germany were some dysenteries. An earthquake was experienced at Naples, and Smyrna was laid in ruins.

In 1689 appeared a comet, and both Etna and Vesuvius discharged fire. The autumn was very rainy, and the spotted fever prevailed in some parts of Germany. In Boston the smallpox was epidemic.

In 1690 the summer was rainy, frogs were in unusual numbers in Italy, and corn was cut short by mildew. Rainy seasons generally succeed great eruptions of volcanoes and earthquakes.

The year 1691 commenced with severe frost, followed by a hot dry summer. The spotted fever prevailed in Italy, in which bleeding was fatal. There was also great mortality among cattle and sheep.

The seasons in this year were peculiarly unfavorable in America, altho I am not able to describe them. It appears from the journals of the assembly of New-York, that upon an address of the house to the governor and council, a monthly fast was appointed to be observed from September 1691 to June 1692; the special reasons assigned for which were, "a burthensome war, and a blast upon the corn." This is a remarkable fact, and not unfrequent, that at one and the same time, the powers of vegetation fail in the most distant parts of the earth. Perhaps we shall be able to account for this instance of a deranged state of the elements by the universal explosions of fire in the two following years. St. Domingo experienced a severe earthquake in 1691, in the year of this blast on the corn.

Description of St. Domingo, by Moreau St. Mery, vol. 1. 142.

On the 7th of June 1692 after a series of dry, hot, calm weather, a most dreadful earthquake suddenly sunk the town of Port-Royal in Jamaica, and demolished most of the buildings on the island, with the loss of 2000 lives. After the earthquake, the heat was still more intense, musquetoes were innumerable, and a malignant fever fell upon the inhabitants in all parts of the island, with which 3000 perished.

In the same year, a similar disease invaded Barbadoes, and afflicted the island for many years. Indeed the whole world was sickly.

On the 8th of September England, Holland, France and Germany were convulsed by an earthquake, and Switzerland felt a shock in October. In the same year was an eruption of Etna, and great snows followed.

The spotted fever continued its ravages; and it was remarked to be much more malignant and fatal in the wane of the moon. During an eclipse in 1693 the sick almost all died. The disease was more fatal in town than country.

I have no account of the diseases in Egypt or the Levant, during this period; but it will be found on examination that great pestilence raged in those places, about this time, or between 1689 and 1693.

On the 10th of January 1693 happened a most terrible earthquake in Sicily and Naples. On the preceding evening, was observed a great flame or light, apparently at the distance of an Italian mile, and so bright as to be mistaken for a fire. The spectators attempted to approach it; but it appeared still at the fame diftance. As foon as the earth began to fhake, the flame difappeared

It is not within my limits to enumerate the miferies occafioned by this concuffion of the earth. Suffice it fay that many towns were laid in ruins and 60,000 people perifhed. During the convulfion a fountain difcharged its waters as red as blood. This calamity was preceded by a ferene fky, and followed by darknefs or vapor of a reddifh or yellow hue.

The effects of this earthquake were remarkable on the human body. Among thefe were malignant fevers, fmall-pox fatal among children; madnefs, dullnefs, fottifhnefs and melancholy, with deliria and lethargy. Are not thefe effects produced by an excefs of ftimulus, occafioned by the fuperabundance of electricity?

The fummer following this convulfion of the earth, was intemperately wet and cool, and corn was mildewed. Another account fays the fummer in Italy was very hot and dry. The fpotted fever, and in fome places dyfentery were very mortal. Wounds degenerated into ulcers, and blifters were followed by mortification which proved fatal to many.

In this year alfo Etna in Sicily, and Heckla in Iceland difcharged fire and lava, a new volcano was opened in Afia, and an ifland, called Sorea, near the Moluccas, was ruined by its volcano.

Moft dreadful ftorms marked the fame year; one in America, on the 19th of October, was memorable for its violence.

An epidemic catarrh began in Europe in October, being preceded by a fimilar difeafe among horfes.

The preceding winter was probably very mild in America; for on the 13th of February, Gov. Fletcher, with a body of troops, failed from New-York for Albany.

Smith's Hift. New-York, 82.

In 1693 the feamen and foldiers, under Sir Francis Wheeler, who was fent to conquer Martinico, were feized with the plague of America, and three fourths of them perifhed. Hutchinfon, vol. 2. 72, relates that this fleet came to Bofton and introduced the difeafe into that town, where it occafioned a deplorable mortality. Douglas relates the fame fact.

This account seems to be contradicted by Mather, in his Magnalia, b. 1. 22. In a sermon delivered on lecture day, April 7, 1698, it is asserted in so many words, that "An English squadron hath *not* brought among us the tremendous pestilence, under which a *neighboring plantation* hath undergone prodigious desolations. Boston, 'tis a marvellous thing a plague has *not* laid thee desolate."

By comparing the date of this sermon, with other events related in it, I find there is no mistake in the date; and as the author lived in Boston, and was cotemporary with those events, and personally acquainted with Sir Francis Wheeler, I conclude it was not Boston, but some other sea port town, which suffered by the arrival of a fleet.

In the 2d book of Magnalia, p. 71, the same author mentions this expedition and the terrible mortality. He says the distemper was "the most like the plague, of any thing that had ever been seen in America, whereof there died *before the fleet could reach to Boston*, as I was told by Sir Francis himself, 1300 sailors out of 2100, and 1800 soldiers out of 2400."

In book 7. 116, the same author says, "there was an English fleet of our good friends with a direful plague aboard *intending hither*. Had they come, as they intended, what an horrible desolation had cut us off, let the desolate places, *that some of you have seen in the colonies of the south*, declare unto us. *And that they did not come was the signal hand of heaven.*" This passage is in a lecture preached on the 27th of September, 1698.

From this authentic history, written by a cotemporary clergyman, we infer that Hutchinson must have made a mistake. Sir Francis Wheeler's fleet arrived at Boston, most dreadfully infected, but no disease was propagated in Boston. Some other fleet, it seems, had introduced the disease into a "colony of the south," perhaps Newport or New-York, but I have no information on the subject.

The great discharges of fire and earthquakes of 1693, were followed, as usual, by an intensely cold winter. The succeeding summer of 1694 was hot and excessively dry in Italy, till October, when the earth was deluged with rain.

In May was a violent earthquake and volcano in Banda, an island in the Indian seas. Fire issued from the neighboring seas, the air was impregnated with the smell of sulphur, and sickness prevailed. An eruption of Vesuvius happened the same year, and violent earthquakes in Sicily and Calabria. In this year the agitations of fire seem to have subsided; and as usual, a series of rainy cool summers succeeded, in which corn perished or was blasted, crops failed, and universal dearth ensued.

One of the most remarkable effects of the late agitations of the elements, was the frequency of apoplexies in Italy. So common were they in 1695, as to be called epidemic, and occasion general consternation. This is not an infrequent consequence of the high excitement that takes place in pestilential times, ending in extreme debility in the brain. Something of this kind has been observed in America, within the last few years.

I have very few facts in regard to the seasons and diseases in America, during this period, from 1689 to 1695. It appears however that the disorders of the elements were experienced in America.

In 1695 prevailed a mortal sickness among the Indians in the eastern parts of this continent.

Hutch vol 2. 87.

A contagious fever prevailed in Bermuda, the same year.

In Europe many malignant fevers prevailed, but no epidemics, except measles and chin cough of a bad type. In Ireland appeared offensive fogs, a thick clammy dew on the herbage, of a yellow color, and consistence of butter. A similar substance was observed at Middletown, Connecticut, on the morning after the earthquake, May 17, 1791.

The year 1696 was cool and wet—summer in Britain, resembled winter, and winter was like summer. Corn was mildewed. Dysentery fatal among children.

In America the winter of 1696-7, according to Hutchinson, was very severe. Loaded sleds passed from Boston to Nantasket. Food was scarce and losses at sea very great. I am not without suspicions however, that the author has here described the following winter, which was as severe as he has represented it.

In 1697 the weather in Europe was moftly cool. An earthquake at Lima in Peru fhook the country with terrible violence.

In a diary kept by Daniel Fairfield, of Braintree, in Maffachufetts, an unlettered man of good underftanding, I have a particular defcription of an influenza that prevailed in America in the fevere winter of 1697-8.* This catarrh began in November and prevailed till February. Its violence was in January, when whole families were fick at once, and whole towns were feized nearly at the fame time. It appears to have been an epidemic of the fevere kind; and the epidemics which followed it in America were of correfpondent feverity.

In the fame winter a mortal difeafe raged in the town of Fairfield in Connecticut, which was fo general, that well perfons could fcarcely be found to tend the fick and bury the dead. Seventy perfons were buried in three months, altho it may be doubted whether the town then contained 1000 inhabitants.

M. S. letter from Dr. Trumbull.

In the fame winter raged a deadly fever in the town of Dover, in New-Hampfhire.

M. S. of the Rev. John Pike.

This difeafe was doubtlefs that fpecies of inflammatory fever, attacking the brain and ending in typhus, which has often proved a terrible fcourge to particular parts of America, during the rage of peftilence in the eaft, and of other epidemics in this country. We fhall hear of it in the following century, and efpecially in 1761.

On the 20th of June 1698 the town of Latacunga, in the province of Quito, nearly under the equator, was laid in ruins by an earthquake, as were Riobamba, Hambato and other towns in the fame diftrict. In one place a chafm of five feet broad and a league in length, was opened, and on a mountain happened a volcanic eruption, from which iffued afhes, cinders and flames.

Ulloa, vol. 2.

* For this and many other articles of intelligence, I am indebted to the late Dr. Jeremy Belknap, whofe value as a man and as a hiftorian many years friendfhip and correfpondence had taught me to appreciate, and whofe lofs to fociety and the republic of letters, I moft deeply lament.

The malignant fever already mentioned, whatever might have been its precife fymptoms, was foon followed by more general ficknefs. In 1699 raged in Charlefton South-Carolina and in Philadelphia, the moft deadly bilious plague that probably ever affected the people of this country.

Mr. Norris of Philadelphia has kindly favored me with a fight of a number of M. S. letters of his grand-father Ifaac Norris, written during the ficknefs, to his correfpondents. This worthy gentleman was then in trade, and well acquainted with the facts refpecting the difeafe, as his own family fuffered a lofs of feveral of its members.

In a letter dated Auguft 15, 1699, he mentions, that a malignant fever broke out about the beginning of Auguft, which he defcribes as the "Barbadoes diftemper," tho he gives no intimations of its being communicated from countries abroad by infection. He fays the patients "vomited and voided blood."

On the 24th of Auguft, arrived the Britannia from Liverpool, which had been 13 weeks on her paffage, fhe had 200 paffengers on board—had loft fifty by death, and others were fickly.

September 1ft, he writes that the diftemper appeared to abate at one time, but afterwards revived. He mentions the fummer to be the hotteft he ever knew; men died at harveft in the field. All bufinefs in the city was fufpended.

During the yearly meeting the difeafe abated, but the meeting was thinly attended. Afterwards the difeafe returned in all its violence.

October 9th, he writes that he had hoped the cool weather would have relieved the city, but it did not.

October 22d, the difeafe had abated. Of this epidemic, died two hundred and twenty, of whom eighty or ninety belonged to the fociety of friends.

The population of Philadelphia at this time, is not exactly afcertained; but as the city had been fettled but feventeen years, the number of people could not have been great. If we confider that the city was thinly inhabited, and that no confiderable artificial caufes of difeafe had been accumulated; together with the fact of the patient's vomiting and voiding blood, we must admit the disease to have been extremely virulent, beyond any thing that has marked its returns in subsequent periods.

In the same letters, Mr. Norris, October 18th, mentions that he had information from Charleston of the great mortality by the same fever—150 had died in a few days, and the survivors mostly fled into the country.

In a history of South-Carolina, lately published, there is a more particular account of the calamities that befel Charleston in this year 1699. A most dreadful tempest, a common event after excessive heat, threatened a total destruction of the town. The sea swelled and rushed violently into the town, compelling the people to fly to the tops of their houses for safety. A fire broke out and laid most of the town in ashes. The small-pox proved fatal to many of the youth, and to fill the cup of calamity, the bilious plague broke out with such irresistible mortality, that the principal officers of government, one half of the members of assembly and multitudes of the citizens fell victims. These calamities came near to dissolve the settlement.

Hist of S Carolina, vol 1. 142

I find no suggestion that any vessels had arrived from the West-Indies at these places, or that any suspicion existed of the importation of this terrible disease. At that time, there was very little intercourse directly between Philadelphia or Charleston and the West Indies.

But it will be remarked, that the disease first appeared about the " beginning of August," as in modern times—that it once abated, as it did in New-York, both in 1795 and 6, so as to be extinguished in the latter year, and that for two or three weeks.—That in 1699 as in later returns of it, it yielded not to cool weather, until late in October. It will be further remarked, that a severe epidemic catarrh preceded this plague, about eighteen months, as it did in 1789-90.

During this period, other parts of the earth did not escape affliction. A comet appeared in 1698 and another small one in 1699; and in this latter year, Lima suffered considerable damage by an earthquake, as did some parts of Batavia in the East-Indies.

In October 1698 began a fatal spotted fever to prevail over all England. In the spring of 1699 a severe and fatal catarrh was epidemic, which carried off the young and robust, together with hard drinkers. A cough was epidemic among horses in England and France. In this period the catarrh in America preceded that in Europe, one whole year.

The seven last years of this century, the period under consideration, were distinguished for a severe and continued famin in Scotland. The general cause was, the wet and cold summers which prevented crops from arriving to maturity. Vast multitudes perished with hunger—the dead bodies lay scattered along the highways. See Sinclair's Statistical account of Scotland in a great number of passages, and especially vol. 6. 132, 189. It does not appear that, during this long period of distress and want, any pestilence prevailed in Scotland.

At the same time, famin afflicted Finland and carried off one tenth of the inhabitants, and a greater proportion in the less fertile provinces of Sweden.

Williams's Obs. on North Governments, vol 1. 638.

The same period was remarkable for failure of crops in America. In a sermon preached in Boston on Lecture Day, Sept. 27, 1698, we have the following account of this subject. "The harvest hath once and again grievously failed, in these years, and we have been struck through with terrible famin.—The very course of nature hath been altered among us; a lamentable cry for *bread, bread*, hath been heard in our streets."

Magnalia b 7 113.

In the preceding page, of this sermon, it is also remarked, that " Epidemical sicknesses have, in these years, been once and again upon us," and it is mentioned that Boston lost, in one year, six or seven hundred of its people, by one contagious disease. The year is not specified.

It will be observed that in the history of the last two centuries few instances of the plague in Egypt and the Levant are mentioned. The reason is, that I have no regular series of accounts of plague in Egypt or Constantinople, for the last two or three hundred years. One remark however I will hazard, on the strength of facts within the present century, that whenever malignant epidemics prevail generally in Europe or America, the plague rages in Egypt and Constantinople, or rather a little before; the commencement of the pestilential state of air in those unhealthy cities being a little anterior to its principal effects in the north of Europe.

At the time of the dreadful bilious plague in Philadelphia and Charleston just before described, the plague was raging in the Levant, and for a year or two after.

During this period, in 1700, the same pestilential constitution displayed itself in a most destructive sore throat in the island of Milo, in the Levant. It is thus described by Tournefort, vol. 1. let. 4. He says it appeared in a "Carbuncle or plague-fore in the bottom of the throat, attended with a violent fever" It carried off children in two days, but spared adults. He calls it the "child's plague." There appears to be some propriety in giving the disease this appellation. It has some resemblance to the true pestis, the ulcer being formed in the throat instead of the glands. The insidiousness of the distemper is another circumstance of resemblance—persons in both diseases often walking about, a few hours before they expire. But this is a most prominent fact, that the ulcerous sore throat, or malignant anginas are rarely or never epidemic, except in periods when the plague and yellow fever prevail in places where they usually appear. In no instance has the sore throat been epidemic in America, except when the plague has been raging in Egypt and Constantinople. At least I can find no exception to this remark, and what is more, the virulence of the one disease in one country, corresponds with the malignity of the other disease in the other countries. Thus, as the plague in Egypt in 1736, was far more destructive than the same disease, at other times, so was the angina maligna of that period in America.

When observation and philosophy shall prevail over the prejudices of men in regard to the origin of these diseases from infection, it will be found that the angina, in its various forms, is only a particular stage or modification of the pestilence, which spreads over the world at certain unequal periods. The milder forms of the peftilence appear in catarrh, meafles and chin cough; wh ch ufually appear together, or nearly fo, at the beginning of the more virulent general contagion ; the later and more fatal ftages are marked by anginas, cynanche maligna, petechial fever, bilious and glandular plague in fummer; and peftilential pleurifies in winter.

There are certain times, when the conftitutions of men in all parts of the world, contract a poifon, which nature makes an effort to expel ; and the different epidemics that accompany or follow each other, in rapid fucceffion, appear to be the different modes by which nature ftrives to rid the human body of the virus. Thefe modes depend on the feafon of the year, the conftitution or age of the patient and a multitude of fubordinate circumftances.—Whether this poifon is a pofitive fubftance inhaled by the lungs and pores, or is the effect of mere debility, which unfits the feveral parts of the body to perform their functions, is a queftion of a curious nature.

It is remarkable that in this year 1700, when this ulcerous fore throat was raging in the Levant Ifles, fmall children in the north of Europe were feized with a fuffocating catarrh or catarrhous fevers. Thefe were followed by mild epidemic meafles.

Short vol 1 418.

In the fame year the fmall-pox was confluent and malignant. The winter of 1700 was very mild.

In this year fell a meteor in Jamaica, which entered the earth, making confiderable holes, fcorching the grafs, and leaving a fmell of fulphur.

Bad Mem. 6. 389

SECTION VII.

Historical view of pestilential epidemics from the year 1701 *to* 1788.

THE year 1701 appears to have been excessively dry in America. Dr. Rush relates that during the dry summer of 1782, a rock in the Skuylkill appeared above the surface of the water, on which were engraven the figures 1701. How little do men suspect the value of this inscription! To this alone I am indebted for the fact of extreme drouth in that year—and the fact is among the proofs of an extraordinary evaporation, before discharges of fire and lava from volcanoes. In 1701 was an eruption of Vesuvius; in 1702 of Etna. It will hereafter appear that a similar dry season in 1782 preceded the great eruption of Heckla in 1783. Indeed it is a general fact, and as far as I can learn, such seasons seldom occur, except during the approach of comets, or antecedent to volcanic eruptions.

This was a pestilential period. In 1701 Toulon lost two thirds of its inhabitants by the plague, and the Levant was severely affected about the same time. See the bills of mortality for Augsburg, Dresden and Boston.

In 1702 appeared a comet; Etna discharged its fires, and in Boston raged a malignant small-pox, attended, in many cases, with a scarlet eruption, which was mistaken for the scarlet fever. It appears from Fairfield's diary that this disease appeared in June and was at first mild, not fatal to any of the patients. In August died one patient—in September it became very mortal, and in this month was attended with a "sort of fever called scarlet fever." In October, many died of the "fever and the small-pox, and it was a time of sore distress," on which account the general court sat at Cambridge. In December "the fever abated;" but the small-pox continued to be mortal, till the month of February 1703, when it began to subside.

I have already remarked that eruptive diseases seem to belong to one family. Physicians will observe the alliance in their symptoms; but I would observe that the progressiveness in this disease of 1702 and the variations in its symptoms, prove it to have been an epidemic, and not the effect of mere infection, or specific contagion.

In this year also the drouth was extreme. In New-York raged the American plague, which was said to have been imported from St. Thomas's. By the accounts, this was more fatal than any disease since that period. It was called the "Great Sickness" and hardly a patient survived. On account of it, the assembly was held at Jamaica on Long-Island.

Smith's Hist N York, p 104. Journals of Assembly, vol. 1. 151.

Such were the epidemics in America which followed the influenza of 1698—malignant pleurisies in 1698—plague in 1699 and in 1702, with virulent small-pox—all of unusual severity. Let the reader compare these facts with the accounts from Europe and the bills of mortality.

The winter of 1702-3 was variable—severe frost and great snows, with intervals of warm weather. In spring catarrh prevailed in England, followed by a sickly summer, with earthquakes.

In January and February 1703 were severe shocks of earthquake in Rome, Naples and other parts of Italy. In October a memorable tempest or hurricane, which did great damage at sea, and injured buildings on land.

In 1704 the summer was very dry, and a most malignant spotted fever raged in Augsburg and in Prussia. Flies were in great abundance, and there was an eruption of Vesuvius. The last eruption of the volcano in Teneriffe was in this year, since which it has discharged smoke, but no fire.

Note. A late arrival from Teneriffe brings an account of the bursting forth of a volcano, in June last, which continued, till the vessel left the island in August.

In December 1705 were many most violent tempests and inundations. The tide rose in the Loir in France 25 feet beyond its usual height. Half of Limerick in Ireland was laid under water. These storms indicated the approach of a comet, which appeared in the following year.

In 1706 coughs and coryzas prevailed, and dysentery fatal among children.

A small shock of earthquake was felt in America in 1705.

In 1707 appeared another comet and subterranean fire was uncommonly agitated. Vesuvius discharged fire, and a new island was thrown up in the Archipelago, with an earthquake and volcano. The seasons in this and the following year were variable.

Buffon's Nat Hist.

In November 1708 began a most severe and universal catarrh in Europe, which was speedily followed by a series of pestilential diseases. Of this catarrh, of the seasons, and the plagues that followed we have from Europe very correct accounts ; but, with the utmost industry, I cannot learn whether the catarrh extended to America.

The explosion of subterranean fire in various places in 1707 seems to have been the commencement of this period ; altho there was a plague in the eastern parts of Europe, most of the preceding years from 1700. A meteor passed over England, near the mouth of the Thames, July 31, 1708, a few months before the catarrh.

The winter of 1708-9 was the severest that had happened, after 1683-4. But it appears that the catarrh commenced two months before the severe cold began. At least this epidemic appeared in the north of Europe, as early as November ; whereas the autumn was one of the mildest, till January, that was ever known. Then the weather changed suddenly to most severe cold and continued for a number of weeks.

Short, vol 1   Lancisius, p 194 and seq.

This catarrh is carefully described by Lancisius as it appeared in Italy. In Rome it commenced in January, but increased afterwards, as the cold abated. It began with coryza, rheumata and slight cough, and was attended with pains in the breast, angina, pleurisies and peripneumonies, which prevailed greatly in the spring, among those who neglected the cough, or used a full diet.

Symptoms of this catarrh were, laffitude, fever with chills, wandering pains in the breaft, continued cough, hard pulfe, flame-colored or turbid urine, fpitting of blood and difficult refpiration. The cheeks were red and the body fuffufed with a yellow color, like that of the jaundice.

Perfons fhut up in prifon, efcaped the difeafe.* Fewer women than men were afflicted, and perfons in eafy circumftances, who could take care of themfelves, fuffered lefs than the poor. Many recovered by means of fweats or hemorrhagy at the nofe, or difcharges from the bowels, or copious difcharges of urine, or by all thefe evacuations, accompanied by fpitting a thick phlegm. Venefection was beneficial, efpecially in robuft conftitutions. On diffection, the precordia appeared of a reddifh color, extending to the diaphragm—and difcolored by fpots of blackifh thick blood—polypuffes were difcovered in the great veffels of the heart.

This difeafe did not entirely difappear till June.

In the fummer of 1708 preceding the fevere winter and catarrh, gnats appeared in prodigious fwarms.

The winter of 1708-9 killed fruit-trees, vines and corn. After this exceffive cold, multitudes of people died of apoplexies, and others were feized with vertigoes, arthritics, pleurifies, inflammatory fevers of all kinds, and confumptions. This feverity of cold extended over America as well as Europe, in the fame winter.

A peftilence raged in the north of Europe from the years 1702 to 1711, of which we have an account in Philofophical Tranfactions, No. 337.

Baddam's Memoirs, vol. 6 p. 5.

It has been obferved already that the plague raged in the Levant, in the firft years of the prefent century. In 1702, the fame year, it will be noted, in which the terrible fmall-pox raged

---

* This has been obferved in one or two inftances in America, and has been alledged as an evidence that the influenza is an infectious difeafe, and that perfons fequeftered from contagion, may efcape it To my mind the fact is rather an evidence that the efcape of prifoners is owing to a different, perhaps a lefs ftimulant condition of the air they breathe. It is hardly poffible they fhould efcape expofure to infection, when every one around them is affected. The contagion of the difeafe however is not denied.

in Boston and bilious plague in New-York, the plague broke out in Poland, near Pickzow, soon after an unfortunate battle between the Swedes and Saxons. No suggestion appears that the disease was caught by infection from a distant country, nor that the fetor of dead carcases was supposed to generate the distemper. On these important points we are left in the dark. All that is recorded is, that it *first began* near Pickzow in Poland, soon after a battle. It spread in 1703, 4 and 5 over Poland, and into parts of Hungary and Russia, sweeping away vast numbers of inhabitants. In 1706 we hear nothing of it. In 1707 it broke out in Warsaw, with great mortality. In 1708 it appeared in Thorn, and parts of Polish Prussia.

This approach of the disease alarmed the people of Dantzick—public prayers were ordered in the churches—all commerce and communication with infected places were forbid—no merchandize from infected or suspected places was permitted to enter the city, and the magistrates neglected no measure that could guard the public safety. All travellers and strangers were strictly examined, and none permitted to enter without sufficient proofs that they came from healthy and uninfected places. These and other strict regulations were enjoined in July 1708; but notwithstanding these precautions, " the distemper gradually insinuated itself, for in March 1709, there died out of one district in the old town seven persons, and another person, being ill, was sent to the hospital, where the disease soon spread." Dr. Gottwald, the author of this account, visited the hospital on the 16th of the same month, and found many persons ill—" some had buboes, others carbuncles, others gangrenous ulcers, which he could not determin to be pestilential, but which he judged to be symptoms, if not of the plague already commenced, at *least of something, but little inferior to it, and certain forerunners of that destructive distemper.*"

In the preceding account, we observe the utter insufficiency of laws and regulations to prevent the introduction of the plague into cities; and the uncertainty of physicians at first as to the nature of the disease. The facts stated prove the disease to have been generated on the spot, and to have been *progressive* from malignant fevers to the real plague. I have no bills of the mortality in Dantzick for the preceding years, but if any such are on record, it will appear, that the approach of the plague was indicated in that city by malignant diseases and increased mortality, for some months or perhaps a year or two preceding.

The disease spread slowly at first, but in July and August became general—it was at its height in September, and gradually declined till the close of the year. The number of victims was nearly 25,000.

From the very accurate history of this pestilence by Dr. Gottwald, the following circumstances are to be collected.

1st. That the distemper first made its appearance in a part of the old town, called Raumbaum. What its situation is, may be seen in Busching; a part of the city built on a stream which falls into the Vistula—low of course—a place of business, and its streets dirty.

2d. The disease, after its first appearance, lay lurking for a long time, in the suburbs of the city, and its progress was not perceivable, for two or three months. This corresponds with its phenomena in London and other places; and proves that cold or favorable weather suspends or checks the action of the pestilential principle.

3d. It was most fatal to the poor—people in good condition mostly escaped. The same was observed at Copenhagen in 1711.

4th. Its decrease was gradual, as well as its increase.

5th. Many of the inhabitants, tho they took never so much care to avoid the distemper, kept at home, suffered no infected person to approach them, and used all manner of preservatives, "yet caught the infection."

6th. The disease was preceded, in 1708, by extraordinary numbers of spiders. The same presage has been observed on other occasions.

7th. While this distemper was raging, on the 11th of August, an offensive mist was observed, like a thick cloud, but of short duration. It returned in the afternoon, from the northwest, so thick as to darken the air. Its color was that of the effluvia from the effervescence of the oil of vitriol with oil of tartar, a blackish yellow.

8th. In the beginning of October appeared over the city a blue fiery globe or meteor, which came from the north west, in the night, shot towards the town rapidly, illuminating the city, and fell to the south.

9th. Crows, sparrows and other birds did not make their appearance during the pestilence.

In 1708 and 9 the plague desolated Livonia. In 1710 the disease appeared in Sweden; 30,000 persons perished by it in Stockholm, and other parts of the kingdom did not escape. Historians relate, that in the latter part of the last century and beginning of the present, the sweating sickness and great plague in Sweden destroyed several hundred thousand lives, in consequence of which Sweden is less populous than formerly.

William's Obs vol. 1. p 638
Universal Hist vol 35 458

In 1710 also the territory of Lithuania was ravaged by pestilence.

In 1711 Copenhagen lost 25,000 citizens by the same malady.

It is proper to remark how extensively pestilence prevailed after the great catarrh and terribly severe winter of 1709.

Nor did America escape the operation of the general principle. A body of troops under Gen. Nicholson, destined to co-operate with a fleet from England, in the reduction of Canada, encamped near Wood Creek in the province of New-York, and in July and August were attacked with a distemper which made dreadful havoc and obliged them to decamp. Some of the men died as if they had been poisoned. This circumstance gave rise to a report which Charlevoix gravely relates, that the Indians had poisoned the water of the creek, by throwing into it all the skins of beasts they had taken in hunting. The disease was probably the lake fever or a malignant dysentery. This happened in 1709.

Hutch. Hist Mass. vol 2. 179.

England also felt the influence of the same general principle, as appears from the bill of mortality for 1710. In France, England and the Low Countries raged a catarrhous fever to which was given the name of Dunkirk rant. In some places prevailed a spotted fever, as at Norwich.

Short on Air. Baddam's Mem. vol. 6. 70, 72.

In 1712 prevailed catarrh in Europe, with sore throats. Whether catarrh prevailed in America also, I can obtain no information. The seasons in England were excessively wet, and corn was rotten or mildewed. The winter was severe, there was an eruption of Vesuvius and an earthquake. From these circumstances, I suspect the approach of a comet, but have found no account of any.*

Short, vol 2. 8.

In October 1712 commenced a mortal sickness in the town of Waterbury, in Connecticut, which raged for eleven months. It was so general that nurses could scarcely be found to tend the sick. What the disease was, I am not informed; but not improbably it was that species of putrid pleurisy, which has so often made dreadful havoc in America.

Trumbull's Hist. of Connecticut, 386.

In the same year, prevailed a sore throat in London, accompanied with dizziness and pain in the limbs.

In 1713 prevailed the measles in America, cotemporary with epidemic pestilence in Europe.

In 1712 and 13, the plague was epidemic in Vienna, Hungary, Stiria and other eastern countries. This disease was preceded by the spotted fever, which gradually changed to plague. At the same time, whole countries were overrun with insects.

Short, vol 2. 10.

In England prevailed a fever which Mead has pronounced to have been of the same kind, as the sweating sickness in the sixteenth century.—He says it was imported from Dunkirk, but how it came to be in Dunkirk, he does not inform us.

During these calamities among men, the beasts of the field did not escape. A fatal distemper among cattle broke out in 1711 and raged with such violence, in Italy, as almost to destroy the species. It spread for three or four years, and horses perished by a similar pestilence. The writers who describe the disease,

---

* Since the text was prepared for the press, I have found an account of a comet in 1712. My suspicions therefore were well founded.

represent it as a kind of plague; and all agree that it sprung from a single infected cow from Dalmatia. How this cow became infected, they do not inform us. The truth is the disease was an epidemic, tho very infectious; and that it did not necessarily originate in infection, is proved by its appearing in many other parts of Europe.

The disease began with rigors, which were followed by violent fever, with eruptions like those of the small-pox, and terminated in five, six or seven days.

Baddam's Mem. vol. 6. 72. Lancisius p. 154.

In 1714 began in Europe a series of dry summers. This year was rather sickly in England, and cattle also perished by an infectious distemper.

In 1715 the small-pox and measles were epidemic in England. In the same year, Plymouth in Massachusetts lost 40 of its inhabitants by a malignant disease, but no particulars are known.

Hist. Col vol. 4. 129.

In 1716 the winter was excessively severe, and a fair was held on the Thames. The rivers in Europe, even in Italy, were covered with ice.

Short, vol 2. 17.

In America, the 21st of October O. S. was so dark that people used lighted candles. Lima, the same year, was shaken by an earthquake.

Mem. Am Acad vol 1. 244 Ulloa. Lima.

In 1717 appeared a comet, and there was an explosion of Vesuvius. Holland and Germany suffered severely the same year by inundations. In America the winter was terribly severe, and remarkable for "prodigious storms of snow," says Mr. Winthrop of New-London in a letter to Dr. Mather, Hist. Col. vol. 2. 12. One hundred sheep belonging to that gentleman were buried in the snow on Fisher's Island, and 28 days after, were dug out, when two of them were found alive; and they both lived and thrived. The snow was accumulated over them to the height of sixteen feet.—This snow storm is distinguished in the Annals of America, as by far the greatest ever known.

This year was remarkable alfo in America for the death of many old people, fays

Hutchinfon's Hift vol 2 223.

In Europe catarrh was prevalent, and malignant fmall-pox among children. At Underwald in Switzerland prevailed a tertain, fo violent as to deftroy life at the fecond attack. The plague made its appearance in fome part of the Turkifh dominions.

See Short, vol 2 20, and Lady Montague's Letters.

In 1718 the winter was cold in Europe, the feafon in England hot, and a comet was feen. The plague advanced.

See Short, vol 2 and Ruffel's Hift Aleppo.

In 1719 malignant fevers were prevalent in many parts of Europe, marking a peftilential principle of great extent. The winter of 1719-20 in America was very cold.

Douglas.

In thefe laft years raged malignant pleurify in Hartford, in Connecticut, with great mortality.

In March 1719 an immenfe meteor paffed the heavens, illuminating the earth and burfting with a tremendous report. Its diameter was calculated by Dr. Halley at a mile and a half.

At this time the plague appeared in Aleppo, and carried off by report 80,000 people. Ruffel agrees that this difeafe came from the north, altho he has given us few particulars. It raged, as ufual, for two or three years.

Hift of Aleppo—paffim.

In 1718, 19, 20 and 21, fays Dr. Rogers, the greater number of thofe who lived near the flaughter-houfes at Cork, died.

In 1720 happened the laft great plague in Marfeilles, on which occafion has been publifhed " Traité de la pefte," a treatife in quarto, by Chicoyneau, under the fanction of the French king, in which great efforts are made to prove the difeafe to have been imported from the Levant.

The proofs of importation ftand thus. " Capt. Chataud left Said in Syria in January 1720, with a clean patent. The plague was not then in Said, tho it broke out foon after. On the paffage, feveral perfons died, and the phyficians at Leghorn, where the fhip ftopped, pronounced their difeafe to be " a malignant peftilential fever."

The ship arrived at Marseilles, and some persons who had concern with the goods, died in May. The suspected goods were subjected to fifteen days retreat and purification—they were forbid to be introduced into the city—the porters were shut up; but all regulations were fruitless. In June, deaths appeared in the city with distinctive marks of the plague."

On such flimsey evidence do the sticklers for the sole propagation of the plague by infection, ground all their assertions respecting the disease at Marseilles!

But it happens in this case, as in most similar instances, that the pretended proofs of infection carry refutation in the very face of them.

In the first place, it is an acknowledged fact, that at the time the ship left Said, the plague had not appeared in that port, or town. It was at Aleppo and in other places far distant in 1719, but had not broke out in Said. How, in the name of reason, could men or goods be infected, when the disease did not exist in the place?

To overcome or rather to evade the force of this objection, the writers on the subject are compelled to resort to *supposition*. They say it is *possible*, the plague might have been in the place, tho not known or generally admitted. And here rests their whole argument!

It is true, that some of the seamen or passengers died on the passage, with a malignant pestilential fever. But in this case, the malady originated on board the ship—and the infection is not traced to the Levant ports. There is an end of the chain—the disease began *without infection*, on board the ship, as malignant fevers have done in thousands of other ships.

Again, it is admitted by Dr. Mead himself, p. 255, that from the time of the sailors' death, after the ship arrived, it was full six weeks before the disease was known in the city of Marseilles; a circumstance that renders it nearly impossible that there could have been any propagation of the distemper by infection. To remove this objection, the advocates of infection again resort *to supposition*. They *suppose* it possible some latent seeds of the disease had been concealed in goods, or clothes—and such ridiculous suggestions are made the grounds of assertion.

But what completely refutes all thefe idle fuppofitions, is, that we have full evidence, that the plague in Marfeilles was generated in the city, and gradually arofe from milder difeafes. In the beginning of the " Traité de la pefte," it is ftated from Mon. Didier and not denied, that " the preceding year 1719 was a barren year—the corn, the wine and the oil, were defective. The heat of fpring was exceffive and followed by great rains, with wefterly winds—the fruits were bad. In this year a peftilential fever appeared in Marfeilles, of which many died, and *in fome, appeared buboes, earbuncles and paroitides.*"

Here we obferve facts that always exift, before the plague, and which demonftrate the uniform operations of the laws of nature. The year 1718 began to exhibit malignant difeafes in greater numbers than ufual. In 1719 the plague broke out at Aleppo, and in the north and weft of Europe, malignant fevers became in many places, epidemic and peftilential. In 1720, the peftilential ftate of the air, arrived at its crifis in Marfeilles. The peftilence in Europe exhibited a *regular progrefs*, from ordinary typhus fever to the plague. A fatal fmall-pox and fpotted fever prevailed in Piemont.

To demonftrate this fact, the reader will only turn to the bills of mortality in London, Amfterdam, Vienna, Drefden, &c. for the years under confideration, and obferve every where the effects of a general unhealthy ftate of air, in the increafe of the number of deaths.—The bills of mortality in Bofton and Philadelphia alfo prove this ftate of air to have extended to this country; and the malignancy of it feems to have abated in America after 1721, in which year the fmall-pox was very mortal in Bofton.

The accounts of difeafes in America, at this period, are few and imperfect. Tradition has preferved the memory of defolating ficknefs, at various times and in various places, fome of which, I fufpect, refer to this period, but I am not able to afcertain the dates, with any certainty.* By accident however,

---

* My father mentions an inftance, which he believes to have been not long before his birth, which was in 1722. An aged lady of 96, who was born in 1702, informs me that a malignant pleurify raged when fhe was 17 years old; this fixes the period in 1719.

I am able to determin positively the pestilential state of air in America in 1720. A genuine letter is extant, from Thomas Hacket of Duck Creek, now in the state of Delaware, dated April 10th 1720, in which he states that a mortality prevailed in that place, which exceeded that in London in 1665, and almost depopulated the village. I have seen the letter in possession of Dr. Rush.

In 1721 there was an eruption of a volcano in Iceland. A dreadful dysentery raged in Upper Saxony.

In 1720 there was a great earthquake in China, and in 1721 shocks were felt in the Mediterranean, by Dr. Shaw who was then on his travels to the east.—In October 1720, fire arose out of the sea near Tercera, one of the Azores, and a small island arose.

Buffon's Nat. Hist.

In 1722, the seasons were cold, wet and rainy. In August happened a most violent storm in Jamaica and S. Carolina. In May an earthquake in Chili.

The winter of 1722-3 was cold and dry in England. In 1723 appeared a comet, and on the 24th of February, O. S. a mighty tempest which is recorded among the memorabilia of America. The wind blew violently from the southward, then veered suddenly to the eastward and northward, bringing in a tide which rose two or three feet above the Long Wharf in Boston, and flowed over all the lower part of the town, filling cellars and destroying property to a great amount. Immense damage was sustained in all the maritime towns.

See Mather's letter. Hist. Col. vol. 2. 11.

The confluent small-pox raged in England See the London bill of mortality for 1723. Dysenteries, pleurisies and other inflammatory complaints prevailed in the different seasons.

The bilious plague prevailed in Barbadoes, said to be imported from Martinico. We are not informed from whence it came into Martinico. In these accounts of infections, we are not led to the end of the chain.

In the same year 1723 prevailed in many parts of the colony of Rhode-Island, a fatal disease called the " burning ague." It was particularly fatal, near Providence, between Pautucket and Pautuxet. In proportion to its patients, no difeafe in America, was ever more mortal. It did not prevail in a large town, but in villages, and perhaps the clearing of fome neighboring fwamps might have been one caufe of the difeafe. The year however was lefs healthy than ufual. A difeafe of the fame name is noted once or twice in ancient hiftory. See the year 1001.

The year 1724 in England was moftly wet and cold; the whooping cough prevailed; but the year was generally healthy.

The fummer of 1725 was alfo wet and cold in England. In January a fevere froft produced many inflammatory complaints. In this year happened violent earthquakes in South-America, and eruptions from two volcanic mountains in Iceland. I have no account of the weather and difeafes in America. I only learn from an old gentleman, that one of the winters between 1722 and 1725 was called, " the hard winter."

The winter of 1726-7 was changeable in England, but moftly cold with great fnows. Remitting fevers prevailed in fummer and inflammatory, in winter, which fwelled the bills of mortality to an unufual degree. At the fame time the plague raged in Egypt.

The fame winter in America was milder than ufual—the fummer of 1727 was very hot and dry. See Dudley's account of the great earthquake.

Philof. Tranf. and Mufeum, vol. 5. 363.

In 1727 appeared a comet—an explofion of fire took place from Vefuvius and a volcano in Iceland. The interior counties of England were fhaken by an earthquake; and on the 29th of October of the fame year happened one of the moft extenfive and violent earthquakes ever known in America. A malignant dyfentery was epidemic in Bern. In America, the fummer was very hot.

Short, vol 2. Van Troil on Iceland Williams on Earthquakes. Memoirs of American Academy. Pennant's Arctic Zoology. Zimmerman on dyfentery. Phil. Tranf. 437. Baddam's Mem vol 10. 110

This was a fickly year; fee the bills of mortality for London and Amfterdam, Bofton, Philadelphia Chrift's Church and Dublin. The prevalent difeafes in London were fevers of a malignant type. What the difeafe was in Philadelphia, I know not; but the greateft mortality was in February, March and April.

In 1728 putrid fevers were frequent—the fummer was cold in England and the following winter fevere. The year 1727 was unproductive; corn in England was fcarce and the fcarcity continued into this year. An eruption of a volcano in Iceland and the plague in Egypt marked this year, 1728. The eruption in Iceland continued till 1730.

This year, 1728, the fummer weather in South-Carolina was unufually hot and dry. The earth was parched and the fprings exhaufted. In Auguft a violent hurricane occafioned an inundation, which fpread over the low grounds and did incredible damage to the wharves, houfes and corn fields. The ftreets of Charleftown were covered with boats; the inhabitants were driven to the upper ftories of their houfes; twenty-three fhips were driven afhore and thoufands of trees were levelled. The fame feafon, the bilious plague raged in Charlefton with great mortality.

Hift. of S. Carolina, vol. 1. 316.

In 1729 appeared a comet, and in autumn a univerfal catarrh in Europe, and perhaps over the globe. This was preceded by meafles. It feized with a flight chill, a flow fever, wearinefs, continual hoarfenefs, pain of the head, and difficulty of breathing. The fuddennefs of the attack was aftonifhing, and it proved fatal to many aged and phlegmatic people. Many pleurifies and peripneumonies followed. Its firft appearance was in Poland, Auftria and Silefia, and it marched over Europe in five months. At the clofe of this epidemic in 1730, Vefuvius difcharged its contents of fire.

In this year 1729 the plague was in Aleppo, and it will be feen that the bills of mortality in the north of Europe exhibit a fickly ftate, through a period of many years at this time. The meafles prevailed in America, and in Farmington, Connecticut, a malignant pleurify.

The fummer of 1729 was in moft parts of England, very wet, in other parts, dry; but this made no difference in the prevalence of the catarrh. The fmall-pox was very frequent in England.

This year alfo is remarkable for the firſt appearance of the yellow fever or black vomit at Carthagena, in South-America, where it made dreadful havoc among the crews of the fleet under Don Domingo Juſtiniani. The fame fate attended the crews of the galleons under Lopez Pintado in 1730.

Ulloa, vol. 1. p 44.—Lond 1772.

The winter of 1729-30 was very mild in Europe. There was a ſmall eruption of Vefuvius in 1730 and in Iceland, and an earthquake in South-America, on the 8th of July totally demoliſhed the towns of Conception and Santiago, in Chili. This dreadful calamity was foon followed by an epidemic difeafe which fwept away greater numbers than the earthquake.

Ulloa, vol. 2. 235, 257.

The plague was in Cyprus about this time, and was preceded by an earthquake.

In January 1729, the rivers and canals in Holland were covered with ice, from 12 to 20 inches thick. Meafles and anginas prevailed, and in autumn the fmall-pox made great havoc.

Bad Mem vol. 9. 314 and fequel.

It will be obferved that thefe eruptive difeafes in Holland were cotemporary with the meafles in America, and the malignant pleurify in winter, which was the predominant fymptom of a peftilential conſtitution of air, in America, until the year 1761.

The winter of 1730-31 was very fevere in Europe.

It appears from the bills of mortality in Boſton and Philadelphia, that the years 1730 and 31 were fickly. What the malady was which fwelled the mortality in Chriſt Church to double the ufual number in 1731, I am not informed; but the greateſt mortality happened in March and April. The fmall-pox was the difeafe which augmented the bill in Boſton in 1730.

In 1731 the fmall-pox fpread in New-York, and occafioned an adjournment of the legiſlature in September.

Journals, vol. 1 p 633.

In 1732 appeared a comet, and in America the following winter was very fevere, continuing from the middle of November to the end of March. In Europe, the winter was mild.

Douglas Sum Short on Air.

Lima in South-America was fhaken, this year, by an earthquake; a shock was experienced also in England; and in November the same was experienced in Canada and New-England. On the 9th of August happened a remarkably dark day.

<blockquote>See Douglas, and Professor Williams Mem. Am. Acad.</blockquote>

In this year, the plague prevailed at Tripoli, Sidon and Damascus; and the American plague at Charleston, S. Carolina.

<blockquote>Lining's letter. Edin. Essays, vol. 2.</blockquote>

Towards the close of the year, in October, commenced in America a severe universal catarrh, which appeared in Europe also in December. It spread over all Europe, in the beginning of 1733, and probably over the earth, as it was experienced at the isle of Bourbon, in the Indian Ocean.

<blockquote>Mem. of Dr. Hunt of Northampton, and the Medical publications in Edinburgh.</blockquote>

This epidemic seems to have been the precursor of the most pestilential period of this century. The summer of 1733, in England, was dry and pleasant. The winter following was very mild. The plague raged at Aleppo.

The scarlatina appeared in Edinburgh; and the chin cough also began in England in 1734, continuing to prevail in 1735.

This period also was noted for meteors. In June 1734, a ball of fire passed through two opposite windows of a steeple at Air, in Scotland, broke one end of the bell joist, and descended to the earth, without doing further harm. A boy in the neighborhood was killed by another ball of fire.

<blockquote>Sinclair's Stat. Ac. of Scotland, vol. 1. 96.</blockquote>

On the 2d of February 1735, Popayan in S. America, was nearly ruined by an earthquake.

The summer of 1735, was very wet and cold. In Europe in 1734 commenced a slow putrid fever. An anginous fever became epidemic among children, and quinsies or swellings of the throat, with contagion, and great mortality. Small-pox of a malignant kind prevailed at the close of the year. The pestilential state of the air is said to have affected birds, which died in the cages. Canine madness prevailed.

<blockquote>Short, vol. 2. Van Swieten, vol. 16. p. 56.</blockquote>

In 1735, prevailed a spotted fever of a fatal kind, and other malignant diforders, with hydrophobia. In Scotland, the meafles became epidemic, and fevers of a bad kind.

Effays and Obf Edin Phil. Tranfac vol. 4.
H xhom, vol. 1.

Earthquakes were felt in England in 1734 and 1736.

In 1736 and 7 a fatal ulcerous fore throat and malignant peripneumonies, prevailed in France.

In 1735 or 6, three or four thoufand people, in the Orkney Iflands, perifhed with famin. The fcarcity there in 1782 and 3 was alfo deplorable, but none perifhed.

Sinclair's Scotland, vol 7 497.

While thefe epidemics were prevailing in Europe, America felt the peftilential ftate of air. In May 1735, in a wet cold feafon, appeared at Kingfton, an inland town in New-Hampfhire, fituated in a low plain, a difeafe among children, commonly called the " throat diftemper," of a moft malignant kind, and by far the moft fatal ever known in this country. Its fymptoms generally were, a fwelled throat, with white or afh-colored fpecks, an efflorefcence on the fkin, great debility of the whole fyftem, and a tendency to putridity.

It firft feized a child, who died in three days. In about a week afterwards, three children, in another family, at a diftance of four miles, were fucceffively feized and all died on the third day. It continued to fpread, and of the firft forty patients, not one recovered.

In Auguft, it appeared at Exeter, a town fix miles diftant. In September, it broke out in Bofton, fifty miles diftant ; altho' it did not appear in Chefter fix miles weft of Kingfton, till October.—It continued its ravages, through that year into the next, and gradually travelled fouthward, almoft ftripping the country of children. Very few children efcaped, for altho' the difeafe was very infectious, yet its propagation depended very little on that circumftance. It attacked the young in the moft fequeftered fituations, and without a poffible communication with the fick. It was literally the *plague among children*. Many families loft three and four children—many loft all.

In fome places, this diftemper was more fatal than in others—

country towns suffered more than populous cities. And it should be here remarked, that the virulence of this species of disease seems at times to be greatly augmented by cold and wet weather—it is most mild in cities where the air is, in a degree, corrected of its rigor and moisture.—To this observation however there are exceptions.

Scorbutic people and those who lived on pork, and of course the poor, suffered most. In some families, it was comparatively mild—in others it was malignant like a plague. This disease gradually travelled westward and was two years in reaching the river Hudson, distant from Kingston, where it first appeared, about 200 miles in a strait line. It continued its progress westward, with some interruptions, until it spread over the colonies. Few adults were affected; its principal ravages were among persons under age, or rather under puberty. For many years after it was epidemic, it frequently broke out in different places without any apparent cause, but did not spread—a striking proof that such diseases will not become *epidemic* by the sole power of *infection*, but that some *general cause* must aid its propagation, or it will perish in its cradle. This is probably true of every species of pestilential disease.

From an elderly lady of great observation in New-Haven, I have learnt that persons who recovered of this distemper, were subject, all their lives, to sore throat and quinsies, and what is perhaps more remarkable, that few or none of them have lived to be old. It is at least apparent, in the sphere of her observation, that those persons have died at an earlier age than others. These facts are striking proofs how much the whole system, and especially the seat of the disease, was impaired in strength and firmness, by that distressing malady. A gentleman still living, who was affected with the same disease in 1742, informs me that his constitution has never recovered from the shock it received from that malady.

The invasion of this distemper was gradual, and for some time before its attack, children appeared to languish. It was not always attended with great prostration of strength, for persons were often walking, an hour or two before their death. The same happened in the angina of 1794.

> See further particulars in Colden's account. Medical Obser. and Enq London, vol 1 211, and in Belknap's History New-Hampshire, vol. 2 118

Diseases among cattle in New Hampshire marked this period.

In 1736, and during the rage of the ulcerous sore throat in America and in England, the plague made terrible havoc in Egypt—authors relate that Cairo lost 10,000 persons in a day.—In Nimeguen raged a malignant dysentery.

In 1737 while the angina maligna was spreading over the northern parts of America, the bilious plague prevailed in Virginia. In England and Scotland, the measles broke out and prevailed in 1735 and 6, cotemporary with the angina in America. Dr. Short relates that the first person seized was a woman in her child-bed illness.

At the same time prevailed miliary fevers in Cornwall, accompanied with glandular swellings Coughs, defluxions and catarrhs were frequent. A pestilential disease in Devonshire swept away cattle and swine.

In 1737 a very severe influenza invaded both hemispheres. It commenced in November.

In 1737 also appeared a comet; Constantinople was shaken and Smyrna half destroyed by an earthquake. A small shock was felt in Boston. In October of this year, a storm or hurricane in the East-Indies, destroyed 20,000 vessels of different sizes, and 300,000 people. There was a great eruption of Vesuvius in the same year. In Iceland also was an eruption between 1730 and 1740, but the year is not specified.

> See Gent Mag and Tablet of Memory, art. Storms.

A most singular meteor in the same year, followed by a very severe winter.

This pestilential constitution did not produce the same diseases in England, as in France and America. The fatal ulcerous sore throat was cotemporary in America and in France in 1737; but that disease did not appear, in its formidable array, in England until 1742. In 1734-5 appeared its sister-malady, the scarlet fever in Edinburg; but it subsided; and the epidemic took the form of measles of a bad type, with hoarseness, defluxions and catarrh. The catarrh prevailed also in Barbadoes in the close of this year and beginning of the next, and in New-England was a great death of fish and water fowl.

In 1738 sudden deaths, vertigoes and apoplexies followed the preceding epidemics in England. The plague raged at Ockzakow, at Barbadoes, and in New-Spain the pestilence was so general and mortal, as to threaten the country with depopulation.

In 1739 the small-pox prevailed in New-York, and some dysenteries, but I hear of no remarkable occurrences in this year; except that angina maligna appeared in England in a few sporadic cases, but did not spread at that time; and an infectious fever prevailed at Charleston.
Journals N. York Assembly, vol. 1. 756.
Fothergill, ac. Sore Throat.

A comet was seen in 1739, and the winter following in Europe was the severest known since 1716 or perhaps since 1709. The cold continued till June and was succeeded by a dry season; then a wet, cold autumn. A dearth succeeded in Scotland, and measles spread over America.

In England spread the whooping cough in December 1740. The small-pox prevailed and in 1741 that disease, with the spotted fever were very mortal.
See the London bills of mortality.

In Bristol and Galway, in Ireland, the fevers fell little short of the plague.
Huxham, vol. 2. Short, vol. 2.

It was computed that in 1740 and 41, Ireland lost 80,000 people by famin, dysentery and spotted fever.
Rogers on Epid.

Amsterdam experienced the same pestilential constitution.
See the bills.

Not less remarkable were the seasons in America. In 1740-41, a year later than in Europe, the winter was of the severest kind. Many cattle perished for want of food.
Journals of N. York Assembly, vol. 1. 799, 804.

During this winter measles prevailed in Connecticut. The American plague appeared in Philadelphia and Virginia. In Scotland many perished by famin.
Sinclair's Scot. vol. 6. 433.

Don Ulloa relates an opinion among the Spaniards in South-America, that in 1740, the black vomit was first introduced into Guayaquil by the galleons from the south seas. They aver the disease not to have been known there, anterior to that year. It was most fatal to seamen and foreigners, but the natives did not escape. Here we have a new source of yellow fever!

In 1742 the ulcerous sore throat of a malignant kind appeared in England, and continued to prevail more or less for many years, and in 1745 became very infectious.

See Short, vol 2. and Fothergill's Works.

The summer of 1742 in England was dry.

In America, the same angina prevailed in 1742. From 1740 to 1744 pestilential diseases prevailed in all parts of the known world.

In Syria, the winter of 1741-2 was very severe. In March began an acute fever in Aleppo, attended with a severe pain in the right hypochondrium. The plague had previously shown itself on the sea coast. In April, says Alex. Russel, some reapers brought the infection into the neighbourhood of Aleppo. In the city, no notice was given of the plague, till the 18th of May; but on strict enquiry, it was found that cases had occurred before that time. Whether the "reapers" introduced the fomites into the city, the author does not inform us.

The distemper made no great havoc in this season. It abated in July, and nothing is said about *infection*, till November, when a few more cases occurred. In February 1743 a few cases appeared and in March an alarm was given. It was more general in this year, but disappeared in 1744.

When the disease subsided in Aleppo, it was followed by diarrhœas and dysenteries with petechiæ; and some obstinate intermittents.

In December 1742 and January 1743 were earthquakes with great snows, violent rains and frost.

In 1742 a mortal fever prevailed at Hollifton in Massachusetts, in which died Mr. Stone, the minister and fourteen of his congregation. In this year was seen a comet.

In the spring of 1743; a smart shock of earthquake convulfed Sicily, Naples and Malta. A catarrh prevailed at the same time. These were the precursors of the dreadful plague which raged, in the following summer, at Calabria, Reggio, and especially at Messina in Sicily, where perished 46,000 inhabitants out of 72,000. The summer was violently hot, and dysentery prevailed in other parts of Italy.

At the same time, New-York was severely afflicted by the bilious plague, where died, in one season, 217 of the inhabitants—a considerable number for the population of that day.*

I know not what diseases prevailed in Boston, but the bill for that year shows it to have been sickly.

The year 1743 was distinguished for a tremendous eruption of fire at Cotopaxi, a mountain in the province of Quito, five leagues north of Latacunga; all the neighboring villages were ruined by floods from the melted snows of the mountain. The eruption was repeated in 1744.

Ulloa, vol. 1.

Venice suffered by an inundation in 1743, and the year was remarkable for violent storms, at Boston, Jamaica, and in many countries.

In December 1743 appeared a comet of distinguished magnitude, which was visible till February of the following year. This was probably the same which appeared in 1401, and in both instances attended with pestilence.

In 1744 severe catarrh spread over Europe. It was at Rome in February; at London in March; and in a few weeks pervaded England.

---

* "New-York, Oct. 24, 1743. By the Mayor of the City. An account of persons buried in the city of New-York,

From July 25th to Sept. 25, 1743.		From Sept. 25 to Oct. 22d.	
Children,	51	Children,	16
Grown persons,	114	Grown persons,	36
	165		52
			165
			217

And I do find by the best information I have of the doctors, &c. of this city that the late distemper is now over.

JOHN CRUGER, Mayor."

New-York at that time contained about 7 or 8000 inhabitants.

In June of this year, was an earthquake of confiderable violence in New-England.

In 1745 Lima was fhaken by an earthquake. An infectious fever broke out among the troops employed in the expedition to Louifbourg. A fimilar fever prevailed at Bofton; and how far the health of the town was affected by the returning troops, I am not informed. This was a time of general ficknefs.

In Charlefton prevailed the infectious yellow fever, while Egypt and Smyrna were fuffering the ravages of the plague. The bilious plague prevailed, at the fame time, in New-York.

In this year, the town of Stamford in Connecticut was feverely diftreffed by a malignant dyfentery, which fwept away feventy inhabitants out of a few hundreds. The difeafe was confined to one ftreet.

The year 1746 was probably ftill more unhealthy. An earthquake laid Lima and Calao in ruins. The concuffion began on the 28th of October, about fix hours before the full of the moon; and at intervals, the fhocks were repeated for four months, in which time they amounted to four hundred and fifty. During thefe convulfions, fire burft forth in feveral places of the diftant mountains. Many days before the fhocks began, hollow rumbling noifes were heard in the earth, at times refembling the difcharge of artillery. Similar founds continued for fome time after the earthquake.

See the melancholy tale in Ulloa, vol. 2 83.

Albany was, in this year, vifited by a malignant difeafe called by Colden, a nervous fever; and by Douglas, the yellow fever. From an old citizen, who was living in 1797, my friend Dr. Mitchell obtained the following particulars relative to that difeafe. The bodies of fome of the patients were yellow—the crifis of the difeafe was the ninth day; if the patient furvived that day, he had a good chance for recovery. The difeafe left many in a ftate of imbecility of mind, approaching to childifhnefs or idiocy; others were afterwards troubled with fwelled legs.

The difeafe began in Auguft, ended with froft, and carried off forty five inhabitants moftly men of robuft bodies. It was faid to be imported.

As this was an unusual disease in Albany, ingenuity was occupied to find out its origin. It was *reported* that a like disease prevailed in New-York, and that it had been imported in a vessel from Ireland. Nervous, yellow fever imported from Ireland! Such are the vulgar tales that disgrace this age of science and philosophy. From what fairy land were imported the malignant diseases, which every where swelled the bills of mortality in the same year?—Not that I would insinuate that diseases of a certain kind are not infectious. A pestilential fever originated in the Chebucto fleet, under the Duke D'Anville, which landed an army on our shores in this same year, and one third of the Indians who visited the cantonments, died. There the disease subsided, without becoming epidemic.

But what I severely reprobate is, the disposition of men to trace all the evils of life to a foreign source; when the sources are in their own country, their own houses, and their own bosoms.

A similar disease raged, the same year, among the Mohegan Indians.

See the postscript at the end of the volume.

At Zurich in Switzerland and in Saxony prevailed a very malignant dysentery. Indeed for a number of years, at this period, dysentery was epidemic in many parts of Europe and America.

In 1747 prevailed epidemic catarrh in America and Europe. In the same year the bilious plague prevailed in Philadelphia.—In 1748, in Charleston. The same years were sickly in Boston.

In 1747 appeared a comet, and Etna, which had been quiet more than forty years, commenced her discharges of fire and lava. In the West-Indies, a tremendous hurricane laid waste the Islands.

Two comets appeared in 1748; the winter was severe, and two or three excessively hot and dry summers succeeded. In England the summer of 1747 was very dry. In 1748 a fast was appointed in Massachusetts on account of the drouth.

In England the angina maligna continued its ravages with increased mortality. The same malady prevailed in France in 1749; and there was an earthquake at London. The 18th of

June was a noted hot day, and Mars was as near to the earth as her orbit will permit.
Almanack for 1749.

In 1749 the dysentery and nervous long fever visited many towns in Connecticut with distressing mortality. Waterbury sustained a loss of about 130 of her inhabitants principally by dysentery. Cornwall, then a new settled village, on high mountains, lost twenty of her citizens. Hartford was severely visited with intermittents, for the last time. The summer was very dry, and locusts or grass-hoppers overrun the fields and devoured the herbage.
Douglas, vol. 2 208.

I am authorized to say that the terrible dysentery in Woodbury did not appear to be very contagious—it excited great alarm; every one avoided the sick, if possible; but many who lived remote and never came near the sick, were seized, and suddenly died.[†]

In 1749 and 50 the dysentery, according to Zimmerman, made great havoc in the Canton of Berne It is remarkable that this formidable disease should be thus prevalent in both hemispheres at the same time, and for a series of years. About this time measles prevailed in America.

In 1750 appeared a comet, and the summer was excessively hot. In Philadelphia, the heat raised the mercury to 100 deg. by Farenheit. The plague carried off 30,000 people in Fez, and one third of the inhabitants of Tangiers.

Violent tempests marked this year, in America, and an unusual swell of the Severn in England. Earthquakes happened in England, Jamaica, Peru, Leghorn, Rome, Sicily and Lapland.

At Beauvais, 50 miles from Paris, broke out a pestilential disease, called la Suete, resembling the sweating sickness, terminating fatally in three days.
See Gent Magazine.

At Bethlem in Connecticut raged a mortal fever, which swept away between thirty and forty of the inhabitants. The exciting cause was supposed to be the exhalations from a swamp which

[†] M S. letter from Z. Bears.

had been drained. It is not improbable that this might have aided the general principles of disease.

Med Repos' vol 1 p 523.

The winter of 1750-51 is mentioned as extremely severe in America Vesuvius discharged fire and lava, in 1751, and on the 7th of March, a most dreadful tempest at Nantz in France, destroyed 66 ships, with 800 lives. On the same day, a tempest at Jamaica did damage to the amount of a million of dollars. A storm at Cadiz on the 8th of December destroyed 100 sail of shipping. On the Adriatic coast was an earthquake.

In this year Constantinople lost 200,000 inhabitants by the plague.—The preceding winter was cold in Turkey, and the old people predicted a severe plague from the quantity of snow that fell in Constantinople. This prediction was founded on long observation; and I am able to confirm the justness of it, by discovering that those years which produce the most violent action or discharges of electrical fire, generate most snow, hail and cold.

Chenier's Morocco vol. 2. 275.

In America the spring flights of pigeons were unusually large. The dysentery was epidemic and mortal, in the same year, at Hartford and New-Haven; probably in many other places.—With this fatal dysentery prevailed a mortal angina for several years. The same concurrence of these diseases will be mentioned under the year 1775.

In England, the summer of 1751 was cold and wet; and a mortal distemper prevailed among horses and cattle, in most parts of the country. In Cheshire died 30,000 cows. In Glasgow the seasons were very sickly.

Gent Magazine.

Great and uncommon inundations occurred in the same year, in France, England and Scotland. In Cork the water was three feet deep in the midst of the city.

The dysentery and ulcerous sore throat were very fatal, this year in Guilford.

In 1752 the summer in South-Carolina, and probably in all parts of America, was distinguished for intense heat. The thermometer, for nearly twenty days successively, varied between

90 and 101.—The effects of this heat were visible in a number of sudden deaths by apoplexies. There were some cases of bad fever, but no epidemic. In September a violent tempest laid the city under water. The dysentery was still prevalent in the northern parts of America.

Museum, vol 3 316 and sequel. Dr Chalmers.

In Ireland prevailed angina of such a malignant type, as to kill the patient sometimes in eight or ten hours. See Rutty on weather. The plague raged in the East.

An Reg. 1766 100.

In this year Adrianople was nearly destroyed by an earthquake. In Hinsdale, on Connecticut river, in the state of New-Hampshire, was an eruption of fire from a volcanic mountain, called west river mountain.

Mem Am Acad. vol 1. 316.

In America the winter of 1752-3 was long and severe.

I have no account of any general epidemic in 1753; but particular places were visited with distressing sickness. A singular instance of a local pestilence occasioned by vapor deserves to be related.

In autumn 1753 after a dry season, arose in Rouen, the chief city of Normandy, a thick fog, with the smell of sulphur, which increased to that degree, that in the evening, lights could not be distinguished at any considerable distance. It did not wholly disappear, till the next day. It was more dense in some streets than in others.

In three or four days after, began an epidemic sickness which seized both sexes, with chills, lassitude, loss of appetite, slight pains in the arms and legs. These symptoms were followed by bilious loosenefs, nausea and vomitings. Most patients bled at the nose, frequently in small quantity. The head-ache then became violent, with a small, hard pulse—a high fever followed. The region of the stomach and hypochondria was tumefied; this symptom was succeeded by a tension of the belly—and a slight delirium followed. The tongue was brown or black, but moist; sometimes with green ulcers or apthæ. The patient died the 5th, 7th, or 11th day; but not in every case. Some were thirty, or forty days in recovery; many were left with a puffiness of the face, hands and legs.

In some other parts of France appeared peripneumony and inflammation of the pericordium, which was called a new difeafe.
Phil Tranf vol 49.

In December 1753 and January fucceeding, the finall town of Hollifton, in Maffachufetts, loft forty-three of its citizens, by a fever. The difeafe began with a violent pain in the breaft, or fide, not often in the head; then fucceeded a high fever, but without delirium. The critical days were the 3d, 4th, 5th, or 6th. Some of the patients appeared to be ftrangled to death. The town contained no more than 80 families.
Hift Collections, vol. 3 19.

The winter of 1753-4 in Europe was very cold. In 1754 was a great eruption of Vefuvius which lafted feveral weeks, and violent earthquakes in England, Conftantinople, and Amboyna, in the Eaftern Ocean. The heavens appeared to be in a flame, and Egypt, which rarely feels earthquakes, was feverely fhaken, and 40,000 of the inhabitants of Cairo, perifhed in the ruins of two thirds of the city.

The gangrenous fore throat was very mortal in Ireland, and prevalent in England. See Rutty on weather. The fame fpecies of angina was, at the fame time, very fatal in America.
See Belknap's Hift. N Hampfhire, vol. 2. 121

In Maryland, the earth was deluged with exceffive rains, and intermittents were unufually obftinate.
Gent Mag 1755

At this time there were two or three very mild winters in America. In 1754-5 and 1755-6 floops failed from New-York for Albany in January and February. Smith's Hift. N. York, 82. In this inftance, America is an exception to the general rule, that fevere winters extend over both hemifpheres, about the time of great volcanic eruptions. The feverity was limited to the other continent.

The year 1755 was remarkable for violent earthquakes, and volcanic eruptions from Etna and the mountains in Iceland. In April, Quito in South-America was demolifhed.

Portugal had fuffered for three or four years, moft exceffive drouth, by which all springs were exhausted. But the year 1755 was rainy. On the first of November, a tremendous convulsion laid Lisbon in ruins, with the destruction of 50,000 lives. This shock was felt on the whole Spanish coast, and 10,000 people perished on one of the Azores. In Mitelene, an island in the Archipelago, 2000 houses were destroyed. The day preceding this concussion was remarkable for a haze or vapor that obscured the sun.

On the 18th of November, America sustained a violent and extensive shock; but its effects were not very calamitous. The fish in the ocean did not escape without injury. Two or three whales, and multitudes of cod were seen, a few days after, floating on the surface of the water.

In the remarkable year 1755, the most prevalent epidemics seem to have been angina maligna, and catarrh, which spread over France and England. The angina maligna was very mortal in some parts of America. In one town on Long-Island, two children only, under twelve years of age, survived.

M S of Mr. Reeve.

In this year also prevailed a petechial fever in Ireland, and according to Baron de Tott, Constantinople lost 150,000 inhabitants by the plague.

See his Memoirs, Fothergill on fore throat
and Rutty on weather

The winter of 1756-7 in Syria was excessively severe; the fruits were destroyed, olive-trees, which had withstood the weather for fifty years, were killed, and thousands of poor people perished with cold.

Lon Mag. 1764.

In the following summer, crops failed, a dearth ensued, and so severe a famin that parents devoured their own children; the poor from the mountains offered their wives for sale in market, to procure food.

Ibim.

This winter was also very severe in Europe. In 1756 appeared a comet and there was an eruption in Iceland. A meteor was seen in France, and earthquakes were experienced in various places.

In 1756-57 the catarrh was very prevalent in America, followed by an earthquake in July. This catarrh preceded the same epidemic in Europe by one year.

In 1758 catarrh spread over Europe, and the plague began to show itself in Egypt and Smyrna. In November, a large meteor was seen in Great Britain, and is described by Sir John Pringle in the Philofophical Transactions.* In this year also, the petechial fever, the precursor of the plague, began to show itself, in Aleppo.—The summer in America was extremely hot.

Letter of Gov Ellis, Museum, vol 5 151

In 1759 appeared two or three comets; and in November a most tremendous eruption of Vesuvius. In August was an earthquake at Bourdeaux—and one at Bruffels. The winter following 1759 was exceffively cold in both hemifpheres. In Leipfic, centinels froze to death; and in South Carolina, the fnow covered the earth to the depth of nearly two feet. In England, the cold was lefs fevere.

The year 1759 was memorable for violent earthquakes, in Syria. Buildings were demolifhed and Damafcus was buried in ruins. The fhocks were repeated for many weeks. In November, Truxillo in Peru was fwallowed up by means of an earthquake. It will be obferved that this happened in the month, when Vefuvius was in eruption. Thefe great phenomena announced a general and fevere peftilence, and the effects of the general principles of difeafe were foon felt over Europe, Afia and America. Annual Regifter, 1761. 96 and paffim. The earthquakes in Syria were preceded by drouth and followed by exceffive rains.

See Ruffel on the plague at Aleppo and Velney's Travels.

In 1759 the plague began to appear in Cyprus, and at Acre and Latakia on the Syrian coaft. In Copenhagen raged fmall-pox with great mortality.

In New-England were fhocks of earthquake in February, at Bofton and Portfmouth. An. Regif. 1759. 88. In Autumn an unufual tempeft and tide at Nova Scotia.

---

* Seen from Dublin, it moved from fouth to north. Annual regifter, 1759 58.

In America, cotemporary with the commencement of the plague in Egypt, appeared the measles, in 1758, and the year 1759 appears, by the American bills of mortality, to have been very unhealthy. The predominant diseases were the measles and dysentery. M. S. letter from Dr. Betts of Norwalk. The measles appeared in 1758, but was most extensive in 1759. This is an instance of the prevalence of dysentery and measles in the same year.

In this year also the scurvy, an endemical disease in Canada, was unusually mortal.

Lind, p. 26.

At Bombay, a meteor of extraordinary brightness was seen on the 4th of April, 1759.

After the severe winter of 1759-60, happened in America, a snow storm on the 3d of May, when the apple-trees were in blossom. The disposition of the elements to generate snow and hail, during pestilential periods, has already been remarked. M. S. of Mr. Whitman. The spring of 1760 in America was very dry.

In 1760 earthquakes were repeated in Syria, and the plague appeared at Aleppo, Jerusalem and Damascus. It continued to extend and increase, until the summer of 1762; after which it declined. In Holland and Belgium were small shocks of earthquake—preceded by flashes of light. Annual Register 1760. 70. Russel on the plague at Aleppo. Indeed earthquakes were felt in most parts of Europe.

Cyprus, which had been free from pestilence for 30 years preceding, lost 20,000 inhabitants by the malady. On the first appearance of the plague in Egypt, the magistracy published an ordinance to prevent the introduction of the disease by infection; but it was of no use. The disease was preceded, as usual, by a petechial fever.

Mariti's Travels.

In England, the summer of 1760 was dry and autumn wet. In this year occurred another discharge from Vesuvius.—A comet was seen in January, and a distemper made great havoc among horses in and about London. Annual Register 1760, 67. Immense damage was sustained by tempests. Ibm. 73.

The principles of difeafe in 1760 began to exhibit themfelves in the Weft-Indies, and the ordinary fever of the climate affumed new and malignant fymptoms, with contagion.

Lind, p. 126.

In this year alfo the northern parts of the American continent, which had been overrun by meafles, began to feel more feverely the violence of the epidemic conftitution.

In November, the town of Bethlem was affailed by an inflammatory fever, with fymptoms of typhus, which in the courfe of the following winter, carried off about 40 of the inhabitants. The difeafe was extremely violent, terminating on the 3d or 4th day; in fome cafes, the patient died within 24 hours of the attack. It feems to have been that fpecies of winter fever, which occurs in peftilential periods, mentioned under the year 1698. During this epidemic, a flock of quails flew over the chimney of a houfe, in which were feveral difeafed perfons, and five of them fell dead on the fpot. This was thought ominous; but was a natural event, which may rationally be afcribed to deleterious gas emitted from the chambers of the fick.

Med Repof vol 1 524.

This difeafe was afcribed to the draining of the pond or fwamp, mentioned under the year 1750. But to this explanation, there are ftrong, if not infuperable objections.

Firft. The fever began in November; but this is the month when the marfh fevers of our climate difappear. I doubt whether the effluvia from marfhes ever act upon the human body, fo as to produce difeafe, without a greater degree of heat than Connecticut ever experiences in the month of November. Cold puts an end to all marfh fevers, but this difeafe continued to increafe in December, and did not ceafe till late in the winter.

Secondly. This difeafe was called a malignant pleurify; but marfh effluvia are not known to produce fevers of that defcription. They are common on high, as well as on low grounds, as I can prove by facts in America.

Thirdly. There is no neceffity of reforting to marfh exhalations for the fource of this malady. The fame fpecies of fever prevailed in that winter and the fpring following, in many other parts of Connecticut, where no marfh exifted. In Hartford it carried off a number of robuſt men, in two or three days from the attack.* In North-Haven it attacked few perſons, but every one of them died. In Eaſt-Haven died about forty-five men in the prime of life, moſtly heads of families. The ſame diſeaſe prevailed in New-Haven among the inhabitants, and ſtudents in college.

It is obvious then that this was an epidemic, very well known in ſickly periods, and not dependent on local cauſes. From Dr. Trumbull of North-Haven I have the following remarks on the diſeaſe.

The blood was very thick and ſizy; often iſſuing from the noſe and ſometimes from the eyes. The inflammation was violent, and ſoon produced delirium. The moſt róbuſt bodies were moſt liable to the diſeaſe. A free uſe of the lancet, in the early ſtages of the diſorder, was the only effectual remedy; where the phyſicians were afraid to bleed, the patients all died.† This malady prevailed from November 1760 to March 1761.

I cannot learn that this ſpecies of inflammatory fever, has ever been epidemic in the northern parts of America, ſince this period. But it is a common winter fever, in the Carolinas, after ſickly ſummers; and in the northern ſtates, ſporadic caſes of it occur with all its formidable ſymptoms. Inſtances will be hereafter mentioned. It is the peſtilence of winter, and rarely, if ever appears, except when peſtilential epidemics are current in ſummer. And I am not without ſuſpicions that the debility occaſioned by marſh effluvia in ſummer may prediſpoſe the ſyſtem to that fever in winter, tho not neceſſary to produce it.

In March 1761 was a ſmall ſhock of earthquake in New-England, and the ſame occurred in Iceland, Hamburg, Syria, England and South-America.

* One of them was my paternal uncle.
† Dr. Hugh Williamſon, in the ſecond volume of the Medical Repoſitory, has deſcribed this ſpecies of diſeaſe, which, he ſays, prevails often in Carolina in winter, eſpecially among thoſe who have been affected by bilious fevers in the preceding autumn. He obſerves that bleeding is uſually pernicious in that diſeaſe. Perhaps a difference of climates may make different remedies neceſſary. But in different periods, the ſame diſeaſe may require different treatment. In New-England, that fever has uſually demanded an early uſe of the lancet.

In the winter and spring of 1761 a severe influenza attacked the northern parts of America. In Bethlem it was cotemporary with the fever just mentioned. In Philadelphia it prevailed in the winter, and in Massachusetts, in April. From Dr. Tufts, a respectable practitioner of medicin in Weymouth, I have the following description of the disease.

"The distemper began in April, and in May ran into a malignant fever, which proved fatal to aged people. It spread over the whole country and the West-India islands. It began with a severe pain in the head and limbs, a sensation of coldness, shiverings succeeded by great heat, running at the nose, and a troublesome cough. It continued for eight or ten days, and generally terminated by sweating.

In May, the aged who had before escaped, were seized with an affection like a slight cold; this, in a day or two was followed by great prostration of strength, a cough, labor of breathing, pains about the breast, præcordia, and in the limbs, but not acute. The countenance betrayed no great marks of febrile heat. The matter expectorated was thin, but slimy. As the disease advanced, the difficulty of breathing encreased; the expectoration was more difficult; the matter thrown off more viscid; at length the lungs appeared to be so loaded with tenacious matter, that no efforts could dislodge it, and the patient sunk under it.

This disorder carried with it bilious appearances—the countenances of some patients were of a yellowish hue. In some, there was an appearance of indifference or insensibility; and at night, a slight delirium."

M S. letter from Dr Tufts

In the spring of 1761 earthquakes were felt in many parts of Europe See an account of them in An. Register, 1761 92. Shocks also were felt in the Azores and West-Indies. These agitations were precisely cotemporary with the epidemic catarrh in America. Scarcely any country escaped the convulsions of nature. During the pestilence in Thessalonica, shocks were felt almost every day. Ibm.

In the summer of 1761, I am informed, the infectious bilious fever prevailed in Charleston, but I am not possessed of the details.

In May happened a most extraordinary typhon or whirlwind, which swept Afhly river to its bottom. Five vessels were sunk and eleven dismasted. Annual Register, 1761. 93. In Italy a woman was killed by a sudden eruption of vapor under her feet Ibm. 95. The summer in America was very dry.

In the spring of 1762 the influenza was epidemic in Europe. It appeared at Edinburgh in April in a few cases; at Dublin in May; and in June was general and severe. It was therefore a year later than in America.

Essays and Obs Edinburgh. Rutty on weather An Reg 1762.

In March was an earthquake in Ireland, and in autumn a considerable shock in Spain. On the 11th of June was seen a meteor, passing from north to south, which met a dark cloud and exploded. Another as large as the moon, and bright as the sun descended slowly on the 4th of December, and dissipated.

Annual Register, 1762.

In 1762 appeared a comet, and in America the heat and drouth exceeded what was ever before known From June to September 22d, there was scarcely a drop of rain, almost all springs were exhausted, and the distress occasioned by the want of water was extreme. The forest trees appeared as if scorched.

The winter following was equally remarkable for severity, both in Europe and America. The Thames was a common highway for carriages, and the poor perished in the streets of London.

Lond Mag. 1763 Annual Register, 1762.

In America the snow fell on the 8th of November and continued till about the 20th of March. These extraordinary phenomena were followed by an eruption of Etna in 1763, of three months continuance.

In the extremely hot summer of 1762, the bilious plague prevailed in Philadelphia. The same disease swept away most of the troops in the expedition to Havanna. The plague raged in Constantinople and in Syria; while the yellow fever spread mortality in Bengal.

In this year the plague in Aleppo came to its crisis. In 1760, died about 500 persons; in 1761, 7000, and in 1762, 11000; after which year it subsided.

See Patrick Russel, Hist. of that plague.

The bills of mortality will best show how severely the principles of disease were felt in London, Amsterdam and Dublin in 1762 and 3.

No part of the earth seems to have escaped a share of unusual mortality in the period between 1759 and 1763. In the latter year, the bilious plague in Bengal carried off 800 Europeans and 30,000 natives. Lind, p. 82. In the year preceding, a violent earthquake occurred at Chitacong in the territories of Bengal.
An. Reg. 1763. 60.

On the 19th of October 1762, happened a remarkably dark day at Detroit, and the vicinity. While at dinner, the inhabitants found it necessary to use candles. The darkness continued, with little interruption, during the whole day.
Phil. Transf. vol. 53. p. 63. Mem. Amer. Acad. vol. 1. 244.

During this pestilential period, fatal diseases carried off the cattle on the continent of Europe, and Toulon lost one third of its inhabitants by an epidemic.
An. Regist. 1761. 161.

The summer of 1763 was a moist and unkindly season. In August the Indians on Nantucket were attacked by the bilious plague, and between that time and February following, their number was reduced from 358 to 136. Of 258 who were affected, 36 only recovered. The disease began with high fever and ended in typhus, in about five days. It appeared to be infectious among the Indians only; for no whites were attacked, altho they associated freely with the diseased. Persons of a mixed blood were attacked, but recovered. Not one died, except of full Indian blood. Some Indians who lived in the families of the whites, escaped the disease; as did a few that lived by themselves on a distant part of the island. I am informed, by respectable authority, that a similar fever attacked Indians on board of ships, at a distance of hundreds of leagues, without any connection with Nantucket.

In December of the same year, the Indians on Martha's Vineyard, distant eight leagues from Nantucket, were invaded by a like fever; not a family escaped, and of 52 patients, 39 died.

In this instance, disease discriminated as nicely between the Whites and Indians, as in 1797, it did between men and cats;

and as exactly as the plague in Egypt, between the Ifraelites and Egyptians.

Some fufpicions were fuggefted that the difeafe at Nantucket might have been received from a fhip which put in there, with fick paffengers, from Ireland bound to New-York ; but there is no foundation for this opinion, as the diforder broke out before the arrival of the fhip.

See Phil Trans and Lond Mag 1764. Hift Collections, vol 3. 158 M S. of Mofes Brown.

In 1764, juft after this fatal peftilence among the Indians, a large fpecies of fifh, called *blue fifh*, thirty of which would fill a barrel, and which were before caught in great numbers, on every fide of Nantucket, fuddenly difappeared, to the great lofs of the Inhabitants —Whether they perifhed or migrated, is not known.

Hift. Col 3 158.

In Europe, the year 1763 was remarkable for difeafes among various fpecies of animals. In Denmark, an epidemic catarrhal diforder affected horfes. In Madrid, a peftilence among dogs fwept away multitudes—900 died in one day. In Genoa, the poultry perifhed in a fimilar manner. In Italy, horfes and fwine fell victims to the peftilential principle. In France, horfes and mules, in Sweden, fheep, horfes and horned cattle perifhed under the influence of the general caufe.

Rutty on Weather.

The fummer was remarkable for hail ftorms, one of which totally ruined 36 villages in Maconnois in France. See the account of thefe and of the earthquakes in that year in An. Regif. Chronicle. Hail ftones fell of fizes from three to ten inches in circumference. Thefe ftorms were numerous and many fire balls fell in various parts of England and a globe of fire was feen in Sweden

Thefe hail ftorms occurred during or near the time of the eruption of Etna. In 1764 was another eruption of Etna. In moft parts of Europe and America, this period of peftilence appears to have clofed with the years 1762 and 3. But in Naples fpread a malignant fever in 1764, preceded by famin, by which difeafe it was fuppofed 200,000 people perifhed. The difeafe was marked by petechiæ and glandular tumors and was a mild species of plague. The season was excessively hot, and the bilious plague prevailed in Cadiz. Lind, 189. 122. An earthquake occured in Portugal and Siberia. In the February following occured a degree of cold, rarely known in England. The mercury in Farenheit fell to 7 deg. and in one place, within the ball. An. Reg. 1765-66. A remarkable high tide in China in May swept away a whole city. The cause is not mentioned.

Ibim. 92.

To the epidemics above mentioned, succeeded a series of dysenteries, in the hot summers of 1765 and 6. In 1765, the malignant dysentery raged in Berne and other parts of Switzerland, in Suabia and Austria. The invasion was, in many cases sudden, says Zimmerman, without any preceding symptom; but more generally its approach was indicated by chills, lassitude and other premonitory signs. In its progress, it exhibited most of the symptoms of the yellow fever of America. It was preceded by a putrid fever, which yielded to the dysentery in June.

See Zimmerman on Dysentery.

This epidemic was followed by violent and malignant pleurisies; a circumstance that marks its alliance with the pestilential fever of America, and probably of all temperate climates, which is also succeeded by pleurisy or peripneumony in winter.

In 1765 were many earthquakes in Italy, and Sweden, and a volcanic eruption at Truxillo in Spanish America. Dysentery prevailed in Scotland, and intermittents in Pennsylvania and Georgia, were universal.

In 1766 the summer was every where hot and in Europe excessively dry. In Germany, the Rhine was lower than in the terrible drouth of 1476, and in many places, was forded. In Scotland, the people were compelled to kill their cattle for want of fodder. The heat and drouth produced great hail storms, and in autumn, were followed by inundations, one of which at Montauban, in France, swept away 1200 houses. Terrible tempests marked the year, and in the West-Indies, those hurricanes which lay the islands waste, and are recorded among the memorabilia of the climate. In August, the planet Mars was nearer to the earth, by two millions of miles, than it had been for many ages, and in the spring appeared a comet.

The winter preceding this remarkable summer, was extremely cold in Europe. At Ratisbon, Reaumur's thermometer was two degrees lower, than in the noted year 1709, and birds perished with cold. At Naples, the snow lay in the streets, to the depth of 18 inches, and Vesuvius began to discharge smoke, the harbinger of an explosion. At Lisbon, Reaumur's thermometer was 3¹ degrees below the freezing point, and at Madrid, people skated on the ice.

These remarkable phenomena preceded and attended a general discharge of fire and lava, from the three well known volcanoes, Etna, Vesuvius and Heckla, which took place in 1766. This is one of the few instances on record, in which these volcanoes have been in eruption, nearly at the same time. The eruption of Heckla continued from April to September. These phenomena account for the excessive drouth in Europe.

See Sinclair's Scotland   Annual Reg.ster, 1766.

In this year 1766 was an earthquake in New-England, and a violent shock at Constantinople. Vegetation failed in some parts of Europe and America, and grain was very scarce in Italy, Great-Britain and the Carolinas. In 1767 a million sterling was paid in England for imported grain.

An. Reg 1768 p. 101.*

The winter of 1765-6 was not severe in America and there was little snow; but in this remarkable period, as in many others, the severity of the seasons commenced in Europe one year before it did in America. The winter of 1766-7 was terribly severe in both hemispheres. The cold was as intense as in 1740; the Rhine at Cologne became a bridge of ice, and supported laboring artificers, as in 1670. In Italy, the poor crouded to the cities for aid, and perished with cold. In Russia, both rich and poor perished. The wolves became ravenous, entered towns and destroyed people. In England, the larks took refuge in hay-carts and the market; the snow fell to the depth of many feet and buried thousands of sheep. In America, the cold was

---

* I am struck with surprise to observe how universally crops fail, about the time of great volcanic eruptions,

very severe, and at Brandywine, the mercury fell in Farenheit to 20 deg. below cypher—an unexampled degree of cold in that latitude. In January happened a thaw, which broke up the rivers in Connecticut, and left scarcely a bridge over the rivers. The cold in France in 1767-8 was more severe than in 1740 and within a degree of that in 1709. In Constantinople snow and hail fell as late as March 16.

See An. Regis. 1767. p. 52, 53, 54, 76. 1768. p. 58, 101.

Every thing indicated uncommon agitations in the elements. Pages would be necessary to enumerate the tempests and hail storms of these years. In January 1769 fell two fire balls in England; one of them on Tower hill. At Amiens, a man his wife and his horses were killed by a discharge of subterraneous vapor. A violent storm in Virginia on the 11th of September tore up trees, stranded ships and demolished houses; Bagdadt was almost ruined by an earthquake, and Cuba was desolated by a hurricane in 1768. An. Register, 1769. 67. 146. These last years in England were rainy.

In 1767 epidemic catarrh prevailed in Europe, and diseases among horses in New-England and New-Jersey. The summer was remarkable for hail storms; Cephalonia was ruined by an earthquake, and Vesuvius, from this year to 1777 never ceased to discharge smoke, and frequently scoriæ, stones and cinders.

An. Reg. 1767. 142, 151. Encyclop. art. Vesuvius.

In 1768 vast multitudes of caterpillars devoured the grass in the fields at Northampton, in Massachusetts.

The summer of 1768 was hot, but I have no account of the diseases in America in this and the preceding year, except of a disorder in the head and throat among horses.

Mem. Am. Acad. vol. 1. 529.

In 1769 the summer was very hot, and in autumn appeared a comet with a vast coma. Venus passed over the Sun's disk on the 3d of June; there was a small earthquake in New-England and a great tempest. Among the diseases in America is mentioned a fatal angina in Boston, and other towns, but I am not furnished with its history. The same distemper prevailed in 1770, and in Jamaica occasioned considerable mortality.

Museum, vol. 1. 35, 430.

In Holland 32,000 cattle perished by a pestilential distemper. An. Reg. 1769. 166. Great sickness prevailed at Rome. Ibm. In America some cases of canine madness were observed. The measles prevailed in America, but I have no details of its origin and progress. The dysentery was epidemic and fatal in 1769.

In July 1770 appeared also a comet. There was an eruption of Vesuvius in 1770, and another in 1771. Flames issued from Heckla in 1771 and 72, but no lava. An earthquake was felt in New-England in 1771, and Italy was repeatedly shaken. On the 17th of July was seen a meteor or fire ball.

These two years were distinguished by the most terrible earthquakes, storms, rains and inundations, accounts of which fill the gazettes of those years. In 1770 the floods in England, Holland and France exceeded any that could be recollected. In France the vintage was greatly injured. In 1771 the territory of Honduras was wasted by locusts and famin.

An. Reg p 163.

In 1771 great rains continued to occasion floods. In Virginia, a flood in the Rappahannock filled the warehouses and ruined the tobacco, which occasioned public prayers to be ordered. Similar inundations happened in Germany.

There were earthquakes in Hispaniola, St. Maure, England, and in Ternate, a Molucca island, where was an eruption of fire.

Gent. Magazine An Regis. 1770, passim 1771. 120.

In 1771 a mortal distemper swept away great numbers of foxes in America.

Mem Am. Acad. vol. 1. 529.

In Italy the harvest failed, and in Sardinia, Holland, Flanders, and some parts of England, the cattle were swept away by an infectious disease. The number of cattle that perished in Holland, was stated, in Sept. 1771, to amount to 171,780.

An. Regis. 1771 147.

In Constantinople raged the plague in 1770; and one thousand bodies were, for some time, buried daily. In 1771 this malady prevailed in Poland and Russia, and 200,000 people perished. The number that died in the Russian dominions was 62,000.

An. Regis. 1772. 155.

In the East-Indies the disorders in the elements at this period produced still more deplorable effects. The excessive heat and want of rain, which usually precede or attend the approximation of comets and volcanic eruptions, occasion a failure of crops in countries, where the grain which is the principal food of the inhabitants, depends on water from inundation. Such is the fact in India and in Egypt, where rice is the great article of food.

The heat and drouth of 1769 cut short the rice crops in the territories of the Ganges The consequence was a famin, which, in 1770, destroyed incredible numbers of the natives. The streets were filled with dead carcases, and such numbers were thrown into the river, as to render the water and the fish unfit for use.

In 1771 disease was added to the calamities of the miserable inhabitants, a million of whom were supposed to perish by the bilious plague.

See Encyclopedia, Art Bengal.

In 1770 the atmosphere at Calcutta was filled and clouded with flies of a large kind, which never descended to the earth, but came so near that they could be distinguished with glasses. It is remarkable that the appearance of these animals was cotemporary with the millions of worms which overran the northern districts of America. Encyclop. Article Bengal. The Bramins mentioned that a similar phenomenon occurred about 150 years before, which must have been during the pestilence among the Indians in America from 1618 to 1622. At this time also began a disease among the potatoes in Scotland, which has been gradually extending itself to this time. The leaves contract and shrivel; and just below the surface of the earth, there appears on the stalk a scar of some length, or groove corroded through the rind, of the color of ocher. The fruit on the roots is small and of an unpleasant taste.

Sinclair's, Scot. 2. 187.

In 1771 anginas, in some parts of America, occasioned a considerable mortality.

Register of deaths in New-Haven.

Catarrh prevailed in 1771, but was epidemic in America in 1772. The winter of 1771-2 was very severe in Europe. In

America the month of March 1772 was diſtinguiſhed for great falls of ſnow, beyond what was ever before known. In Bohemia, it was computed that 168,000 perſons periſhed in that year by epidemic diſeaſes. An. Reg. 152. A tempeſt in China deſtroyed 150,000 lives in Canton River.

An. Reg. 1773. p. 102

In 1770, cotemporary with the clouds of flies in India and a moſt fatal peſtilence among men and cattle in Europe, appeared in America a black worm about one inch and a half in length, which devoured the graſs and corn. Never was a more ſingular phenomenon. Theſe animals were generated ſuddenly in the northern ſtates of America, and almoſt covered two or three hundred miles of country. They all moved nearly in one direction, and when they were intercepted by furrows, in plowed land, they fell into them in ſuch numbers as to form heaps. They ſought ſhelter in the graſs, a hot ſun being fatal to them. They diſappeared ſuddenly about the cloſe of June and beginning of July.

New-England Farmer, Art. Inſect.

This ſpecies of worm has been ſeen at other times, and in 1791, in great multitudes. No account can be given of their origin and they ſeem not to have regular periods of return. In July 1791, the late governor Huntington, a gentleman of careful obſervation, informed me, he had expoſed ſome of theſe animals to a hot ſun on a dry board, and in a few hours, found them diſſolved into mere water. They ſeem to be generated by ſome elementary proceſs, and to be the harbingers of peſtilence; at leaſt they have preceded diſeaſes in America.

In February 1772 prevailed in America epidemic catarrh.

M S letter from Dr. Tufts

In this year, the meaſles appeared in all parts of America, with unuſual mortality. In Charleſton, S. Carolina, died 8 or 900 children.

Public prints, Oct. 1772.

A mortal fever prevailed alſo in Wellfleet on Cape-Cod, which proved fatal to forty of its inhabitants. Hiſt. Col. vol. 3. 118. The mortality in Bohemia has been mentioned, and the ſickneſs in London appears by the bill of mortality.

This year, 1772, was distinguished for a great hurricane in the West-Indies, like those of 1766 and 1780.

An. Reg. 1772. 140

The anginas of the preceding year continued to prevail in 1772.

The winter of 1772-3 was moderate in England, but on the continent more severe. In February, occurred in America, a remarkable day, still known by the name of the cold Sunday.

This year, 1773, was in general sickly. In America, the measles finished its course and was followed by disorders in the throat. After the measles left the patient, came on a secondary fever, which, in some cases, proved fatal. Those who survived, lay ill a long time, troubled with an excessive expectoration. It seemed as if the patient discharged the amount of his weight.

But the most mortal disease, was, the cynanche trachealis or bladder in the throat. In general, there was little canker, but an extreme difficulty of breathing; the patient being nearly suffocated with a tough mucus or slime, which no medicin could attenuate of discharge, and which finally proved fatal. All medical aid was fruitless, and scarcely a child that was attacked in some towns, survived.

This disease was speedily followed, in some places by the dysentery of a peculiarly malignant type, occasioning mortification on the third day. This disease was prevalent and very fatal in New-Haven and East-Haven, in Connecticut, and in Salem, Massachusetts.

M S. letters from Dr. Trumbull and Dr Holyoke.

In Philadelphia, the measles appeared in March, attended with efflorescence about the neck; at the same time, catarrh which could hardly be distinguished from the measles.

Rush's Works, vol. 2. 238.

Cotemporary with these diseases in America, were the small-pox and a fatal fever in some parts of Scotland, and a plague which carried off 80,000 people in Bassora, a town in Persia, near the Euphrates.

In this year, an earthquake sunk the town of Guatimala in New-Spain.

The year 1774 was more healthy than the preceding; but the scarlatina anginosa began to show itself in Edinburgh, and in some parts of America, especially at Philadelphia. On the 4th of May was a fall of snow.

Rush, vol. 1 94, and the British Med Publications in that year.

The winter of 1774-5 began on the continent of Europe with unusual severity. The rivers in Germany were frozen, early in December, and there was deep snow at Bologna in Italy in October. But in England, the winter was not severe—an instance which is sometimes observed in both hemispheres, that cold and falls of snow run in veins.*

An. Register, 1775. 87. and 1774 173.

In 1775 happened a great eruption of fire from a volcano in Guatimala. An. Reg. 136. The summer was remarkable for thunder and lightning.

A halo and mock suns were observed in England, and a meteor in America. In Sweden and England, the summer was dry. In Holland happened a great tempest and high tide, Nov. 14th.

An Register, 172.

In 1775 prevailed in England epidemic catarrh, preceded by mild serene weather.

In America prevailed cynanche maligna, with considerable mortality. It seems to have invaded all the northern parts of America, and in many places it continued to be current with dysentery for three years. This was the case in Middletown on Connecticut river. In other places, it disappeared in the winter following.

M. S letter from Dr. Betts.
Registers of the first society in Middletown.

This pestilential period seems to have commenced with the great agitations of the elements in 1769 and 70, and to have been first displayed in the drouth and famin in India, the plague in Turkey, and the insects and distempers among cattle in Europe and America; to which may be added anginas. The process was marked by a comet, volcanic eruptions, earthquakes and tempests, with measles, influenza and angina, and a series of most fatal dysentery closed the period.

* A remarkable instance has happened, the last winter, 1798-9—the weather being very cold, with immense quantities of snow from the Atlantic to the mountains, but very mild in Canada and the western country, until the close of winter.

In 1775 an eruption of water took place from mount Etna, and Lipari, a neighboring island, discharged fire.

Encyclopedia, art. Volcano and Lipari.

In this year began or very much increased the mildew of oats in Montquitter in Scotland. About the beginning or middle of August, the plant assumes a fiery red color; then black spots burst forth near the roots, and ascend to the fibers that support the ear; circulation then ceases, and the grain advances no further in maturity. Sometimes it yields a little fruit; at other times none. This disease of the oats still continues to be very injurious to the parish; but in 1789, a year of unusual commotion in the elements in the north of Europe, as will hereafter be related, it spread to a greater extent than was ever before known. This phenomenon has been a subject of great research among farmers and philosophic men; but no satisfactory cause has yet been discovered.

Sinclair's Stat. Acc. of Scotland, vol. 6. 131.

It is remarkable that the prim in America began to decay and perish about this period; and near the same time, the wheat insect first appeared on Long-Island.

I would just observe that the disease among the oats, and the death of the prim, with the wheat insect, may be new phenomena in the natural world; or certain revolutions which unusual causes may have induced in animal and vegetable life.

About this time, for the year is not recollected, there was an eruption of fire at Derby, in Connecticut, a few rods from Naugatuck river; the only instance ever known in that place. It happened on a steep bank where it made a large excavation in the earth, throwing trees and stones to some distance. A light was seen on the spot in the evening before the explosion. It was accompanied with a loud report, and some fossil substances were ejected, which were analized by Dr. Monson of New-Haven, and found to contain arsenic and sulphur.

In 1775 also perished a bed of excellent oysters in the harbor of Wellfleet, on Cape-Cod, twenty leagues south of Boston. These oysters had been in great plenty, and furnished the inhabitants with no small portion of food; but in this year from fome unknown caufe, they fickened and perifhed, and have never fince grown in that harbor.

Hiftorical Collections, vol. 3. 119.

During this fickly period alfo, the oyfters on the fhores of Connecticut were in an unhealthy ftate, and fometimes excited vomiting in thofe who ate of them.

It is remarkable alfo that in 1776 the lobfters in the vicinity of York-Ifland, all difappeared. This event has generally been afcribed to the firing of cannon in the fummer of that year. But the place where they lived being many miles from the Britifh fhipping, this explanation is not fatisfactory. It is more probable that they perifhed, or abandoned the ground, on account of the bad ftate of their element.

The winter in 1776 was fevere in Europe. The cold exceeded that of 1740. In Denmark the found was frozen and croffed on fledges. The Thames was alfo frozen.

An. Regifter, 1776. 114.

The fummer of 1776 in America was hot and in the northern ftates rainy. The dyfentery was prevalent in all parts of the country, and was terribly fatal to the American troops in New-York and at Ticonderoga. I was at Mount Independence in October, and witnefs to the ravages of the difeafe. Of thirteen thoufand troops, it was faid that one half were unfit for duty.

It has been cuftomary to afcribe the prevalence of this mortal difeafe to infection fpread by the foldiers who returned home from the armies. It is certain that the difeafe was thus introduced into particular families; but infection was the fmalleft among the caufes of the epidemic. In moft places, it originated without any communication from the army; and I was a witnefs of fuch inftances. The difeafe was the effect of a particular ftate of the atmofphere, aided by the feafons.

To prove how unfounded is the opinion that the difeafe originated in the army alone, and fpread from that as from a focus, it will be fufficient to mention two facts. The firft is, that this epidemic commenced in 1773, *two years before the war*, in which year it was more malignant and fatal, in fome places, than in any fubfequent year. Witnefs New-Haven, Eaft-Haven and Salem in Maffachufetts

In 1775 a remarkable fact occurred. About one hundred men belonging to Danbury, in Connecticut, went to join the army on Lake Champlain; they performed their duty and all returned in good health. While they were absent, the dysentery invaded the town and carried off more than one hundred of the inhabitants. In this instance, not a soldier returned from the army, until the disease had subsided.

The second fact is, that the same disease has before raged generally in this country, with all its horrors, in time of peace. Witness the epidemic at Georgetown in Maryland in 1793, at Derby in 1794 and at New-Haven in 1795. In an especial manner, I ought to mention the distressing dysentery, between 1749 and 1753, a time of profound peace, when not a soldier was seen in the country; a period when the disease was as mortal and as general, as between 1773 and 1777. A like epidemic prevailed in many counties in Europe at the same time.

I have also taken pains to enquire of physicians in the country, as to the propagation of this disease from the army, and am informed that the disease was as fatal in villages where no intercourse was had with the troops, as where there was intercourse.

The acquiescence of all descriptions of men, learned and unlearned, in the opinion that epidemic diseases are to be ascribed solely to infection or specific contagion, has proved extremely injurious to philosophy and to medicin.* The disease is infectious, but it originates in any place, in particular seasons, whether in peace or war; and ends at the command of the elements and seasons. It ceased at the close of 1777 in the army as well as country, and without any effort which had not been made in preceding years. It may be observed further that the dysentery was and always is, most prevalent among old people and children who have least intercourse with the sick, especially in the country, where no artificial causes of disease exist.

* A man in my father's neighborhood, was drafted to perform a tour of military duty at New-York, during the revolution-war. He was so much terrified by the apprehension of *catching* the dysentery in the army, that he hired another man as a substitute. The latter went to New-York, performed the duty and returned in health. The drafted man remained at home, was seized with the distemper in a few weeks after, and died.

In 1777 there was a small earthquake in the interior of England, and the London bill of mortality was higher than usual. A volcano in Ferro discharged discolored water, but no lava. The measles appeared in some parts of America, the same year.

The summer of 1778 was excessively hot in America, and fevers of a typhus kind were frequent. In Philadelphia an infectious bilious fever marked the summer and autumn after the British army left the city. Rush, vol. 3. 162. In general however the year was more healthy than the preceding summers.

In 1778 the plague was severe in Constantinople. It was preceded by a great earthquake at Smyrna. An. Reg. 1778. In the same year an epidemic angina was mortal at Manchester in England.

In the beginning of the winter succeeding 1778, there occurred some cold weather; but the latter part was the mildest ever known. In February 1779, many people along the river Connecticut plowed their fields; and in Pennsylvania the peach blossomed. The summer succeeding was one of the healthiest ever known in America.

In August 1779 happened a most tremendous eruption of Vesuvius; and about the same time, the ships of Capt. Cook, then in a high northern latitude between Kamschatka and America, were covered with ashes which were supposed to be discharged from a volcano on the neighboring continent. In the succeeding winter, Tauris, the capital of Persia, was laid in ruins by an earthquake.

See Encyclopedia, art Vesuvius, Cook's voyage, 1779.

The winter following these eruptions and commotions was, in America, the severest that had been known since 1741. From Nov. 25th to the middle of March, the cold was severe and almost uninterrupted. The following was the state of the mercury in January by Farenheit's scale—at Hartford in Connecticut, lat. 41. 44.

AT SUNRISE.

January,				
1	2 deg.	19	13 below 0
2	7 below 0	20	5
3	14	21	6 below 0
4	16	22	5
5	6	23	9 below 0
6	10	24	6
7	9	25	16 below 0
8	1 below 0	26	6 below 0
9	5	27	2 below 0
10	19	28	8 below 0
11	26	29	20 below 0
12	11	30	15
13	8	31	4 below 0
14	9	February, 1	2
15	15	2	3
16	10	3	0
17	17	4	15
18	12	5	8 below 0

Mean temperature in January at sunrise 4 deg.—almost 20 degrees below the temperature of the same month in ordinary winters.

See Connecticut Courant, January 1780.

Not only all the rivers, but the harbors and bays in the United States, as far southward as Virginia, were fast bound with ice. Loaded sleds passed from Staten-Island to New-York; the sound between Long Island and the main land was frozen into a solid highway, where it is several miles in breadth. Chesapeek bay at Annapolis, where the breadth is 5 and an half miles, sustained also loaded carriages.—The birds that winter in this climate, as robbins and quails almost all perished; and in the succeeding spring, a few solitary warblers only were heard in our groves.

The snow was nearly four feet deep, in Atlantic America, for at least three months. The winter was severe in Europe also; and on the 14th of January, the mercury at Glasgow fell to 46 deg. below 0.

On the 19th of May 1780 occurred a day of fingular darkness, in New England, and it was perceived, in a smaller degree, as far south as New-Jersey. The heavens were obscured with a vapor or cloud of a yellow color or faint red. The cloud which occasioned the principal darkness, passed over Connecticut about the hours of 9 and 10, and continued till after twelve. In the greatest obscuration, a candle was necessary to enable persons to read. For some days before, the atmosphere was filled with vapor.

Mem. Amer. Acad. vol. 1. 234.

On the same day that this lurid vapor overspread several hundred miles of country in America, Etna began to discharge lava from a new mouth, between two and three miles from its crater. The lava divided into three streams of a quarter of a mile in breadth, and in a few days ran fourteen miles. Violent earthquakes accompanied and followed the eruption. The coincidence of these events, in point of time, well deserves notice. The great discharges from Vesuvius and a volcano in the Arctic regions in 1779, the terrible earthquakes, severe cold and eruptions of fire that followed, may perhaps lead us to a rational solution of the phenomenon of the *dark day*—which has not hitherto been explained.

Courant, Oct. 24, 1780.

The plague broke out in Smyrna in the spring of 1780 but I have no account of its progress.

The spring was cool and dry, and catarrhous complaints were prevalent among children, says Dr. Rush, vol 1. 123. The summer following was hot,* and a bilious remittent was epidemic in Philadelphia, accompanied with such acute pains in the back, hips and neck, as to obtain the name of the *break-bone-fever*.

In the midst of summer, but I do not recollect the precise time, appeared the most singular halo about the sun which I ever beheld. I wrote a particular description of it, at the time, which is mislaid, and therefore I shall not attempt to describe it

---

* At Hartford, July 8th, the Thermometer at half after 11 A M. was at 102, at 2 P. M. 99 and an half, two degrees higher than it had been since 1772.

from recollection.—Haloes are among the moſt certain forerunners of tempeſtuous weather.

On the 2d of October the leeward Weſt-India iſlands experienced a moſt dreadful hurricane; and on the 11th the windward iſlands were almoſt laid waſte by a ſimilar calamity. Barbadoes which is leaſt ſubject to theſe tempeſts, was laid deſolate; and it was eſtimated that 6000 ſouls periſhed. Houſes, plantation-buildings, wharves, piers, ſhipping were all overwhelmed in one general ruin. It is ſaid that, during the tempeſt, ſome of the iſlands experienced an earthquake. Courant, Dec. 12, 1780. Jan. 9, 1781 and Jan. 23, 1781. As hurricanes are occaſioned by diſcharges of electricity, ſome trembling of the earth almoſt always attends thoſe which are violent, and flaſhes of fire are viſible. Indeed the atmoſphere appears to be a ſheet of fire. Similar diſcharges of electricity attended the tempeſtuous earthquake that deſtroyed Nicomedia in 358—that which defeated Julian's attempt to rebuild Jeruſalem in 362—the hail-ſtorm in Egypt, in the time of Moſes—and that which happened at Mantua in 1785, to be hereafter related.

The canker-worm made extenſive ravages in this period; but I cannot ſtate their riſe and decline in different parts of the country. The winter of 1780-81 exhibited nothing worthy of particular notice.

In the ſpring of 1781 prevailed the influenza, or epidemic catarrh. It began with a ſevere pain in the head, proſtration of ſtrength, coldneſs and chills, the pulſe not quick nor tenſe. The pain in the head laſted about twenty-four hours, and was ſucceeded by a pain in the ſide, not pointed nor acute, extending to the hips, accompanied with a ſoreneſs, and reſembling a rheumatic pain. The cough was troubleſome, full, and the matter diſcharged of the glandular kind, not well concocted. Reſpiration was difficult, and a conſiderable defluxion on the lungs. In a few caſes, the diſorder terminated in 7 or 8 days; but uſually not till the 13th or 14th; altho the patient was ſeldom confined to his bed. The diſeaſe left a ſoreneſs and weakneſs in the ſide, which continued after the ſtrength was recovered. Veneſection had little effect on the pain in the ſide. Epiſpaſtrics applied to the part gave relief. The diſorder was ſeldom fatal, but its effect were very vifible in the multiplied cafes of pulmonary confumption, in the following year.

M S letter from Dr. Tufts.

In the fummer following no particular phenomena occurred; the elements were in their ufual ftate, fo far as my information extends; and in general the country enjoyed good health. A malignant fever prevailed, in fome degree, in New-York, but excited no great alarm.

One year after this influenza in America, the fame difeafe pervaded the eaftern hemifphere. Its progrefs was from Siberia and Tartary weftward; and it reached Europe in April and May 1782: I have no account of its courfe in America, but it feems to be probable, that it took its direction from America weftward, and paffing the Pacific in high northern latitudes, invaded Afia and Europe from the eaft. This muft have been the cafe, if the epidemic in Europe was a continuation of that in America. For an account of this epidemic, fee the publications of that year.

In 1782 happened confiderable earthquakes in Calabria, during which the mercury in the barometer in Scotland funk within the tenth of an inch of the bottom of the fcale, and the waters in many locks in the highlands were greatly agitated.

Sinclair's Statiftical account of Scotland, vol. 6. 622.

In Britain the fummer was univerfally wet and cold, and crops failed, in confequence of which a diftreffing dearth afflicted Scotland in the following year.

In America alfo the fummer was cool. Two or three tornadoes happened in Vermont and New-Hampfhire, with deluging rains, and in one place hail of enormous fize—the gazette accounts fay, pieces of ice were found of 6 inches in length.

The latter part of fummer was exceffively dry. In New-Jerfey, a cedar fwamp of 20 miles in length and 8 in breadth, taking fire by accident, was totally confumed. The fire penetrated among the roots to the depth of 6 feet.—Corn, grafs, and the very forefts withered. The air was loaded with a thick vapor, for fome days in September *

Mem Am. Acad vol. 1. 356 Courant, Oct. 8, 1782.

* The reader will judge how far this extreme evaporation and drynefs, indicate the action of the internal fires or electricity which produced the tremendous difcharges from Heckla in the following year.

In autumn happened the violent tempest which difperfed the Englifh fleet from the Weft Indies, and in which two or three of the French fhips, taken by Admiral Rodney, foundered.

The winter of 1782-3 was more variable than ufual; and extreme drouth cut fhort the crops in the Weft-Indies.

Courant, May 20, 1783. Mem. Amer. Acad. vol. 1. 360.

On the morning of the 5th of February 1783, a thick vapor or fog was obferved over the ifland of Sicily, indicating the agitation of the element of fire or electricity; and about 12 o'clock, a violent fhock of earthquake laid many houfes in ruins. This was but a prelude to more terrible calamities; for about feven o'clock P. M. a tremendous fhock laid in ruins the greateft part of Meffina, Calabria and many towns and villages. From 30 to 40,000 perfons perifhed in the ruins. On fubfequent days, many fhocks were felt, but of lefs violence. During the convulfions on the 5th, flames were feen to iffue from the neighboring fea.

Courant, June 3, 1783, &c.

On the evening of the 10th, a denfe fog or vapor fpread over fome parts of New-England, having the fmell of burnt leaves. The ground, at the fame time, was covered with fnow.

Mem. Amer. Acad. vol. 1. 361.

About this time, for the gazette accounts are not particular as to the month, commenced a moft diftreffing famin in the Carnatic, which afterwards extended to moft of the European fettlements in the Eaft-Indies. At Madras hundreds of the natives perifhed daily, and the ftreets were filled with dead bodies. The caufe was a four years drouth; for during the approach of comets, and the action of fubterranean fire in other parts of the world, that country is fubject to exceffive drouth, as happened in 1769 and 70.

Courant, June 24, 1783, and July 1, Dec. 5, 1785.

In the evening of the 29th of March the heavens were illuminated with a moft fplendid lumen boreale.

The fummer of 1783 was variable in the northern parts of America; in England, it was hot.

In June commenced a moft formidable difcharge of lava from Mount Heckla in Iceland, which continued till the middle of

August. The country around the mountain was covered with burning fluid, to the extent of 40 miles, and in some places, to the depth of 40 feet. The lava spread over 3600 square miles.

Previous to this eruption, all the springs and streams of water in the neighborhood had been dried up; a sure forerunner of the discharge of fire; and for some months before the eruption, the atmosphere over the island was filled with a dark, bluish, sulphurous vapor or cloud, which was stationary in calm weather, but which was sometimes dispersed by winds, and spread over Europe. See Encyclopedia, article Iceland. During this eruption, a new island was thrown up, at some distance from Iceland. On the 18th of August, soon *after* the eruption of Heckla ceased, an immense meteor or globe of fire shot through the heavens, from north to south, passing the Orkneys and the island of Great-Britain, and bursting with a loud report.

Encyclop. art Iceland   Sinclair's Scot. vol 6 623.

A part of the summer was excessively hot in America. No less than thirty persons in Philadelphia, killed themselves by drinking cold water. Many putrid fevers were the consequence of the heat in various parts of the country; as also tornadoes and thunder gusts of unusual violence, with hail of uncommon size, in all parts of America. Rarely indeed has so much injury been done by hail in the same space of time.

On the 31st of May a large meteor or fiery globe was seen at Richmond in Virginia, shooting from north to south. It burst with a heavy report. It will be remarked that this meteor occurred about *two weeks before* the eruption of fire from Heckla, but while the fires or electrical causes were in agitation, as appears from the cloud of vapor, that was suspended over the island.

Courant, Sept 2, and June 24, 1783, and Aug 5, and 12.

During the immense discharges of fire and lava from Heckla, all parts of Europe, Great-Britain, Italy, Sicily, France and even the Alps were overspread with a haziness in the atmosphere. This caused universal consternation, as a similar appearance had preceded the earthquake in Sicily on the 5th of February. The churches were crouded with supplicants. The French astronomer La Lande attempted to quiet the popular fears, by ascribing the phenomenon to a superabundance of watery particles in the earth, from the moisture of the preceding year, which were then exhaled by the summer heats. But this solution is not satisfactory. It was more probably the smoke from Heckla, wafted by northerly winds and difperfed over Europe, in an attenuated form.

Courant, Oct. 28, 1783, and Nov. 11th, and 25th.
Franklin's Meteorol. Obferv. Mufeum, vol. 1. 473.

It is ftill more probable that this vapor was the effect of infenfible difcharges of electricity, combined with aerial fubftances; as in Sicily on the 5th and in America on the 10th of February.

In October occurred tremendous gales of wind and high tides which did no fmall damage in the feaports of the United States. The firft, on the 15th and 16th, occafioned the higheft water at New-Haven, which had been known in 40 years. Many other tempefts occurred in September and October; and from Vermont to Georgia, the gazettes were filled with accounts of difafters from the violence of the winds and rains.

Courant, October 21, 1783.

On the 29th of November, a confiderable fhock of earthquake was felt in all the northern ftates; and New-York experienced two or three fhocks in the morning of the next day.

Some of the Weft-India iflands were feverely fhaken, about the fame time, and efpecially on the 4th of December.

Courant, Dec. 16, 1783. March 9, 1784.

In autumn 1783 fome parts of Europe were deluged with continual rains, and at Rome 5 or 6000 children died of the fmall pox. About Grenoble raged an epidemic fever.

A diftemper among the cattle in Derby in England, occafioned no fmall alarm, and a royal proclamation was iffued enjoining certain precautions to prevent the propagation of the difeafe.

Cotemporary with thefe convulfions of nature, was a moft defolating plague in Egypt, the Grecian Ifles, Dalmatia, Conftantinople, Smyrna and in the Crimea. It is not poffible, with the *general* accounts given of fuch an epidemic, in the public prints, to ftate, with any precifion, its origin and progrefs in the eaft. It is mentioned to have appeared in Smyrna, in the fpring of 1783, and it certainly raged in Conftantinople, and many other parts of Turkey in the following summer, as well as on the north of the Euxine.

Courant, Jan 17, 1784. July 6. Sept 21, and 28, 1784.

In Egypt the same disease committed most terrible ravages in 1783-4 and 5. It began in November 1783. To this calamity was added a severe famin; the inundation of the Nile, in the summer of that year, having proved insufficient. So severe was the plague, that in the winter after 1783, fifteen hundred dead bodies were carried out of Cairo in a day; and the plague and famin of that and the succeeding year, was supposed to carry off one sixth of the inhabitants of Egypt. See Volney's Travels, vol. 1. 192 and 3, and Courant, Oct. 28, 1783, and Oct. 17, 1785, in which it is said that in Cairo 3000 perished in a day in April, 1785.

We have then an exact general view of the phenomena which introduce and accompany pestilence in Europe, Africa and Asia —terrible earthquakes and eruptions of volcanoes; excessive drouth in America, India and Egypt, failure of crops and famin —meteors, great heat and deluges of rain, in other countries. Let us now see what followed these abovementioned agitations of the elements, in our country.

See Courant, April 27, 1784, and Jan 27, 1784, and June 8.

In August 1783, the scarlatina appeared in Philadelphia and in September it became epidemic. It appeared about the same time in Salem, in Massachusetts. It was in Charleston, South-Carolina in 1784, in which year, it appeared in the interior of the northern states, as in Vermont and New-Hampshire, and in Middletown, on Connecticut river. It continued to prevail about five years; but was not severe in general and many towns wholly escaped its attacks.

Rush, vol 1 141. Museum, vol. 2. 562.
Mem Amer Acad. vol 1. 369.
Belknap's Hist New-Hampshire, vol. 2. 121.
Register of deaths at Middletown

In 1787 the cynanche maligna was epidemic at Northampton, in Massachusetts.

M S. letter from the Rev. Mr Williams.

The measles appeared in America in 1783; at Salem as early

as May. I find it in all parts of America, in that year, but cannot trace the progress of the epidemic.

During this period neither dysentery nor pestilential autumnal fevers made any considerable ravages in America, as far as I can learn; except at Fell's-Point in Baltimore, where the bilious pestilential fever occasioned a mortality in 1783. Many sporadic cases of a similar fever appeared in various parts of the country, and almost a whole family in New-Jersey perished by it in the autumn of that year. Fortunately however the constitution of the elements was corrected, without producing its most fatal effects. Even the scarlet fever, with the exception of a few places, was less malignant than it has been in the last period.

This pestilential constitution was felt also in the north of Europe. The scarlatina broke out in Edinburgh in the winter of 1782-3, a few months before it did in America; but of its progress I have no account. It appears to have been epidemic in London in 1786; so that its period was of about the same duration as in America. The cotemporaneousness of this species of disease in Great-Britain and America, deserves particular notice.

In December happened a fog in Amsterdam of such density as to occasion complete obscurity for three hours in the middle of the day. It was not possible for persons to find their way in the streets, and many passengers and some carriages fell into the canals.

Courant, March 9, 1784.

The severity of the winter succeeding these phenomena, both in Europe and America, corresponded with their extraordinary number and violence. The weather was less uniformly cold than in 1780, but the frost, in some parts of the winter was most intense. The following was the state of Farenheit's thermometer, at Hartford.

February 10th, 1784, . 19 deg. below o.
   11 . . 12 do.
   12 . . 13 do.
   13 . . 19 do.
   14 . . 20 do.

February 15 . . 12 deg. below 0.
16 . . . 16 do.
17 . . 16 do.

On the 20th of January was discovered a comet in Pisces, which was involved in a luminous atmosphere. It was visible about four weeks.

The severe cold commenced early; the Delaware at Philadelphia was closed at the beginning of December, and continued bound with ice till the middle of March; notwithstanding a relaxation of cold and a heavy rain in January. The gazettes state that such intense cold had not been known in that city, since 1750-51.—The Mississippi was reported to be covered with ice, as far south as New-Orleans. At the breaking up of winter, the thaw was sudden, and immense bodies of ice, floating down the rivers, which were greatly swelled, spread ruin along the low lands on their banks. Great damage was sustained on the banks of the Schuylkill, Susquehanna, Potomack and James rivers.

Courant, May 11, 1784. Feb. 24. March 30. April 11.

In Europe, the winter was no less severe—an instance in which a severely cold winter in Europe coincided in time, with the same in America. It may be remarked also that this winter was just one century after the coincidence of like events; the winter of 1683-4 being equally severe in both hemispheres.

In 1783-4 the river Liffey in Ireland, the Thames in England, and all the rivers in the interior of Holland, were covered with solid ice. In Holland, the ice gave way about the first of March, and the rivers being greatly swelled, the adjacent country was inundated, with immense loss of lives and property. The river Waal, near Nimeguen, broke through its dikes and overwhelmed 34 villages. The Rhine from Cologne and Manheim, exhibited similar scenes of devastation.

Courant, April 27, 1784, and May 18.

In January a terrible tempest spread desolation along the coast of France from Rochelle to Bourdeaux; vessels at sea shipwrecked, and houses on land blown down. This happened on the night of the 17th. Its violence extended along the coast of Spain and Portugal. An earthquake accompanied this hurricane. The coast of Italy did not escape, and so high was the swell of the ocean, that fish were lodged on the houses in Syracuse.

Courant, May 18, 1784, and June 1.

This remarkable tempest happened just before the appearance of the comet.

The spring was wet and cold; and repeated snows fell in April.

The heat of some part of the succeeding summer in America was extreme. The following observations were made at Hartford.

See Courant, June 29.

June 24th at 2 P. M.	97 deg. by Farenheit.
25	2 P. M.	96
26 at sunrise,	80
at 10 A. M.	96
at 2 P. M.	100
at 3 P. M.	101
at 4 P. M.	100
at sunset,	91
at 10 P. M.	80
27 at sunrise,	82
at 7 A. M.	91

This extreme heat, as usual, produced most violent hurricanes or thunder gusts, with hail of unusual size. In May, pieces of ice fell in South-Carolina of nine inches in circumference. On the 17th of August the southern part of Connecticut was swept by a tornado, which levelled trees and buildings and did great injury. The beginning of summer was very dry; but frequent showers afterwards refreshed the earth, and good crops succeeded.

Courant, August 10, 1784. August 24 and 31. See also Appendix to a Sermon preached at Hartford on the death of Israel Seymour, who was killed by lightning.

A great eruption of Vesuvius happened on the 10th of May. Sickness prevailed in Leghorn and other parts of Europe. The plague raged this year also at Smyrna, Constantinople and in Dalmatia. Spolatro was nearly dispeopled. The heat in Europe was great and Hungary was overrun by locusts, which devoured the fields of grass and corn. A severe earthquake at the same time, shook the country of Armenia, and its vicinity, and a town was demolished with the loss of 6000 inhabitants, on the 21st of July. The plague raged also in the regency of Tunis on the African coast.

Courant, Aug 31 Supplement to do Nov 9.

On the 30th of July a tremendous hurricane laid waste a considerable part of Jamaica, sweeping away buildings, canes, fruit-trees and overwhelming all the shipping in the harbors.

Courant, Sept 28, 1784, and Oct. 26.

In October, according to the public prints, Barbadoes was severely shaken by an earthquake.

On the 25th of November was a very violent tempest from the N. E. and S. E. by which means, a most extraordinary tide was brot into our harbors from the St. Lawrence to New-York, and probably further to the south. Great injury was sustained by loss of shipping, and of property stored near the wharves.

Courant, Dec. 7, 1784.

The great rains swelled Connecticut river to the height of usual spring floods

A meteor was seen in New-England on the evening of December 13, 1784, passing rapidly from south-east to north-west, and bursting with a loud report.

The winter following exhibited nothing very worthy of remark. In Europe it was colder than usual, and in America, it produced great snows, the melting of which in the spring swelled Connecticut river to an unusual height.

On the 13th of March 1785, there was an eruption of fire in the river Majuro, in the province of Palermo, in Sicily, which occasioned a large chasm in the earth.

Courant, July 4, 1785.

In America canine madness began to rage and spread in all parts of the northern states. The gazettes of 1785 abound with accounts of the dreadful effects of this singular disease. It will be remarked that epidemic madness of dogs is one of that series of diseases which belong to every pestilential period. Whenever the human race are generally afflicted with epidemics, the canine species rarely escape the effects of the general principle; and not unfrequently foxes, wolves and other wild animals, experience its malignant effects, and run mad. In 1785, the scarlatina anginosa was prevalent in the northern states. This was in the midst of the period, and almost every gazette announced some new case of hydrophobia.

See Courant, Aug. 1, 1785. Aug. 8 and 29.

The wheat-insect, which has been ignorantly and improperly named the Hessian Fly, committed uncommon ravages in this year. The precise time when this insect originated, is not ascertained, probably about the year 1776, or a year or two earlier. Little notice was taken of it, for two or three years. In 1780, Mr. Underhill of Long Island lost his wheat crops by the insect; and in subsequent years, it penetrated into New-Jersey, travelling, according to common opinion, about 15 or 20 miles in a year. In 1785, it occasioned unusual destruction of wheat—and such was the alarm in England, for fear it should prove *infectious*, and be introduced into that country, that the King issued a proclamation dated June 25, 1788, prohibiting the importation of American wheat.—This event excited no small uneasiness in America, especially in the states, whose staple is wheat. Whereupon the Supreme Executive Council of Pennsylvania requested the opinion of the Agricultural Society, as to the manner by which that insect is propagated. To this request, the Society returned for answer, their decided opinion that it is the plant alone which is injured by the insect; that the grain is sound and good, and that the insect is not propagated by sowing wheat which grew on fields infected with it.

See Museum, vol. 4. 244. Am. Magazine.

The prohibition by the King and Council of Great-Britain was deemed a judicious precaution; but was the fruit of an error that pervades the world, respecting the powers of *infection* and *contagion*. The opinion of the Agricultural Society is well founded, but it remains for time and the force of truth to convince the people of Philadelphia, that the yellow fever can no more be transplanted and rendered epidemic by infection, than the wheat-insect. Both are *diseases*, originating where they have a suitable aliment, and ceasing to exist, when that aliment fails.

The prohibition of the British government was repealed the next year; under the apprehension of a dearth.

The summer of 1785 was excessively dry in France and England and fevers very prevalent in France. In Holland such a drouth could not be recollected by the oldest man living. The canals, rivers and wells were almost totally exhausted. In the first part of summer, there was not a drop of rain for three or four months, and cattle were fed upon the leaves of the trees. The drouth was nearly as severe in the West-Indies.

Courant, August 8, 1785, and 29th—also Sept 12 and 19.

In North-Carolina, the fields were overrun with bugs, which threatened a destruction of the grain.

Courant, August 29, 1785

The summer contained some excessively hot days in America, as well as in Europe.

Courant, Sept 5.

On the 25th of August happened in the West-Indies one of the most dreadful hurricanes ever known, and equal to that of 1772 or that of 1780. This tempest was preceded by very sultry heat, and the phenomenon called *looming*, by which distant objects at sea appear to be raised higher or brot nearer than at other times. I have often noticed this singular effect of the powers of refraction in the air, previous to storms, of which it is the usual forerunner. Guadaloupe, St. Croix and the other windward islands were laid desolate by this tempest. On the 27th of August, the leeward islands suffered a similar calamity. On the 24th of September, an easterly storm brought into the rivers in the southern states, as high a tide as ever was known.— Norfolk was inundated, with great loss.

Sickness was very general in many parts of the United States. The scarlatina was prevalent, and the gazettes mention a precinct in Ulster in which died almost every child under six years of age. Many adults also fell victims to this or other maladies.

See Courant, Oct. 3, 1785, and Oct. 10.

On the 9th of August happened a memorable tempest at Mantua, in Italy, and the neighboring country. The wind was a hurricane, and accompanied with rain and hail-stones of the weight of 18 ounces. The accounts state that visible flames issued from the earth, and scorched people's legs and clothes; other accounts mention that the fire ran along on the surface of the earth. The reader will call to mind the relation of the like fact, in the terrible hail-storm which constituted one of the ten plagues of Egypt in the reign of Pharaoh.

Courant, Nov. 28, 1785.

The autumn was uncommonly sickly in Jamaica. Kingston was a general hospital.

Courant, Jan. 30, 1786.

On the 9th of October there was an uncommon darkness in Canada; while the atmosphere was of a fiery luminous appearance. This was followed by squalls of wind and rain, with severe thunder.

On the 15th occurred a still greater obscurity, succeeded also by lightning, thunder and rain.

On the 16th the morning was calm and foggy. At 10 o'clock arose a wind from the east, which partly expelled the fog; and soon after, commenced the darkness of midnight. The people dined by candle-light. Soon after the darkness fell a meteor or fire-ball.

See Mem. Am. Acad. vol. 2, and the Gazettes of that month.
Courant, Dec. 12, 1785.

A slighter degree of obscurity on the 15th extended over New-England: but the 16th was a fair day.

The year 1786 exhibits fewer of the great phenomena of nature, than the preceding year; but it commenced with a degree of cold rarely known in this country. State of the thermometer at Hartford,

<pre>
        Jan. 17 at sunrise,   14 deg. below 0.
             18   do.   20   do.
             19   do.   24   do.
                at noon,   0
                at 2 P. M.   3   above 0.
             20 sunrise,   17   below 0.
</pre>

The frost of the whole winter was however far less severe than in 1784. The summer following was cool.

One or two violent tempests occurred during the summer, particularly one on the 23d of August, which passed over Woodstock, in Connecticut, with fatal violence.

The scarlet fever and hydrophobia continued to prevail in this year.

The plague prevailed on the Barbary coast; and several thousand people in Carthagena and Malaga, in Spain, perished with yellow fever.
Town's Travels, vol 3.

In June 1786 was a smart shock of earthquake in the north of England. In August a second shock of confiderable extent. In January 1787 a shock was felt in Scotland, on the night preceding which, a piece of ground, near Alloa, on which was a mill, suddenly sunk a foot and a half. The waters of rivers receded and left their channels dry, before the concussion.
Sinclair, vol 6.

The winter of 1786-7 began early and with great severity.— On the 28th of November, the temperature at Hartford was at 10 deg. by Farenheit, through the day. At sunrise on the 29th, it was at cypher, and the cold continued to be extreme for two weeks. It did not rise above the freezing point till the 13th of December. The cold then abated, but the winter, on the whole, was more severe than usual. Courant, Dec. 4, 11 and 18. The winter was also severe in Europe.

The sore throat was fatal in some parts of the eastern states. One man in Newton, Mass. lost three children after 30 hours illness.
Courant Feb. 20, 1786.

The plague continued to prevail on the Barbary coast, and in this winter and the spring following seventeen thousand inhabitants of Algiers perished. It made great havoc also in the dominions of Morocco, as it did in Aleppo.
M S of Mr. O'Brien Courant, April 16, 1787 and July 23.

The wheat infect continued its ravages in the United States.

Two or three violent tornadoes are recorded to have occurred in the summer of 1786—one at Wethersfield, which overset a house and killed several persons; and another at Northborough in Massachusetts.

About the close of August a celestial phenomenon of a singular kind appeared at Portsmouth, New-Hampshire. A small light cloud was feen, from which iffued repeated reports, like the burfting of crackers, or an irregular difcharge of mufquetry—fuppofed to be the explofion of a meteor or fucceffion of meteors. The wind was high at north-weft, with flying clouds.

Courant, Sept. 10, 1787.

A dreadful hurricane almoft deftroyed the fettlements at the bay of Honduras on the 2d of September. The hurricane was followed by fatal difeafes.

About the clofe of 1787 Vefuvius difcharged a large quantity of lava. In the fame year was an eruption of Etna, in the month of July.

A moft extraordinary tempeft and inundation defolated the Coromandal coaft on the 20th of May. Whole towns were overwhelmed, and more than 10,000 people perifhed.

Courant, May 26, 1788, and Aug. 4.

This year was in general healthy in America and in the north of Europe. In fome towns in New-England prevailed angina, but it was not general.

SECTION VIII.

Historical view of pestilential epidemics, from the year 1788 to 1798 inclusive, comprehending the last epidemic period in America.

THE winter of 1787-8 was colder than usual in America, but not of great severity.

In Europe prevailed epidemic catarrh in 1788. It appeared at Vienna in April—was in Poland and Russia in May—at London in June—and at Paris in August. In St. Luke's Hospital, it began on the 16th of July, and a few cases occurred till Nov. 10th; but only twenty five persons out of 190 were affected; a proof that it has little contagion. Gent. Mag. 1789. 346. The invasion of this epidemic was less sudden than usual.

On the 22d of July was a violent tempest from the N. E. which occasioned a very high tide in the Chesapeek, and no small damage. This is a singular occurrence. A north-east gale in June or July on the American coast, must be attributed to some extraordinary cause; and perhaps this may be ascribed to the approach of a comet, which appeared in October and November following. This comet was predicted by Mr. Herschel, who made previous preparations for examining it.

Courant August 11, and 25, and April 28, 1788.

The summer was remarkably tempestuous. On the 29th of August, a severe gale of wind did great damage in many of our ports. Of 30 sail of vessels, in certain rivers and bays of North-Carolina, 26 were destroyed. A tempest in the beginning of the month had been terribly destructive. No one event is more certain, than a vast increase of tempestuous weather during the approach of comets. The tempest of the 19th extended over the whole face of the country, penetrating to Vermont, levelling buildings, trees and corn. Many cattle and one child was killed by falling timber and trees. To enumerate the particulars, would fill many pages.

Courant, Sept. 1, 1788, and 8.

It is remarkable that this tempeft in the United States was but two or three days after a tremendous hurricane among the windward iflands, which was fuppofed to do more injury than the great tempeft of 1766. At the leeward alfo the fame calamity befel the iflands. In Martinico the barometer fell nearly to 27 inches.

Courant, Oct. 27, 1788.

About the fame time fimilar difafters befel France and England. A tornado of great violence occurred about Paris, in which, the gazettes declare, fell hail-ftones of 8lb. weight. During a tempeft in London, a fire ball entered a houfe and ftruck down two perfons.

Courant, Oct. 27, 1788.

In the Weft-Indies hurricanes were repeated in September with deftructive rage.

On the evening of the 17th of October 1788 was feen, at various places, in Connecticut and New-York, a meteor or fire ball, whofe apparent diameter was equal to that of the fun in the meridian. It paffed from the eaftward to the weftward with amazing rapidity, illuminating the earth, and approaching near the weftern horizon, it burft with a heavy report.*

Courant, Oct. 27, 1788.

The comet already mentioned firft appeared about this time. It rofe about 3 o'clock in the morning in the north-eaft. A violent north-eaft gale occurred on the 11th of November.

Courant, Nov. 3 and 17.

This fummer in America was very rainy; earthquakes happened in Italy and Mexico; and a fhock was felt in July in the ifle of Man.

Sinclair's Scot. vol. 6. 625.

The thermometer on one day in July rofe to 103 in Columbia College, in New-York; but the general heat of the fummer was not exceffive.

Mufeum, vol. 7. 36.

---

* This meteor was feen at Poughkeepfie, on the Hudfon, nearly in the zenith. In Suffex county, weft of Cape Henlopen, it appeared to be about ten degrees above the horizon. *Courant, Dec. 8, 1788.*

In November 1788 appeared the measles in New-York. On its first invasion, it appeared with great malignity. The same distemper appeared in the northern liberties of Philadelphia, in December; and spread till it became epidemic in February and March.

Courant, Nov. 24, 1788, and Rush, vol 2 234.

The eastern parts of Europe were sickly during the summer of 1788. The immense armies on foot, in the war between the Austrians, Russians and Turks, contributed to increase the mortality. It was estimated that 80,000 Austrians perished, mostly by disease. The year however was generally healthy.

The winter of 1788-9 was colder than usual in the United States. On the morning of the 2d of February, the mercury in Farenheit fell to 28 deg. below cypher; 4 degrees lower than had before been observed in Hartford. The season however was on the whole less severe than in 1780 and 1784.

Courant, Feb 2, 1789, and 9th

In Europe, the winter appears to have been unusually severe. The frost penetrated to the southern parts of Spain and Portugal; and the rivers in Estremadura and Alantejo were covered with ice. The Pyrenees were involved in deep snow in March.

Courant, Aug 3, 1789 Univ Mag. 1789

It should have been related under the year 1788, that almost all the cod-fish taken on the banks of Newfoundland, in that year, were thin and sickly; when dried, they were of a dark or bluish color, little better than skeletons, and not well received in foreign markets. This condition of that fish was confined to those banks; as the cod taken at other places were in their usual state.

M S letter from Dr. Holyoke.

On the 28th of May 1789, appeared in Connecticut a most singular halo, of which the public prints contain a particular description. This phenomenon seems to indicate the approach of tempestuous weather, and was in this instance, followed by a heavy wind and rain. But when this appearance is of singular brightness or extent, it indicates a state of the atmosphere highly electrified perhaps and certainly tempestuous, and storms are numerous and violent. Thus the remarkable hurricanes of

1780 were preceded by as remarkable haloes. The halo of May 28th was preceded by a most splendid lumen boreale.

The instance under consideration was surprising and to gloomy minds, awful. A clergyman, since dead, wrote a moral essay on the occasion in which he predicted great calamities to happen; and he mentioned other events, of that period, as unusual numbers of flies, caterpillars, locusts, and dearth of corn, in confirmation of his opinion that the arm of the Lord was extended in wrath over our land.

Courant, June 8, 1789, and June 15.

It is true that our crops had been thin, in the preceding year, and the northern states, in the spring of 1789, experienced a dearth, approaching to famin. In Vermont, people were reduced to the necessity of feeding on tad-poles boiled with pea-straw. In one instance four potatoes sold for nine pence. None of the human race were actually starved to death, but a few died of a flux in consequence of bad diet.* Cattle however perished in considerable numbers. Such were the gazette accounts of the day. It is certain that a similar scarcity had not been experienced in America for many years. Whether the failure of crops and the sickly state of the cod-fish marked a derangement of the elements, let the philosopher determin.

Courant, June 15, 1789, and June 22.

The spring of 1789 was cold and vegetation tardy, beyond what could be recollected by the oldest persons living. Part of the summer succeeding was excessively hot. For nine or ten days successively, in August, the heat was above 90 deg. and in the midst of the day, it rose nearly to 100 deg. The mean temperature of the summer was however not much above what is usual. Rush, vol. 2. 234. Courant, Aug. 24 and 31. On the 4th of June ice at Wioming was as thick as window glass.

Courant, June 22.

The failure of crops in the Carnatic in 1788 occasioned a severe famin, by which thousands perished in the succeeding year.

Courant, April 27, and Sept. 28, 1789.

The hydrophobia showed itself in America early in 1789.

* In old settlements, there was food enough for men, but the failure of a surplus in this country, is a rare event.

A man in Coeyman's precinct, state of New-York, died in July of that dreadful malady, taken as was supposed, by skinning a cow that died of the disorder in the April preceding.

Courant, Aug 3, 1789

In Maryland, the autumn was distinguished by an unexampled mortality among horses.

Courant, Dec 31, 1789.

In Europe also crops had failed, and England, Holland and France apprehended the most calamitous effects In Paris the cry of *bread, bread* was every where heard, and many riots and mobs marked the distress of the inhabitants.

Courant, Oct 12, 1789.

The empire of China experienced the same calamity, and the people suffered indescribable distress from famin and disease. In Madras died 30,000 people by famin in 1788. *Courant, April 27, 1789.* In this instance, crops failed over the whole earth, in the same year.

On the 10th of July a most tremendous earthquake convulsed Iceland. Large chasms were opened in the earth, and some mountains were rent asunder. Several shocks happened on subsequent days, and a violent shock in September is mentioned in the 6th volume of Sinclair's Statistical works, 625.

Courant, January 21, 1790.

On the 30th of September occurred a violent earthquake in Tuscany, by which some villages were destroyed and several thousand lives. On the same day, but not at the same hour, a small shock was felt at Edinburgh. On the 5th of November, a shock was felt at Crieff, 50 miles from Edinburgh; and on the 10th and 11th, severe shocks were felt at other places.

Courant, Dec 7, 1789 Sinclair, vol 6 625

On the 4th of December arrived at Lieth, Capt. Stewart of the ship Brothers, from Archangel in Russia; who informed that on the coast of Lapland and Norway, he sailed many leagues among multitudes of dead haddock floating on the water. He spoke several ships which also passed among them.

Sinclair, vol. 6. 627.

Whether these fish were killed by an earthquake or a discharge of subterranean vapor or heat, or died by sickness, is not known.

If they were killed, it would seem probable that other fish in the same seas, would have shared the same fate ; which does not appear to have been the case ; for the accounts make no mention of the death of other kinds. And what renders it probable that they died of disease, and a disease peculiar to that kind of fish, is, that for some years after, no haddock came to the markets in Scotland, as before that mortality. That species appeared to be almost extinct ; whereas there is no mention made of a failure of other kinds of fish. Careful observations and precise dates would assist our researches into the causes of these wonderful phenomena.

In October, Vesuvius was in a state of eruption for several weeks, and discharged small streams of Lava. The plague prevailed at Constantinople and Smyrna.

Gent. Mag. 1789.

On the 29th of October from 2 o'clock P. M. to half after 4, Kentucky was enveloped in thick darkness, so that people were obliged to use candles.

Courant, January 14, 1790.

It will be observed that this darkness, and the beginning of the influenza in America coincide nearly in time with the eruption of Vesuvius, and many earthquakes.

Such universal disorders in the elements never fail to produce epidemic diseases ; and those here related were the heralds of the most severe period of sickness that has occurred in the United States for 30 years.

The first appearance of that series of epidemics to be hereafter described, seems to have been in the measles at New-York in November 1788, and at Philadelphia in December following. This disease became epidemic over the northern states in 1789, but I have not the means of describing its progress. I find, in bills of mortality, from various places, deaths by measles are mentioned in 1789 and 90.

In autumn 1789 appeared the influenza or epidemic catarrh. The precise time and place of its appearance, are not ascertained. Some accounts say, it originated in Canada. But I shall confine my observations to its progress in Atlantic America. It was first observed about the close of September 1789, in New-York and Philadelphia. Dr. Rush informs me, that it was brought to Philadelphia by the members of Congress, who returned from New-York, about the first of October. Another account, written by one of the faculty in Philadelphia, and published in the 7th volume of the Museum, mentions its first appearance there, about the time of the Friends Yearly Meeting, in September. The precise time is probably not ascertainable; the opinion of its propagation by infection is very fallacious, as I know by repeated observations. It probably appeared in detached cases, some days before it became a subject of observation.

Museum, vol 7 231.

From the middle states, it moved rapidly over the whole country. It appeared in Hartford, where I then resided, about the middle of October. On the 19th of that month, I left Hartford for Boston and arrived the next day in good health. I was seized with the influenza on the 23d, and by the aid of a diluting regimen, recovered in four days. No person who attended me was seized with the distemper, sooner than the other inhabitants of that town. I mention this to disprove the common opinion of its infection; not that I deny it to be in a degree, infectious; altho my own observations do not warrant that concession; but I aver that its propagation depends almost entirely on the insensible qualities of the atmosphere. Two ladies who left Boston with me on the second of November, before the disease had appeared in their family, and before it was a subject of conversation, were seized with it in Hartford, at the same time, that it became epidemic in Boston, one on the 8th and the other on the 12th.—The disease had then passed Hartford, and there is no evidence of their being exposed to any person infected. This fact shows a regular progress in the state of air producing the disease—as persons leaving Boston and travelling one hundred and twenty miles distance, were effected precisely at the time the disease became epidemic in that town.

This disease pervaded the wilderness and seized the Indians—it spread over the ocean and attacked seamen a hundred leagues from land, and as to infection, entirely insulated—it appeared in the West-Indies nearly at the time it did in the northern states. It overspread America, from the 15th to the 45th degree of latitude in about 6 or 8 weeks; and how much further it extended, I am not informed

It should have been mentioned that, in September, anterior to the invasion of the catarrh, the scarlatina anginosa appeared in Philadelphia; but in October it yielded to the influenza, the controlling epidemic. The scarlet fever re-appeared in December, and became epidemic; often blending itself with the influenza. It exhibited one predominant feature of the whole series of succeeding epidemics, a prevalence of bilious matter, which was often discharged by purging and vomiting. This disease continued to prevail in Philadelphia, and if my information is correct, in some parts of New-Jersey, till the spring of 1790. The measles occurred in some cases, but was not epidemic.

Museum, vol. 7. 120, 175.

It is remarkable that the scarlatina anginosa was cotemporary in Edinburgh with the epidemic measles in America in 1789, and nearly so, with the death of the haddock on the coast of Norway.

It will be observed that the scarlet fever, tho epidemic in Philadelphia, did not spread over the country in 1790. It was little known in the northern states, till two years after—this is among the proofs that this disease does not depend on infection for its propagation. If infection was its only or principal means of propagation, the fomites existed in great abundance, in particular places in 1790, and sufficient to have spread it over the United States. But a disease however infectious, will not spread far in an atmosphere that will not generate it. Indeed scarcely a year passes in which sporadic cases of scarlatina, or anginas of other kinds do not appear in particular places; but they never spread without some uncommon concurrence of causes.

The winter of 1789-90 was one of the mildest that is ever known in this country; there being little frost, except for a few days in February. There fell frequent snows and in great abundance; but they were immediately followed by warm southerly winds, and dissolved.

Early in the spring of 1790 we had a second epidemic catarrh. I was attentive to its origin and progress. I found it at

Albany in the laſt week in March, and heard of it in Vermont about the ſame time. I returned to Hartford, but altho expoſed repeatedly to its infection on my journey, I was not ſeized earlier than others in Hartford, where the difeaſe appeared about the middle of April. It ſpread to the ſouthward, arrived at Philadelphia near the cloſe of that month, and diſappeared in that city about the middle of June. In the northern ſtates, as far as my knowledge extends, the difeaſe was more violent, than in the preceding autumn. Many plethoric perſons of firm habit almoſt funk under it; while confumptive people and hard drinkers fell its victims.

Muſeum, vol 8 65.

The ſpring and ſummer of 1790 were moſtly rainy; but otherwiſe feaſonable weather. No remarkable epidemics prevailed, except thoſe already deſcribed, but an increaſe of mortality, in ſome places, is viſible in the regiſters of deaths. Severe earthquakes occurred on the African coaſt.

Let it be obſerved that the meaſles appeared in autumn 1788, juſt after great volcanic eruptions, and a moſt tempeſtuous ſummer, when the element of fire appeared to be in univerſal commotion; juſt after the meteor, and during the appearance of the comet.* Let it be obſerved alſo that the harveſt failed, at this time, in China, India, Europe and America, and let any man deny the all-controlling influence of the elements in producing theſe events.

The winter of 1790-91 commenced early and with ſevere weather. The laſt week in November was cold, Connecticut river at Hartford was cloſed with ice on the 9th of December, and not open till the 12th of March. On the whole, the ſeaſon was not of unuſual ſeverity. The ſpring and early part of ſummer were, in moſt parts of the country, very dry, until the middle of June.

On the 15th of January, a confiderable ſhock of earthquake was experienced at Richmond in Virginia. At the ſame time catarrhs were ſo prevalent in that ſtate and in Pennſylvania, as to excite an apprehenſion of another viſit of the influenza.

* In 1732 a dark day occurred in Auguſt *preceding* the influenza. In 1789 a darkneſs at Kentucky occurred, *during* the epidemic catarrh.

Inflammatory diseases were very frequent during the winter. In Philadelphia the scarlatina anginosa appeared late in January and was very prevalent in February. In the interior of Carolina it was sickly, but I have no particulars. The whooping cough prevailed in many parts of the country.

Courant, Jan. 21. 1790. See Museum, vol. 9. 65.

In the month of April, some fishermen at the Narrows, near New-York, caught fourteen thousand shad at a single draft; to secure which, it was necessary to add several seines, one upon the other. This circumstance is mentioned, because several medical authors have related that an extraordinary abundance of fish is among the precursors of pestilence. It will be noted that the pestilential fever, which has prevailed for many years past, first appeared in New-York, in the autumn succeeding this singular draft of fish.

Courant, April 25, 1790.*

On the 16th of May, at half past 10 o'clock P. M. in a serene, moon-light night, an extensive earthquake was felt in the northern states. It was preceded, a few seconds, by a rattling sound; its duration was short; its course as usual in America, from N. W. to S. E. No injury was sustained.

Courant, May 23.

On the morning after the earthquake, was observed at Middletown in Connecticut, a substance like honey or butter, covering the grass and earth for a considerable extent. See an account of a similar phenomenon in Ireland under the year 1695.

To these phenomena succeeded in Connecticut the generation of millions of that species of black worm, described under the year 1770. I believe they were far less numerous than in 1770; they however appeared in Hartford and in Norwich, and disappeared at the same time. They were very destructive to the grass and corn, but their existence was short; all dying in a few weeks.

---

* It may excite surprise that there should be supposed a connection between an uncommon abundance of fish and pestilence. But the theory that resolves this into the unusual powers of excitement, is rational. That state of the elements that causes pestilence, always produces unusual numbers of insects; and often the human race is more prolific than at other times. See the London Registers of births and deaths. Main. Hist. Lond.

A paragraph in a Maryland paper dated June 1, 1791, mentions animals, there called *caterpillars*, but evidently the fame fpecies of worm. They are reprefented as marching in legions from place to place, and devouring the grafs.

About the fame time appeared at Lanfingburg on the Hudfon, a fpecies of worm that greatly injured the fruit-trees.

Courant, June 25, 1792.

But the moft extraordinary phenomenon was the exiftence of the canker-worm, in numbers before unexampled. Whether thefe animals had made their appearance in the preceding year or not, I do not recollect. But in 1791 they devoured the orchards over the New-England ftates ; and their ravages were repeated in the two following years. Orchards, ftanding on ftiff clay and in low grounds which are wet in fpring, efcaped ; but on every fpecies of light and dry foil, the trees were as dry on the firft of June, as on the firft of January. Many trees have never recovered from the effects of their ravages.

Another worm of a diftinct fpecies, and called at the time, *palmer-worm*, overfpread our forefts in this or the next year, devouring the leaves of oak and other fpecies of wood.

It is a prevalent opinion that uncommon flights of wild pigeons in America, indicate the approach of a fickly feafon. I am not inclined to credit any popular opinion, without good grounds ; but this feems to have been formed on a long feries of obfervations. Certain it is that pigeons in the fummer of 1791 were unufually numerous. In Maine, there were tracts of foreft of miles in extent, the trees of which were covered with their nefts.

Courant, July 11.

The fummer of 1791 was exceffively hot. At Salem the thermometer was at and above 80 deg. no lefs than 55 days, and above 90, twelve days—an inftance that had not happened in many years, in that cool place ; altho it often happens in the middle ftates.

Mem. Am. Acad vol. 2 91.

On the 27th of November Lifbon fuftained fevere fhocks of earthquake.

Courant, April 2, 1792.

In autumn, bilious remittents assumed, in Philadelphia, the inflammatory diathesis, so predominant in the last pestilential constitution. Dr. Rush, in his public lectures, mentioned this fact at the time, altho he little suspected what effects that constitution was to produce in subsequent years. It was found necessary to bleed from one to three times. In most cases, the liver was affected with all the symptoms of Hepatitis.

M. S. letter from Dr. Rush.

At this period the pestilential or epidemic constitution of the atmosphere began to show itself in the infectious yellow fever. It appeared in New-York, in autumn, along the east river, and carried off about 200 persons. This gave some alarm, which soon subsided.

It must be noted that the measles in 1788, the disease which marched in the van of this series of epidemics, appeared first in New-York—this was probably the fact also in regard to the influenza of the succeeding year—and the scarlatina anginosa at the close of 1792. The scarlatina of 1789 and 91 in Philadelphia was local, or if it appeared in a few other places, it did not spread over the country. All the last great epidemics have originated nearly in the same longitude between Connecticut and Pennsylvania. It is not to be concluded from this fact that they have been propagated by infection from one spot, as from a center; we know this is not the fact; the same diseases originating in remote places.* But it serves to show that the cause or principle of disease in the elements is of various force, and will first show its effects in places where it has the most strength.

In the same summer of 1791, the pestilential principle began to exhibit its effects in the increased malignancy of the tropical fevers. The "unusual epidemic fever" in Grenada, described by Dr. Chisholm, in the Edinburgh Medical Commentaries for 1793, and which was the occasion of no small surprise, was the commencement of that series of fatal diseases, which, in subsequent years, made dreadful havoc in the Islands. This fever became so violent and infectious, contrary to the common fever

---

* The mild scarlatina, the herald of the epidemic, appeared at New-York and at Bethlem in Connecticut, in 1792, in the same month.

of the tropics, that a labored attempt was made to trace it to fomites from the coast of Africa. The truth is, the fever was nothing more than the common fever of the climate, with the superadded malignancy derived from the existing constitution of the elements. The same fact took place on the African coast; that is, the usual fevers of the climate became more malignant.

This idea is suggested by a series of similar events in other climates; all the diseases of America, at the same time, assuming a similar augmented violence, and sporadic cases of malignant fever appearing in all parts of our country. Such has been the fact in all other epidemic periods.

To confirm this idea, let it be observed that in the same year, when this malignant fever appeared in the African Seas on board of ships, in Grenada, and in New-York, as well as in sporadic cases in other parts of America, the plague carried off two or three hundred thousand people,[*] in Egypt, and raged in Constantinople with great mortality. In all these distant countries, the same or similar effects were nearly cotemporary. The plague in Egypt continued into the next year; but I have no details of its progress and termination. The same general principle was experienced in Great-Britain, and the bills of mortality in London continued to swell, till the year 1793.

The winter of 1791-2 was somewhat colder than usual. The month of January was remarkable for severe weather of three weeks duration. In March a slight earthquake was felt in the middle states, but I have no particulars.

Courant, March 19, 1792.

The spring months were very rainy in the southern states and the islands, which experienced distressing inundations.

Courant, May 28, 1792

In the northern states there was a period of singularly cold weather in the beginning of June, occasioned by a dry N. E. wind. Some persons used fires as late as the tenth day of that month. The heat of the following summer, in general, was not extreme.

---

[*] These numbers are to be suspected of exaggeration.

In May and June, a species of locusts appeared in the northern parts of the state of New-York, which committed ravages among the grain. The wheat-insect continued its ravages, and appeared this year as far southward as Elk Ridge in the state of Maryland. On Long-Island the destruction of wheat was great and distressing.

Courant, June 25, and July 2, 1792.

In July happened at Philadelphia a violent tornado; but the summer was not distinguished for the number of this species of tempest. In one instance, in Vermont, the hail-stones which fell are said to have been from 3 to 6 inches in circumference.

About this time, a malignant fever began to rage in Charleston, South-Carolina, carrying off the patient in three days, and occasioning a considerable mortality.

Courant, August 6, 1792.

In the following winter, Egypt was a prey to famin; and the streets of Cairo were filled with dead bodies.

In November 1792 several smart shocks of earthquake were felt in Perthshire, a county in Scotland.

In Philadelphia appeared an insect in the form of a fly, which generated a small worm or caterpillar, that attacked the tree, called Lime Tree, which is there used for shade. From that year to the year 1798, this insect has ravaged those trees, and destroyed some of them. Just philosophy will not hesitate to believe the cause of this phenomenon and of the pestilence succeeding, to be connected.

In this year, 1792, commenced that scarlatina anginosa which became epidemic, with great mortality. I regret that a want of exact registers, will not permit me to trace it to its sources with the precision desireable in all such cases. I am informed that well defined cases of the disease were observed in New-York, as early as the month of August. But it occasioned no considerable mortality in that city, until the following winter.

At Bethlem, in the western part of Connecticut, there were five deaths in this year by the cynanche trachealis. I have not heard of any other instance. In August, there were seven or eight cases of the scarlatina anginosa, but so mild as *not to prove mortal*. The reader will note the last circumstance; for I am able to prove, that this difeafe in Connecticut, was progreffive in a remarkable manner, and from the fact, which I believe is not uncommon, will be drawn moft important confequences.

The autumn was one of the mildeft ever known. November was fo warm that we fat with open windows, at Hartford, on the 19th of the month. This moderate weather was fucceeded by fevere cold, and Connecticut river was clofed by ice on the 10th of December. The latter part of winter however was not very fevere, except a week or two in February.

'On the 11th of January 1793 appeared a comet in the conftellation of Cepheus. It was feen for the laft time by Mr. Rittenhoufe on the 8th of February.

Phil Tranf Phil vol. 3.

In the courfe of this winter and the fpring fucceeding, the fcarlet fever raged in New-York, with confiderable mortality. It became epidemic alfo in Philadelphia, in the courfe of the fpring months.

Catarrh was very prevalent in the northern ftates, at the fame time; and the fmall-pox by inoculation at Hartford proved unufually obftinate and fatal; indicating an infalubrious ftate of the atmofphere.

In February 1793 the fcarlet fever invaded the town of Bethlem, like "an armed man," fays Mr. Backus, Medical Repofitory, vol. 1. 524. He calls the difeafe angina maligna, and it doubtlefs put on the fymptoms of it in many places. It feized almoft every family and child. It abated in May, difappeared in November, and re-appeared in January 1794 with nearly its former violence. Nineteen children died in the firft invafion, and fourteen, in the fecond.

We have here diftinct marks of progreffion. The difeafe in a mild form appeared in Auguft 1792, then difappeared. In February following, it invaded the town in its worft form. Six months therefore intervened between its precurfor, or mild form, and its invafion with full force.

The fame difeafe appeared in the neighboring diftrict of country and in diftant parts, in nearly the fame longitude, in the courfe of this year; but I have not materials for a detail of facts.

I find however, it prevailed in Litchfield in 1793, and was supposed to be *imported* into that town from Vermont. It was also very mortal in New-Fairfield, the same year. I therefore presume the disease to have been very general through the western districts of Connecticut, Massachusetts and Vermont, and to have prevailed as far westward as Pennsylvania, in this year. Of its progress beyond that state, I have no information.

In September and October of this year, about the time the distemper subsided in Bethlem, it began to exhibit appearances of approach, in the maritime towns of Connecticut. Its precursors at New-Haven, as described by Dr. Monson, a good judge of the subject, were " slight influenza, stinging pains in the jaws and limbs, soreness in the muscles of the neck, with a slight fever."

In November and December following, several cases of ulcerous sore throat occurred, but they had a favorable issue, and the symptoms were not alarming.

In January 1794 arrived the crisis of this disease; it put on its malignant symptoms, and in the course of the six following months, seized more than seven hundred persons, principally youth, of whom died fifty two.

See Dr. Monson's account in my Collection, p. 173.

Here again is distinctly marked a regular progression of symptoms from September to January; the precursors being four or five months in advance of the disease in its most violent form.

In Hartford, on Connecticut river, about thirty miles east of Litchfield and Bethlem, I had an opportunity to make personal observations on the origin and progress of this epidemic.

I do not know the date of the first case; but in my own memoranda, its appearance in my eldest daughter, then in the 3d year of her age, is noted under the 12th of May 1793. The attending physician informed me, that the disease was then epidemic. Its first appearance therefore must have been a week or two earlier.

This disease was a mild scarlatina anginosa. The patient had considerable fever—the paroxisms were daily, and terminated in profuse sweats—there was a partial efflorescence of the skin about the neck and breast, and some affection of the throat. Its crisis, if I do not mifremember, was about the eighth day. I was informed that in no cafe, did this difeafe prove mortal, during this invafion.

The reader will obferve the dates—this mild angina invaded Hartford in April and May, about the time, the feverity of the difeafe began to abate in Bethlem.

Nine months after the invafion of this mild angina, that is, in February 1794, this difeafe appeared in Hartford in its formidable array, and many children became its victims.

Nothing can prove more clearly that infection had no concern in the origin of this diftemper, than this gradual augmentation of its fymptoms. If any fact were neceffary to demonftrate the all-controlling influence of the elements, in the propagation and termination of the difeafe, this *progreffion* alone would be fufficient. The mild epidemic of May 1793, was the fame fpecies of difeafe with that which was then deftroying life, in the weftern parts of the ftate, and in New-York and Pennfylvania ; but the condition of the atmofphere at Hartford was not, at that time, fitted to give the difeafe its full degree of violence. The fummer feafon perhaps fufpended the operation of the general caufe, by means to us unknown. In February following arrived the crifis of the difeafe.

I know not whether other epidemic anginas have been characterized by the fame progreffivenefs in the fymptoms. It is not improbable that they have ; and that age after age has paffed away, without noticing the circumftance ; a circumftance that throws more light on the origin, caufes and fphilofophy of epidemics, than all the differtations on the fubject, fince the days of Hippocrates.

My own children were affected with the mild angina in May. I removed, with my family, to New-York in November 1793, *before* the fatal angina invaded Hartford, and *after* it had finifhed its courfe in New-York ; my children efcaped its violence, and probably in confequence of this removal. This was an accidental circumftance in my family, but I fufpect a fimilar removal of children, during the progrefs of that malady, might fave a multitude of lives ; altho the circumftances of many people will not permit them to avail themselves of the expedient; and in some cases probably it would fail of success. It however deserves consideration. The angina had completed its course in New-York in 1793 or nearly. It did not invade Boston till 1795. A removal of the children from the atmosphere of Boston in 1795, to an atmosphere where the disease had ceased, would probably have secured most of them from an attack.

The summer of 1793 was excessively hot, after a dry spring, and produced a great number of violent gusts, with rain and hail. The autumn was very dry. A fatal dysentery prevailed in Georgetown, on the Potomak, and in the vicinity, which swept away many hundreds of the inhabitants. The same disease prevailed in Coventry, in Connecticut, and killed almost every person whom it seized. A nervous or long fever prevailed in Wethersfield. In short, in most parts of the United States, the pestilential principle exhibited its effects, in some form or other, and every where swelled the bills of mortality. It extended to the West-Indies, and so violent was the epidemic at Grenada, that the physicians and inhabitants, unable to account for it, really supposed it an imported disease. The treatise written by Dr. Chisholm to prove it imported, is satisfactory evidence to me that the disease was an epidemic. The disease corresponds in its principal character, with the pestilential fevers of this country, many of which are known to be generated in our own climate.

In August 1793 commenced in Philadelphia that dreadful pestilence which alarmed the United States, and spread terror and dismay over that city. The spring diseases, which ushered in this malady, were influenza, scarlatina and mild bilious remittents. See Rush's Treatise on that fever. These are the most certain and immediate precursors of pestilence, in this country; and the influenza seems to be so, in all countries.

During this epidemic, the weather was very sultry and dry. About the 12th of September, fell a meteor between the city and the hospital. The number of victims to this disease was 4040.

A controversy arose among the physicians in Philadelphia, relative to the origin of the plague; one party tracing the disease, as they supposed, to infected vessels from the West-Indies;

the other afcribing it to exhalations from damaged coffee and filthy ftreets. This controverfy has occafioned an unhappy fchifm among the medical gentlemen, and the citizens of Philadelphia.

It is greatly to be regretted that gentlemen of the faculty committed themfelves, by prematurely giving pofitive opinions on that important queftion, and thus laying the foundation for permanent evils to the country. It would have been wifer to have inftituted a regular enquiry into hiftorical facts, relating to peftilential difeafes, antecedent to any pofitive decifions on the fubject.

By an account of the deaths in Algiers; kept by Capt. O'Brien, while a prifoner, I perceive that 4893 perfons died in 1793 by the meafles and plague. There was a confiderable increafe of mortality in that year; and we obferve the meafles and plague prevalent in the fame year—an evidence that on the Barbary coaft, as well as in Europe and America, thefe epidemics are allied.

By this account alfo it appears that in 1789 a number of perfons died by the *afthma*. It is not probable this was epidemic, and I fufpect by this name was intended catarrh or influenza. As this difeafe was then epidemic in the United States, it would be gratifying to know whether the fame epidemic prevailed on the African coaft, at the fame time.

It is remarkable that in the fpring of 1793, when the fcarlatina anginofa had firft commenced its progrefs in America, it began alfo in England. It appeared firft in the villages about London, and afterwards defcended into the city. Med. Mem. vol. 4. It continued to prevail for feveral years, with different degrees of violence, at different times. See the Monthly Magazines.

The winter of 1793-4 was milder than ufual in America. The thermometer in New-York, in a northern expofure, defcended no lower than 13 deg. above 0, and but twice to that degree.

On the 17th of May was a fingularly fevere froft in the northern ftates of America, which deftroyed garden vegetables and the leaves of trees. The wheat, oats and flax in many places turned yellow, and fruit was deftroyed.

This froſt was preceded by a few remarkable hot days, ſuch as we uſually have in June; and ſpeedily followed by a long ſeries of rains, with eaſterly winds.

This froſt has been ſuppoſed to kill the canker-worms, which had ravaged the orchards, for ſome years preceding. Another opinion is, that a hard froſt in April, deſtroyed them, juſt after they were hatched. A third opinion is, that they had run thro their period of exiſtence, and periſhed in a natural way. In confirmation of which opinion, it is ſaid they were evidently declining in the preceding year. There is probably truth in both the latter opinions.

The ſummer of 1794 was, on the whole, not intemperate. We had hot weather, but frequently was the earth refreſhed by ſhowers, and cool weſterly winds. The whooping cough prevailed in New-York.

The ſcarlet fever, in the courſe of this year, ſpread over Connecticut. Its effects are very apparent in the bills of mortality.

It appeared in 1795 in Boſton, in the ſpring or early in ſummer, and continued to prevail in Maſſachuſetts and New-Hampſhire in 1796. Its progreſs from New-York to Maine, about 300 miles or perhaps 400, was run in about four years. It travelled therefore about 100 miles in a year. Such alſo was the fact in the preceding period; as well as in 1735. It ſhould be obſerved alſo that its direction, in the two laſt epidemic periods, has been oppoſite to that of the diſeaſe of 1735. The latter began in New-Hampſhire and marched to the weſtward; the former began in the middle ſtates, and advanced to the eaſtward.

On the 10th of June 1794, the bilious plague made its appearance in New-Haven, a ſeaport in Connecticut. The perſon firſt ſeized with the diſeaſe was, the wife of Iſaac Gorham, living on the wharf, and the nature of her complaint was not underſtood, nor ſuſpected, till near the time of her death, on the 15th.

No ſooner was it known that a peſtilential fever was in the city, than the inhabitants took the alarm, and directed an examination to be made into the cauſes. On enquiry, the following appeared to be the ſources of the diſeaſe, or were reported to be the probable cauſes.

In the beginning of June, Capt. Truman arrived from Martinico, in a sloop, which was hauled up by the store of Mr. Elijah Austin, a few rods from the house of Mr. Gorham. This sloop was *supposed* to be infected with the pestilential fever of the West-Indies. From this sloop was landed a chest of clothes, which had belonged to a seaman who died with the fever in Martinico; which chest was opened and the contents inventoried by Mr. Austin, in his store, in presence of Capt. Truman, of Henry Hubbard, a clerk in the store, and of Polly Gorham, a niece of Isaac Gorham. Mr. Austin and his clerk were seized, a few days after the opening of this chest, (but how many days is not stated) and died about the 20th of June. Polly Gorham was seized on the 12th and died on the 17th of June.

These circumstances appeared to the people at that time, to be clear and decisive evidence of the importation of the fomites of the disease; and especially the fact, that Mr. Austin and his clerk were attacked with the symptoms, nearly at the same time. This acquiescence in an opinion so important to society and truth, renders it necessary to state the result of more careful enquiries.

In the first place, the opinion that the sloop could communicate the infection, is unfounded; for it does not appear that any person, ill with yellow fever, had been on board—there certainly had not been any sick on board, after her leaving Martinico. The sloop was taken by the British troops, when they took that island, and lay in port some weeks, unoccupied; until Capt. Truman had an opportunity to purchase her. In the mean time, some of the crew, to keep themselves employed and procure bread, went in the business of *droging*; that is, transporting goods from place to place. One of them died with the fever, but on shore, and he had not been on board of the sloop, after his illness. On the passage home, the seamen were all in good health. There is therefore not the least ground to suppose the sloop contained any infection, and no part of her cargo was supposed to be in a bad state. The external parts of a vessel or house cannot retain or communicate infection.

Secondly As to the chest of clothes, it is probable it contained no infection from diseased persons, for by the affidavit of

Capt. Truman, taken before Alderman Furman of New-York, at the requeſt of Dr. Baily, the Health Officer of that port, which affidavit I have conſulted, it appears that the clothing, worn by the ſeaman who owned the cheſt and died at Martinico, was all wrapped in his blanket with his body and buried. As Capt. Truman is a man of good character and has made his affidavit, four years ſince the diſeaſe at New-Haven, when all apprehenſions of injury from declaring the truth, have ſubſided, there ſeems to be no reaſon to queſtion the fact.

But as men, who have not attended to the great operations of nature in producing epidemic diſeaſes, naturally look for the cauſes among viſible and tangible ſubſtances, they ſtill found a reſource in a Britiſh regimental coat, which was in the cheſt, and which, it was *ſuppoſed*, might have belonged to a ſoldier who *might have died* of the yellow fever. In conſequence of theſe ſuſpicions, the contents of the cheſt were all burnt.

On examination it appears that the coat was new—and the mate of the ſloop has ſworn that he ſaw the coat plundered by the ſeaman from a bale of goods, and he believes it had never been worn. It was taken by the ſeaman in the buſineſs of droging, from among the packages of clothing ſent by the Britiſh government for the uſe of the troops. But had we no ſuch evidence, common ſenſe might inform us, that a man, *laboring under a fever in the ſultry climate of the Weſt-Indies*, would not wear his regimentals.

In the cheſt therefore, as in the ſloop, we can find no infection of yellow fever. If Mr. Auſtin and his clerk received the ſeeds of diſeaſe from the clothing in the cheſt, as it is poſſible they did, the ſources of the diſeaſe muſt have been the fetid effluvia of dirty clothes, which had been kept a long time, cloſe packed in a cheſt, in a ſultry climate. It is not neceſſary to ſuppoſe the clothes to have been worn by a diſeaſed perſon. The ſweat and filth from a body in health, if confined in the hot ſeaſon, will ferment and produce a poiſon injurious to health, and productive of yellow fever or other diſeaſe.*

* It is a well authenticated fact, that Mr. Daniel Phenix, treaſurer of the city of New-York, and his ſons, were infected with a violent yellow fever, by means of the fetid effluvia from packages of bills of

But as some reports have been circulated, in contradiction of the testimony of Capt. Truman, and as there is a possibility that he might have mistaken the facts, I lay out of this question all the evidence respecting the sloop. For whether the trunk contained infected clothes or not, is wholly immaterial; and without any reference to that point, the evidence that the fever in New-Haven did not spring from any imported source, is complete.

Mr. Austin went on business to New-York, was seized with fever and died. His body was conveyed in a sloop to New-Haven, and buried. It is an agreed point, that no friend, nurse or other person took the fever from him.

Mr. Hubbard went on business to Derby, ten miles distant, was taken ill and died. His body was carried to New-Haven, and buried. It is agreed that no person took the disease from him.

It is not known that Polly Gorham was ever near the trunk of clothing—the report of her being present rests on the story of a child. But if she was, it makes no difference, for no person who attended her was affected, except her mother, who had a slight fever. She lived and was ill, a mile from the wharf, and no person in that neighborhood was afterwards affected. In short, it is not pretended that the infection proceeded from either of these persons—the *only persons* who could possibly have taken the disease from the trunk of clothing.

It is admitted on all hands that the infection must have proceeded from the house of Isaac Gorham. Now it happens that Mrs. Gorham who was *first seized and five days before Mr. Austin and his clerk*, had never been near the trunk of clothing, nor was an article of clothing from the sloop carried into the house. For this assertion, I have the authority of Mr. Gorham himself, who is admitted to be a man of veracity.

Had the origin and phenomena of epidemic diseases ever been understood, the people of New-Haven would have foreseen, with

credit, which had been returned into the treasury, after being long used, passing through dirty, sweaty hands, and then being close packed for some weeks, in a hot season The fact is related to me by Mr. Phenix himself The attack in the first case, was severe; and on a subsequent occasion, a second attack passed off with a nausea.

a good degree of certainty, that they could not escape pestilence. This will appear from the following facts.

In the winter and spring of 1794, the scarlatina anginosa prevailed generally in New-Haven and the neighboring towns; manifesting a highly pestilential condition of the elements. One case of bilious fever, attended with a vomiting of black matter, occurred as early as the last week in March.

For many months preceding the invasion of the fever, the oysters, on the coast of Connecticut, were in a very sickly state. Many people can testify to the truth of this fact; but I have an account of it recorded at the time by the late President Stiles. In a letter to his son-in-law, the Rev. Mr. Holmes, of Cambridge in Massachusetts, dated Sept. 25, 1794, he writes, that for twelve months past he had eaten very few oysters, as they were diseased, poor and dropsical. He remarked this of the oysters from New-York to Boston. Those caught on the shores of Branford, Killingworth, and at Blue-Point on the south side of Long-Island, were intolerable. At the date of the letter they were recovering and becoming more palatable. This is a striking proof of the derangement of the elements.

Further evidence of this fact was furnished by the multitudes of caterpillars which overran the city of New-Haven, in the summer of 1794.* In such numbers were these insects, that they almost covered the trees, fences and houses to the tops of chimneys. The preceding history furnishes many instances of this phenomenon, preceding and accompanying pestilence.

Had these phenomena been understood, the people of New-Haven would have had no occasion to appoint a committee to examin into the causes of the fever. It was hardly possible, in the nature of things, that the human race should escape the calamity of epidemic diseases, under the operation of causes so general and powerful.

But these were not all. Mr. Gorham, whose family first suffered by the fever, had, in the month preceding the invasion, cleaned a great number of shad, upon the wharf by his door,

* Some persons say, this was in 1793, but it is not material.

and thrown the garbage, to the amount of a cart load perhaps, into the dock.

The alternate washing of the tide, and action of a hot sun, had rendered the putrefaction of this mass of filth extremely rapid; and there being no current to remove it, the stench became intolerable. On the other side of the wharf, a few rods distant, a boat load of clams had been deposited on the mud, that the water, during the flux of the tide, might preserve them; but a great part of them were soon spoiled, and added to the fetor of the atmosphere.

To complete the list of nusances, some barrels of damaged pickled cod-fish had been thrown from a store into the dock, and the whole was left uncovered during the recess of the tide. So noisome was the air of the place, for sometime before the fever appeared, that the proprietor of the wharf desisted from his usual morning visits before breakfast. For all these facts I have the declarations of the persons concerned and eye witnesses.

The putrefaction of flesh, from thirty years observations, I can testify, will not always produce disease. But in a pestilential state of air, the dissolution of flesh is unusually rapid, and the acid evolved, peculiarly noxious. In such circumstances, putrescent substances of all kinds appear to be powerful auxiliary causes of disease. The condition of the elements accelerates putrefaction, and that putrefaction in turn increases the deleterious quality of the air.*

Under the operation of so many causes of disease, instead of being surprised at the appearance of a pestilential fever, we are rather to wonder that its ravages were not more extensive.

That the putrefaction of the fish was an exciting cause of the fever in New-Haven, is probable from the early appearance of it in summer. The first cases occurred about the 10th of June, which is earlier than the epidemic pestilence of America usually occurs; and which indicates the existence of strong local causes. What further confirms this opinion, is, that after a few weeks

---

* I may add to these causes of the fever, the water of the well used by the people living on the wharf, which happened at that time to be covered over with dead rats in a state of putrefaction. This was discovered by the offensiveness of the water.

the diftemper was nearly or wholly extinct. In July died only three perfons, and for about two weeks, no new cafe occurred. But in Auguft, the ufual time of the appearance of this difeafe in this part of America, it broke out with frefh violence. It is probable therefore that the *morbid local* caufes induced the fever in one fmall fpot, before the proper feafon for it to prevail. Thefe caufes being gradually extinguifhed by the tides and a hot fun, the difeafe fubfided, until the ufual feafon for fuch fevers. The fame took place in New-York in 1795—in 1796—and 1798.

That the plague in New-Haven was the effect of a condition of the elements united with local caufes, is proved by fubfequent events. In the following year, a malignant dyfentery originated and prevailed in New-Haven, deftroying more lives than the bilious plague of 1794. This difeafe is acknowledged by able phyficians to be of the fame fpecies as the yellow fever. See Lind on that point, and Rufh's Works vol. 5. 5, where it is ftated, on the authority of Dr. Woodhoufe, that feveral perfons took the yellow fever from foldiers, laboring under the dyfentery. It is well known alfo that an epidemic yellow fever has been converted, by a fudden change of weather, into an epidemic dyfentery, and *vice verfa*; as at Baltimore in 1797. It is alfo true that the yellow fever in autumn paffes off in dyfentery, as in New-London in 1798. The fame is at times true of the plague in Afia.

This difeafe in 1795, as well as a fimilar dyfentery in Derby in 1794, demonftrated the deleterious condition of the elements in that region or vicinity.

If further evidence was neceffary, we have it in the bad ftate of the water in fome of the wells in New-Haven, during the prevalence of thefe difeafes, in which, one of the phyficians of the city has informed me, were animalcules vifible to the naked eye. This fact correfponds with what occured in Athens, during the plague, where the badnefs of the water, it is fuppofed, led the people to afcribe the difeafe to the poifoning of the wells by the Lacedemonians. A fimilar fact probably led the Germans, in 1349, to fufpect the Jews had poifoned the wells, and on fufpicion alone to maffacre them without mercy. This ftate of the water, and the ficknefs of the oyfters alone decide the point, that the principal fources of the epidemics of 1794 and 5, were in the elements.

It has been afferted that no perfon in New-Haven was affected by the fever, without intercourfe with the fick or with infected clothing. On careful enquiry, I find this is not true. Several perfons were affected who were not in the rooms, nor even in the houfes of the fick, and who could not be expofed, otherways than by paffing along the ftreets. But fuch perfons could not take the fever from the effluvia of the difeafed. Men who fuppofe this, are unacquainted with the powers of infection. Dr. Chifholm ftates exprefsly that the infection of that difeafe in Grenada never exceeded *ten feet* ; that it was eafy to avoid it, and many who lived in the houfes of the difeafed, efcaped. Med. Repof. vol. 2. 288. Dr. Lind, the ableft writer on the fubject, who fpent his whole life in jails and hofpitals, has advanced the fame doctrin. A great number of fick in a narrow clofe built ftreet, may render the air of it infectious, but a few difeafed perfons in the wide ftreets of New-Haven could not produce this effect. In general however the difeafe in this place was propagated by infection ; the pollution of the atmofphere being confined to a fmall diftrict on and near the wharf, on low ground, to the leeward of the putrid fubftances before mentioned, and near the creek.

But there is one fact that will decide the queftion relative to the origin of the peftilential fever in New-Haven, and every other place. It is ftated by the phyficians that all other difeafes yielded to this fever. After it appeared in June, the fcarlatina fubfided, and " in September, when the fever was moft prevalent, the inhabitants in general were almoft entirely free from every other complaint."

See Dr. Monfon's account of the fever, in my Collection, p 178.

Here we have an infallible criterion by which to determin whether a difeafe is an epidemic of the place, or introduced and propagated folely by infection. A difeafe of mere infection can never extinguifh other difeafes of the place. The fmall-pox introduced by *variolous matter*, and communicated to every family would not abforb a dyfentery or fcarlet fever prevailing in the fame place ; every hofpital will demonftrate this principle. A difeafe of mere infection would not affect another difeafe even in the next house. Every disease that extinguishes another disease current in a town, is an epidemic originating in that place. It not only proves that the atmosphere will produce that distemper, but it proves that it will produce no other. On this principle I will rest the question, as it regards not only the fever in New-Haven, but every pestilence that ever existed.

The summer of 1794 was, in most places, less sickly than in 1793 and 1795; yet the scarlatina extended its ravages over Connecticut, and Philadelphia and New-York experienced the predominant epidemic constitution. In Philadelphia died from 70 to 100 persons of the bilious plague; in New-York twenty or thirty cases of the same disease indicated the same condition of the atmosphere. It was the general opinion in New-York, that the city was remarkably healthy; but this opinion, so flattering to the people, was a fallacy. The bills of mortality were higher than in healthy years, and this augmented mortality was a prelude to the epidemic of the succeeding year.

On the 15th of June was a great eruption of Vesuvius, nearly equal to that of 1779. The lava ran down the mountain on the west and extended to the sea, overwhelming the town of Tome del Greco.

See Universal Mag. for Aug. 1795.

In this year the bilious pestilence prevailed in Baltimore. No suggestion has been made that it was imported, and the physicians and inhabitants seem to admit the disease to have been only a more malignant form of the ordinary autumnal remittent.

In the succeeding winter, the epidemic of the summer and autumn changed, in Philadelphia, into the form of catarrh or pleurisy, and in many cases, was attended with delirium and mania. See Rush on this subject.

Pestilential epidemics, or rather the state of the atmosphere which produces them, usually affects the brain, in a most sensible degree. This is obvious from the vertigo, so frequent during sickly periods; pains in the head, dizziness and nervous debility often complained of by studious men. In some periods, this affection of the brain has appeared in epidemic madness. See the years 1355; 1373 and 4.

A few cases of a disorder of this species appeared in New-Haven and its vicinity in the winter after the pestilence. The patient was seized with a violent pain in the head, between the Os frontis and the Coronal Sutures, which was periodical, commencing about 11 o'clock A. M. and increasing till 2 P. M. In some cases, the paroxism was accompanied with delirium; but the pain was limited to the head, and unattended with fever. Bleeding, purging and opium produced no alleviation; but a blister on the forehead or temple, soon relieved the patient, and effected a cure. This account is taken from Dr. Hotchkiss, the attending physician.

The winter of 1794-5 was very cold in Europe, and in January 1795, the French troops marched into Amsterdam, over the rivers and canals, on the ice. This severity was to be expected from the great eruption of Vesuvius in the preceding summer.

The catarrh was epidemic in January and February, in the British channel fleet. In one ship it assumed the symptoms of a pure typhus.

Trotter's Med Naut p 366.

In America, the same winter was milder than usual. Persons walked on the battery at New-York, for pleasure, on Christmas day, with no covering but their ordinary autumnal clothes; and vessels sailed up the Hudson and Connecticut till January. In the latter part of the winter, we had some cold weather, and a cool late spring.

About the 20th of July, began a series of hot, damp, rainy weather, with light southerly winds; a season answering to the description which Hippocrates has given of a pestilential constitution. Heavy rains were followed by a humid, close, sultry air; no thunder and lightning; no north-westerly winds to cool and refresh the fainting bodies of men. For many weeks the atmosphere was so loaded with vapor, that no electricity could be excited with the best instruments. Fruit perished on the trees and fell half rotten and covered with mold. Sound potatoes from the market perished in my cellar in thirty-six hours. Cabbages rotted off, between the head and the stalk, as they stood in gardens. The moisture penetrated into the inmost recesses of desks and bureaus, covering books, papers and clothes with mold, under two locks. The walls of houses, and the paper of inner apartments became white with mold and required scraping. This state of the air produced also musketoes without number; while flies disappeared. It is observable that these two kinds of insects thrive in different conditions of the air—flies in a hot, dry air; musketoes, in a hot, moist air.

It is necessary here to correct a mistake of Dr. Currie on bilious fevers, page 12, where he mentions the years 1795 and 7 as " wetter and cooler than many preceding seasons." The truth is, the latter part of the summer of 1795, was on an average three degrees by Farenheit, warmer than the weather had been in the ten preceding years. See a letter from Professor Kemp in Dr. Bailey on yellow fever, p. 54. In the course of my life, I never experienced a state of air so debilitating and unfriendly to animal spirits, as the month of August 1795. The effects of it are very visible in the bill of mortality for that year in Philadelphia, which contains double the usual number of deaths.

In July of this year appeared the bilious plague in New-York. The first case that excited public attention was that of Dr. Treat, the Health Officer of the port, who fell a victim, on the 29th of the month. His disease has been ascribed by some persons, to infection taken on board a vessel from the West-Indies, the brig Zepher in which a person died, whom Dr. Treat assisted in burying. But it is not probable, that this was a just opinion; as many other persons visited the same vessel, and the wardens of the port were on board, while a part of her cargo, some damaged coffee, was thrown into the stream, without the least inconvenience to their health. The plethoric habit of Dr. Treat, and his great fatigue in an open boat and in a burning sun, are sufficient to account for his disease.

But admitting him to have taken his disease from the fomes of a sick or dead person, or from the foulness of the brig, the fact does not in the least aid the advocates of infection, for no person, nurse, attendant or visitor, received the distemper from him, nor did the difeafe prevail, in the ftreet where he died, during the fubfequent feafon.

It was faid that three or four feamen, belonging to the fhip William, were feized with the diftemper in confequence of vifiting the brig Zepher. But on enquiry, it was found, that thefe men only came along fide of the brig and purchafed fome fruit. To fuppofe thefe men fhould all take a difeafe from the brig, when two or three wardens of the port, who were fome hours on board, while a damaged cargo was difcharged, efcaped without the leaft affection, is ridiculous.

But what cuts fhort all controverfy on this fubject, is, that fourteen days at leaft before the death of Dr. Treat, a man in the hofpital died of a fimilar fever; and the late Dr. Pitt Smith, informed me in the autumn of 1795, that he vifited another patient a blackfmith, with a fimilar difeafe, early in July. In fact then, the difeafe was in New-York before the arrival of the fuppofed infected veffels; and the cafes which occurred early in July, were *precurfors* of the epidemic which was to follow.

It muft alfo be obferved that the difeafe in New-York never fpread over the whole city. It ran along the low ftreets on the Eaft river, in what was formerly the fwamp and in the narrow alleys. The high grounds in the center of the city, and the weftern fide of the ifland, were healthy as ufual; and the difeafe, when carried from the infected ftreets, upon the elevated parts of the city, exhibited no contagion, but difappeared.—A fmall part only of the citizens fled; moft of them remained, and purfued their occupations, in the greateft part of the city, with perfect fafety. The deaths were about feven hundred and thirty; among which at leaft five hundred were foreigners, moft of whom had recently arrived from Scotland and Ireland.[*] The mortality in New-York was moftly owing to this influx of foreigners, not feafoned to our climate.

This fever in New-York was preceded in fpring by epidemic meafles, which difappeared totally during the three months, when

[*] Four hundred and fixty two belonged to the Catholic Congregation under the Rev Mr O'Brien, moft of whom had been fo fhort a time in the country, that he did not know them.

the fever was the ruling disease, and re-appeared in November—a decisive evidence that the fever was produced and controlled by the same cause, as the measles.

In this year also appeared the same disease at a landing, called Mill-river four miles from Fairfield, in Connecticut, and about sixty miles from New-York—a small village, near the water. It was reported that this distemper was propagated at Mill-river, by infected persons from New-York. I have taken pains to enquire carefully of both the attending physicians and the clergymen, who visited the sick, who all agree, that one man from New-York had died of the fever in the village, that summer, and he was dead, *three weeks* before, Mr. Tharp, the first man seized, was taken ill.

The disease affected others of his family, but spread no further; and the gentlemen abovementioned do not believe it to have been derived from imported infection.

The bilious remittent fever, is annually the disease of autumn in some parts of the southern states; and strangers, visiting that country from the Delaware to Florida, in the hot season run the hazard of a fever. Drs. Taylor and Hansford, two old practitioners in Norfolk, Virginia, speaking of the yellow fever of 1795, say, " The same fever, with all its malignant and uncontrollable symptoms, occurs every year, in scattered instances, and about the same season."

See my Collection on Bilious Fevers, p. 151.

But during pestilential periods, this disease in that unhealthy country, takes a wider spread, and becomes infectious.

In 1795 this was the case at Norfolk—a town that is situated on low flat land, a few feet only above high-water, and subject to autumnal fevers. The disease prevailed most in the narrow streets and poor small houses, and was most fatal to strangers.

Two remarkable facts occurred there and are related in the account last cited, to prove that the disease was occasioned solely by a general state of the atmosphere in and about the town, without a dependence on infection. The first is, that traders who visited the port, altho they were not known to have had intercourse with the sick, took the disease and died on their return into the country. But a more remarkable fact is, that the seamen of a ship from Liverpool, which did not approach nearer than five miles distance from the town, and which had no communication with the shore, except by means of the healthboat, were almost all attacked with the disease, in ten days after their arrival. This was late in the season, and when the disease had nearly disappeared in town.

In the year 1794 several cases of the same disease had occurred in Norfolk. In 1797 the disease was again frequent. In 1795 and 7, the disease was supposed to have been augmented by the great rains and floods which had preceded, and which had brought down the river and spread on the shores, large quantities of vegetable substances.

The extreme unhealthiness of the summer of 1795, was manifested by unusual mortality in various other parts of the country. On the level plains of Duchess county in New-York state, prevailed a mortal dysentery and typhus fever. At Coxsakie on the west of the Hudson, raged similar diseases with fatal effects. In some western parts of the state, near the marshes which border the waters of the country, a malignant bilious fever was more terribly fatal, than the fever in New York.

In Sheffield, a western township of Massachusetts, near two large ponds which form marshy grounds, bilious fevers, which had not been known there for many years, before, prevailed and in some cases were mortal.

See Dr Buel's account of these diseases, in my Collection, p 53.

In that town, the progressiveness of the morbid principle of this pestilential period, was clearly discoverable. Many cases of intermittents occurred in 1793; and a few instances of bilious remittents. This was during the plague in Philadelphia. In 1794, early in spring, inflammatory diseases of the pneumonic kind, were unusually frequent. These were succeeded by intermittents, which were more frequent than in the preceding year. In July, the bilious remittent appeared, and 80 inhabitants out of 150, who lived within a mile and a half of the south pond, were affected. In 1795, of 200 inhabitants within three fourths of a mile distant from the north pond, 150 were affected with the same disease—but few died.

In 1796, the dysentery, which had not appeared in many preceding years, began its attacks on children, and not long after adults were taken either with the same disease or with the bilious remittent. Of one hundred families living within a mile and a half of one of the ponds, not ten escaped sickness—more than half of the inhabitants were, in the course of the season, attacked with one or other of the above mentioned diseases. Of 150 persons who lived nearest to the pond, not ten escaped. The deaths by these diseases were forty-four. Here then was a regular increase of malignancy in the autumnal diseases, from intermittents, to the worst form of dysentery and bilious remittent.

Med. Repos. vol. 1. 456.

In the preceding period, great mortality prevailed among the geese in some parts of our country; and in the year 1796, a similar mortality among other fowls. I have not been able to obtain a particular description of the symptoms, but it was observed the transition from apparent health to death, was very rapid.

In 1796 the measles which commenced in New-York in 1795 was epidemic in Connecticut; and unusually prevalent in London.

In 1796 also the bilious plague again appeared in New-York, but in a different quarter of the city from that which was principally affected, the year preceding. In 1795, it began and was most general in the north-eastern part—in 1796, in the south-western part, near the battery; and in both summers, its seat was along the wharves on the East river, and in the adjoining streets and alleys. All this part of the city is a level, formed by extending the land and wharves into the East river. The land is of course loose and porous, admitting, in many places, the water of the sea into the cellars of the houses; some of which are penetrated, on every flux of the tide. These artificial streets, Front and Water streets, are not easily washed clean, on account of their level position, and they receive the filth washed from the higher grounds of the city. To these streets, and similar ones in the swamp on the north-east, was the malignant distemper principally limited.

In 1796 a new wharf below Exchange slip, which had been timbered the preceding autumn, and left unfilled, had become a reservoir for all kinds of putrid, filthy substances, and was supposed to be a powerful cause of disease.

Besides, the quarter in which the disease raged this year, is almost wholly covered with old wooden houses, and many of them, built before the raising and paving of the street, have their lower floors two or three feet below the surface of the pavements. In this district appeared the yellow fever in June; but a series of rainy weather and cool westerly winds, suspended its action, in the beginning of July. Succeeding hot weather renewed it, and in the limits above described, extending about forty or fifty rods, about seventy persons fell victims. The other parts of the city remained in the usual autumnal state of health, with only a few scattering cases of the plague.

At Wilmington, North-Carolina, prevailed a similar disease. It was preceded by the dysentery, in July, after a very wet spring. When the bilious fever commenced in August, the dysentery declined, and those who had been affected with it escaped the fever. About one hundred and fifty deaths, by these two forms of disease, occurred in 130 families. Different opinions were entertained about the origin of the fever; but the physician who gives this account has no doubts of its domestic origin. He informs us further that a few cases, in that town, occur annually, which assume all the symptoms of a violent yellow fever.

Med. Repos. vol. 2 153 Dr Roffet's letter.

In this year, the disease occasioned a considerable mortality in Charleston, South-Carolina, and in Newburyport, in Massachusetts. It appeared in Boston also, but was not general nor severe.

In Charleston, it succeeded one of the most destructive fires, ever known in that city; and was in part ascribed to the stagnant water which accumulated in the open cellars.

In Newburyport, there was no plausible pretext for ascribing the disease to imported infection; and the general belief was, that the immediate exciting cause, was, the remains of large quantities of fish which had been left to corrupt on the wharf, near which the distemper originated, and which occasioned an intolerable stench. But in that town, a previous increase of mortality indicated a sickly state of the elements; as in all other places, where the peſtilence has made its appearance. In none of the northern ſtates, which are uſually healthy, has the bilious plague occurred without other diſeaſes for precurſors.—The diſeaſe in Newburyport was confined to a low ſtreet or two, and when carried upon the high grounds, it exhibited little or no infection, but diſappeared with the death or recovery of the patient.

M. S. Letter from Nicholas Pike, Eſq.

In Boſton, the diſeaſe ſpread only in a ſmall part of the town, adjoining the water. The phyſicians were unanimouſly of opinion, that it was not occaſioned by any fomites from infected articles imported, but generated in the town.

See Dr. Warren's Letter in the Medical Repoſitory, vol. 1. p. 136.

The peſtilential ſtate of the elements was ſtrongly marked, this year, by the poorneſs of the ſhad brought to market in New-York. Theſe were all thin, lean and ſmall; and for this reaſon, I purchaſed none for my own uſe, during the ſeaſon. Other perſons obſerved the fact; and I am ſince informed that ſuch of thoſe fiſh as were pickled, periſhed in defiance of all human care to preſerve them. The ſame ſtate of the ſhad was obſerved in Connecticut.

Some caſes of yellow fever occurred in Philadelphia in 1796; catarrh was frequent in the winter, followed by meaſles of a moſt inflammatory nature. A remarkable halo appeared on the 25th of July.

Ruſh, vol. 5. 9.

It has been already obſerved that the winter of 1795, was remarkably ſevere in Europe. In America the ſame winter was as mild as uſual. But in the ſummer and autumn of 1796, the northern ſtates experienced a moſt ſevere drouth.

The following winter was very ſevere; the cold exceeding what is uſual, and being of long duration. The ſummer of 1797 was cool and wet. The winter of 1797-8 was ſevere—and the cold of very long duration. It commenced early in November and continued till March. The Hudſon and Connecticut were cloſed in November; a very rare occurrence. For ſeveral weeks in November and December, the wind, without much ſnow on the earth along the Atlantic coaſt, was from the north-weſt and intenſely dry and cold.

In August 1797 appeared a comet, which, according to calculations of astronomers, passed near the earth, altho it was of small apparent magnitude, and seen by few people.

The influence of this species of bodies in occasioning great tides, and violent storms, has been already mentioned, and of that influence, in the present instance, I was a witness. In 1797 my residence was, as it had been the preceding year, on a height of York Island near Corlaer's Hook to the northward of which is a flat, which is never covered with water by a common tide, but is overspread by spring tides, or any unusual swell in consequence of easterly winds. I observed, as early as the last week in May, high tides were unusually frequent and the swell extraordinary. In the city of New-York, the same fact was observable; and the inhabitants about Beekman slip will recollect how often the wharves and street were covered with water. These tides were not to be accounted for, on any known principles of lunar influence, and I frequently mentioned the phenomenon to my friends, but without suspecting the cause. The same phenomenon was noticed at other places. In Norfolk, the epidemic fever was, in part, ascribed to unusual tides; as I was afterwards informed. On the Delaware, the overflowing of the low lands, below Philadelphia, was extraordinary, and some physicians ascribe to this cause the yellow fever, which swept away most of a family by the name of Whitall.

I was lately mentioning these events to a respectable gentleman in Stamford,* who instantly recollected a fact which confirms the foregoing account. He remarked that the common practice in that town, is to mow the salt meadows, at the quadratures of the moon, on account of small tides; but in 1797, the calculations failed, and the people were much troubled to collect their hay, on account of high tides—a circumstance that was very surprising to him at the time, but he did not advert to the probable cause. This was in August; about the time that the comet was first observed. The fact then of the influence of comets, in raising the waters of the ocean, is well established; and the

* The Hon. John Davenport, now representative in Congress.

appearance of a comet in autumn explained the phenomena of the tides to my satisfaction.

The influence of comets in augmenting tempests is equally certain and remarkable.

On the 19th of August, a storm and whirlwind in South Prussia tore up forests carried trees along like sheaves of wheat, and levelled several villages.

In Rome and Naples happened a most extraordinary tempest on the 25th of September, such as the oldest man could not recollect. It took up men and carried them some distance. The astronomers were consulted and they ascribed it to the approximation of the comet.

A storm of hail in the province of Macconnois, in France, and on the borders of Burgundy, destroyed the vines and fruits of the earth in thirty-four villages. In the appropriations made afterwards by the councils of France, four millions were granted to repair the losses by hail, inundations and other disasters.

On the 7th of September, a considerable shock of earthquake was felt in the Western Pyrenees. On the 28th of the month was a volcanic eruption in Guadaloupe; and many earthquakes occurred during the autumn.

In England, the summer was so rainy and wet, as to injure the corn and threaten the inhabitants with scarcity. It would require pages to relate all the accidents by floods in Great-Britain from August to the close of the year.

During the autumnal months, the Black sea also was unusually tempestuous, and the loss of shipping alarmed Constantinople, with apprehensions of a scarcity of provisions.

In February, 1797, South-America was terribly convulsed. Quito and the neighboring provinces suffered, by the destruction of almost every house. Mountains were detached from their stations and rolled against each other, burying villages in ruin. Volcanoes emitted fire, lava, and rivers of water. It is said, that 40,000 inhabitants perished.

On the 11th of January 1798 a shock of earthquake was felt in Lancaster, Pennsylvania, and the neighboring towns, during which appeared to issue from the earth a flame or blaze, like the burning of a chimney.

In this month, the severe cold reached the West-Indies, and frost appeared, for several mornings, on the windows in Port Royal Parish, in Jamaica. A small earthquake was felt there in January.

Royal Gazette, Jan 29, 1798

In February 1797 also violent earthquakes were experienced on the western coast of Sumatra, in the East-Indies.

This year, 1797, was remarkable for other singular phenomena in Europe and America.

In England a pestilence among cats swept away those animals by thousands. It seems that this disease began as early as April, and succeeded an epidemic catarrh among the human race. The same cat-distemper was afterwards epidemic in France. A society at Montpelier instituted an enquiry into this remarkable phenomenon.

The cat-distemper appeared in Philadelphia, as early as June, and proceeded northward and eastward, like the catarrh of 1789. In August it was very fatal in New-York, and in the course of the summer and autumn, it spread destruction among those animals over the northern states.

In August, dead fish, in great numbers, were seen to float down James' river, in Virginia, for many days in succession.

Canine madness, during the same year, was unusually epidemic and attended with fatal effects, of which full accounts may be seen in the first volume of the Medical Repository.

These phenomena indicate an unhealthy state of the elements. But it is a remarkable fact that, in some places and seasons, the principal force of the epidemic constitution seems to be spent on *one* species of animals, while others are exempt. Thus in England, the catarrh, which had affected mankind in 1797, ceased, before the epidemic seized the cats. In America, the northern states, with the exception of a few places, were remarkably healthy, in 1797, while cats died in multitudes. And it is a frequent occurrence in Europe, that while the plague or some other malignant disease is afflicting the human race in one country; in another country, mankind will escape, and a most terrible mortality will occur among cattle, horses or sheep.

In 1797 the bills of mortality in the northern states, which had been swelled very high by angina and malignant fevers, fell nearly to the standard of health. There are a few exceptions.

The plague appeared in Philadelphia, Baltimore, Norfolk and Charleston. In the two latter cities, it is confidered, as the ufual autumnal fever, with aggravated fymptoms, from feafon or other local or temporary caufes.

In Baltimore, the difeafe appeared firft in the form of a common remittent, but increafed in malignancy till late in autumn and became infectious. The hiftory of this epidemic is minutely ftated by the magiftracy of Baltimore, and is too interefting to be paffed with a flight notice. The following is a correct abftract of the ftatement made and publifhed by authority.

The commiffioners ftate to the mayor of the city;

That the firft appearance of the fever was near the end of June in two young men, Parkin and M'Kenna, who occupied a warehoufe in South-ftreet and who died in a few days. The warehoufe was examined, and was found to contain nothing which could be the fpecial caufe of the fever; nor is it fuggefted that they were infected from abroad. No perfon received the difeafe from them. From this time till the clofe of Auguft, Weft Baltimore remained in a ftate of unufual health.

In Eaft Baltimore (Fell's Point) a bilious fever had fhowed itfelf early in the feafon, and gradually fpread and grew worfe; but was fuppofed to be no other than the common ficknefs of the feafon. It therefore excited no alarm, till the 26th Auguft, when a rumor prevailed, that the fever was fomething *more than common.* The chairman of the board addreffed a letter to each of the phyficians in that part of the city, requefting to be informed whether any cafe of contagious difeafe had come under his obfervation.

Dr. John Coulter wrote for anfwer that fince the third week in June, a fever had prevailed and become epidemic, affecting all defcriptions of people, but moftly thofe who labored hard, in the heat of the fun, intemperate perfons and thofe who expofed themfelves to night air after the labors of the day. The difeafe was violent, and unlefs fpeedily affailed with powerful remedies, proved fatal. It had on that day, August 26th, become general, and " assumed to itself the sole government of the diseases," in that part of the city. " During the wet weather, in the last of July and beginning of August, it yielded, for near two weeks, to the dysentery," which afterwards gave way to a recurrence of the yellow fever. [The reader is desired to note that fact.]

Dr. Coulter calls the fever an epidemic, in contradistinction to imported contagion, and says, " it is in the locality of our atmosphere, the source of which I can perceive in every ten steps I take in our streets, ponds of stagnant water, and sinks of putrid animal and vegetable matters, exhaling perpetually under a hot sun the most offensive effluvia." The conclusion he draws is, that the disease was *not individually infectious*. He then mentions the uniformity of the symptoms, and the correspondence of the fever with the diseases which have prevailed in that city and in other parts of the continent for a number of years past. He enumerates the symptoms, which are exactly the same, as observed in New-Haven, New-York and Philadelphia.

Doctors Alexander and Jaquitt agree in the facts that the disease was not imported nor specifically contagious.

The board of health then called a meeting of the physicians in West Baltimore, and inquired whether any contagious sickness had come under their knowledge. They answered in the negative. Three of their number, at the request of the meeting, went to East Baltimore and visited a number of the sick. They reported on the 29th of August, that the disease was not a malignant, contagious or yellow fever, but the bilious remittent. Their report quieted the alarms of people.

On the 2d of September the commissioners were alarmed with the opinion of the physicians in that part of the city, that the *disease was something more than common*.

Five members of the board, with Dr. Moores, went to the point to examine for themselves. They found the disease had spread, chiefly among the poor, who lived in confined dwellings —a few persons were dangerously ill; but on the whole, were convinced that the disease was *not contagious*.

The next week, the diforder affumed a more threatening afpect. The launching of the frigate on the 7th of September, collected many people together, who were expofed to a hot fun and fatigue, which fpread the difeafe to Weft Baltimore. The next day the board of health received regular information that there was *contagion in the difeafe*. A meeting of the faculty was called, and fuitable directions given to check and alleviate the calamity.

The whole number of interments in the city and precincts from Auguft 1 to October 29th—Adults 408; children 137. Total 545. Number of inhabitants at Fell's Point (where the difeafe principally raged) who removed during the ficknefs 671. Thofe who remained were 2679. Total 3350.

This plain and candid narrative of facts, which is certified by the prefidents of both branches of the city council and by the mayor, Mr. Calhoun, does great honor to the integrity and diligence of the commiffioners ; and *if the laws of nature are to be relied on as uniform in their operation, this report alone will decide every difputed point relative to the origin and phenomena of the yellow fever.*

It is here decided by unequivocal evidence; evidence that precludes the carping of prejudice and the cafuiftry of intereft, that the yellow fever and the bilious remittent are the *fame difeafe*, differing only in degrees of violence ; and it is agreed on all hands that the remitting and intermitting fevers are the fame difeafe, with a fimilar difference in violence.

The difeafe began at Baltimore early in the feafon, in June, and for more than two months, prevailed as a remitting fever of the common kind, without infection, and it is agreed on all hands not to be of imported origin. During a wet feafon, the damp weather caft the difeafe upon the inteftines, and it appeared in the form of a dyfentery—a moft important fact, which proves what Dr. Lind has afferted, that a dyfentery is a yellow or malignant fever feated in the bowels. The wet weather ceafing, the fever refumed its former appearance, and gradually increafed, till it exhibited its *worft forms and became infectious.*

Had the advocates for the domeftic origin of this fever *contrived* and directed a feries of facts, to prove their own doctrines, it would not have been possible to collect stronger evidence in their favor, than the report of the board of health in Baltimore.

In Philadelphia, the disease in 1797 appeared, in a few cases, as early as June—one on the 5th—one on the 9th—one on the 15th and another on the 22d. These cases, instead of being considered as proofs of a pestilential air, and precursors of more general sickness, are thrown entirely out of the question, by the advocates of imported fomites. The division of opinions, which originated in 1793, relative to the causes and origin of that disease, was revived with asperity. One party among physicians contended that the distemper was introduced into the city by the ship Arethusa, which arrived from Jamaica and Havanna, on the 23d of July. Another party believed the sources of the disease to have been, noxious exhalations from putrid substances in the city, with an augment from the foul air of the snow Navigation from Marseilles. The evidence to support each of these opinions, is published in the proceedings of the College of Physicians, and of the Academy of Medicin.

The city of Philadelphia was deserted by a great proportion of its inhabitants, and thus the mortality was limited to about one thousand victims. It prevailed principally in the suburbs.

This epidemic was followed as usual by the influenza.

By foreign publications, it appears that the catarrh was epidemic in England in the four first months of 1797. I have no particulars of the violence or extent of this disorder; but if it was severe and general, no event is more certain than that sickly seasons will follow.

What confirms this opinion, is, that in the following summer, the plague raged in Constantinople, on the Barbary coast, and in Corsica. It appears by an official letter of the French minister Sotin, that there was a difference of opinion in regard to the epidemic in Corsica—some calling it the plague; others, a malignant fever. Those who called it the plague, were prepared to account for it, by the tale of a Turkish vessel wrecked upon the island, with diseased people on board. But the disease subsided without very extensive ravages.

This malignant fever however occasioned no small alarm in England. The government sent orders to ships cruising in the

Mediterranean to have no communication with veſſels from Corſica, and a proclamation was iſſued ordering ſtrict quarantine to be performed by all veſſels from Corſica, Minorca, Gibraltar and Spain within the Mediterranean.

In 1797 the bilious plague carried off forty-five of the inhabitants of Providence. Of this diſeaſe, I have a minute and judicious account from Mr. Moſes Brown, which is here abridged.

In 1791, the year when the diſeaſe firſt appeared in the Weſt-Indies and New-York, ſeveral perſons died of a ſimilar fever in Providence. Two women died in one family, near the centre of the town, after three days illneſs. They vomitted bilious matter, and were yellow, with livid and purple ſpots. The ſecond, being ſeized two days after the death of the firſt, might have taken the diſeaſe by infection ; but no ſuſpicion exiſted that the firſt had acceſs to any infecting cauſe.

On the 14th of Auguſt died another perſon in a different part of the town, and on the 21ſt of September, a fourth, with ſimilar ſymptoms. As no alarm had then been excited by yellow fever, little notice was taken of theſe caſes ; but the attending phyſician, a reſpectable character, who viſited many patients in 1797 and was affected with the diſeaſe himſelf, has ſince pronounced the diſeaſe of 1791 and of 1797 to be the ſame.

A caſe very ſimilar to theſe occurred in September 1792 ; and on the weſt ſide of the river, prevailed a ſingular epidemic, in which perſons became yellow, with black urine, coſtive bowels, pains in the right hypochondrium, without fever. Some had petechial ſpots, and one perſon, petechia, vibices and hemhorage, yet the diſeaſe was not mortal, nor malignant.

In 1793 a perſon from Philadelphia was ill and died of the yellow fever in Providence, but no other was infected.

In 1794 ſeveral perſons had the ſame diſeaſe, but they took it probably in Carolina, where they had been on a voyage ; the diſeaſe did not ſpread by infection.

On the 11th of July 1795, died Capt. J. Gifford, a reſpectable man, of the ſame diſeaſe. No infection was ſuppoſed in the caſe—he was buried under arms, but no inconvenience was experienced from it, at the time. Yet two years after, viz. in

1797, his family were affected with the diforder, at the time when it became epidemic in the neighborhood.

Several other cafes occurred, in the fame year, and one of them exhibited infection.

Thefe cafes demonftrate a peftilential principle exifting in that town, in every feafon from 1791 to 1795 inclufive; at the time when other parts of the United States were more feverely afflicted. They were the diftant precurfors of a more general calamity in that town, which did not arrive till 1797.

Sporadic cafes of peftilential fever do not render it *certain* but *probable*, that the difeafe will, in a future feafon, become epidemic. In 1796 cholera infantum and dyfentery were prevalent.

In 1797 the hydrophobia was prevalent in the ftate of Rhode-Ifland, as well as in other ftates. One T. Lyon was bitten by a dog, the wound healed, and he was feized four months after, and died. The peftilence among cats prevailed alfo in Providence.

In this year alfo prevailed at Weftport in the fame ftate, and on Nantucket ifland, a very malignant epidemic dyfentery. At Weftport died 30 patients of 79 who were feized. On Nantucket the difeafe was lefs mortal; about 100 died out of 2000 patients. On examination, it was found that under the houfe of the family firft feized, there were fome barrels of putrid fifh, and other naufeous matter.

It was fuppofed alfo, that the difeafe might have been augmented by the effluvia of a large pond, at fome miles diftance, which had become ftagnant, filled with grafs, and the fhores ftrewed with dead fifh. A number of men, on this difcovery, opened a trench to drain off the water, and let in the tides, after which, it was fuppofed, the difeafe affumed a lefs malignant afpect.

The peftilential condition of the air at Providence in 1797, manifefted itfelf very early in the feafon; the firft death occurring as early as May 5th—the next on the 25th of June—the third on the 4th of July—the fourth on the 27th—the fifth on the 29th, and the fixth on the firft of Auguft. The fymptoms in all thefe cafes, were the predominant ones of the true yellow fever; and the bodies exhibited more or lefs petechiæ and vibices. Thefe cafes occurred *before* the arrival of the fchooner, to which popular clamor afterwards imputed the whole evil. Thefe were the fcattered precurfors, which, had the fubject of peftilence ever been inveftigated, with philofophical ingenuity and Chriftian candor, would have rendered the epidemic a probable event to the citizens of Providence, as early as July and would have taught them to ufe all human means to avoid or mitigate the calamity.

On the 8th of Auguft arrived the fchooner Betfey, Capt. Barton, from the Mole of Cape Nicholas, after 24 days paffage. Her cargo was only a few hogfheads of coffee. She lay at the wharf, till the 20th, when an increafing alarm from new cafes of the fever induced the police to order her to be removed and cleanfed.

On enquiry, it was found that three of the fchooner's people had been ill in the Weft-Indies, but no one died. One of thefe only had been ill on the paffage, but had recovered fo as to do duty, feven days before her arrival. There were five perfons on board, during the paffage, none of whom were affected by difeafe from infection or other caufe.

The death of Mr. Arnold, the cuftom-houfe officer, who was faid to have vifited the fchooner, and feveral of his family, gave rife to the report that the fever began from fomes on board of her. This point will be hereafter difproved. Certain it is, that another officer of the cuftoms flept on board of the fchooner *feven* nights; another *five*, and another young man *two* nights, with Brown, the owner of the blankets hereafter to be mentioned; all of whom efcaped difeafe of any kind.

It was alfo faid that the woman who wafhed two blankets, belonging to a difeafed feaman, took the fever and died. On inveftigation, this proved to be an idle tale. The blankets were owned by one Brown, who had not been fick; and not having any ufe for them in warm weather, they had lain in his cheft. On his arrival, they were carried home, fpread out on the fence to air; they were then carried to his fifter's to be wafhed and lay two days before the work was undertaken. The day after the wafhing, the women were taken ill; which was two early for the operation of infection, unlefs highly concentrated. But in fact the blankets were not infected; never having been ufed by any difeafed perfon; and the mother and others who handled them, when fiift opened, never had the difeafe.

But ftronger circumftances attended this cafe. The blanket belonging to Rophy, the only fick man, on the paffage, and his other clothes, worn during his fever, and colored yellow, by his perfpiration, were carried to his houfe; the blanket fpread out for children to play on, before it was wafhed, afterwards wafhed by his wife; and no perfon took any difeafe from his clothes or blanket.

Such are tales of imported difeafes, raifed by ignorance and propagated by intereft, pride or credulity, to which the bufinefs of the merchants and the commerce of the country are to be facrificed!

Many other reports were fpread about the infection from this fchooner which, upon ftrict enquiry, were found to be equally groundlefs. Such as the introduction of the fever into Warren, where the veffel ftopped, on her way to Providence. The cafe was, one Cole, an officer of the cuftoms, fculled a large boat a mile or two, againft the tide, in a foggy evening; went on board, wet and fatigued; without refrefhment or change of clothes, flept in a cabin with broken windows, took a fevere cold; repeated his vifit to the fchooner the next day; on the third day went to Providence, a diftance of ten miles in the rain; tarried two nights without a change of clothes; returned on foot, and was taken ill of a bilious fever and died in about feven days. Yet after all this fatigue and imprudence in the man, enough in all confcience to kill him, men are found weak enough to charge his difeafe to the fchooner.

But it happens, that other fimilar cafes of fever occurred in Warren, in perfons who had never vifited Cole or the fchooner; and one at the diftance of three miles from the town. The whole tale therefore comes to nothing.

One fact more, and I will quit the fubject of correcting the popular errors on this head. The men belonging to the fchooner were difmiffed at Providence and returned to their families, with their fea clothes of courfe. My informant took pains to enquire of every family, whether any of them had been infected; and he found not one inftance, altho the families confifted of about forty fouls!—The cafe of the unfortunate family of Mr. Arnold would afford fome flight ground to fufpect the infection to be communicated from the fchooner to him or his fon, the latter having vifited her;* but it happens that Mr. Arnold's wife, who had *not* been on board, nor otherwife expofed, was feized fifty-fix hours *before* her fon and more than three days *before* her hufband. Thus the reports of infection from abroad, when well fifted, vanifh into fmoke; and I am perfuaded this would generally be the refult, if men would be faithful to themfelves, to truth and their country.

On the 12th of Auguft, the fever took a more rapid fpread, probably from a fudden alarm by the burning of two tons of hemp, by means of a fpark from a blackfmith's fhop, as it was paffing the door. This was four days after the arrival of the fchooner, and occafioned the popular clamor which was raifed about her infection. But the appearance of the difeafe long *before* her arrival is decifive of the queftion.

This difeafe had its own atmofphere; raging moftly in a part of Providence much expofed to the effluvia of great collections of filth in vaults, from a diftillery, and in other places. Some cafes however occurred in other fituations; and many parts of the ftate exhibited the peftilential principle, in fporadic cafes, or local epidemics, as at Briftol, Warren, Greenwich, Indian Point, Gloucefter, Warwick, &c.

In Providence, the difeafe affected fifty-fix families—8 before the arrival of the fchooner, and 48 afterwards. In 33 of thefe families, only one perfon in each, had the fever; and as fome of the families are large, the infecting principle could not have been very powerful. In the large houfe, where lived the women who were firft taken ill, after the fchooner arrived, refided 9

---

* It is not rendered certain that the father had been on board, but that the fon had, is not queftioned, fo had at leaft one hundred others, who were not afterward affected with the difeafe.

families, confisting of 37 persons, only 12 of which were affected. In the hospital the nurses and attendants *all* escaped.

Some instances of this disease appeared in the following winter; and there were cases also of the ulcerous sore throat. In the north part of the town, some cases of the yellow fever occurred in the last summer—1798.

In 1797 a malignant fever is said to have been introduced into a village in Chatham, on Connecticut river, by a vessel from the West-Indies. I understand that it was confined to a cluster of houses by the water; but I have not been able to collect the facts in detail, altho I have written letters for the purpose.

During the late pestilential period, the state of the atmosphere produced its usual effects in winter; which appeared in the extraordinary symptoms of pleurisy and peripneumony.

It has already been remarked that in periods when plague and other mortal epidemics rage in summer, the diseases of winter assume new symptoms. The pleurisy, at such times, has often become epidemic and even infectious. It is in fact a modification of the same pestilential principle, as that which renders bilious fevers in summer epidemic and infectious. The fatal effects of this species of pleurisy in Connecticut, in the winter of 1761, have been mentioned.

In the winter of 1795-6, after the epidemic in New-York, several cases of a similar kind occurred, and an able physician of plethoric habit and strong fibres, fell a victim to a peripneumony, with anomalous symptoms.

In the following winter, a similar disorder attacked many people in Connecticut. Three men in Hartford, of one family, two brothers and a cousin, all men of robust health, were attacked and carried off in the compass of a few days. Others of the same family, and several persons of a similar habit were affected, but recovered. It was far less general than in 1761.

This species of pleurisy appeared in Philadelphia as early as September 1791, the month when the malignant fever prevailed in New-York. A patient of Dr. Rush had a "red face, inflamed eyes, a perpetual tossing and sighing, strong animal powers, but weak pulse and sizy blood." In February 1792 many cases of similar pleuritic fevers occurred in Philadelphia—diseases affumed the inflammatory diathefis which has remarkably characterized the epidemic of the laft peftilential period.

In the fpring of the year 1798, a mortal fever raged in Fredericktown, Maryland, beginning with laflitude, chills and pain in the head, and producing, on the third day, vertigo and fpafm in the breaft.

Letter from Dr Baltzell to Dr. Rufh, dated May 2, 1798

In fummer and autumn of 1797, a malignant fever, attended with dyfentery, was epidemic in Portland and its vicinity, in the diftrict of Maine. The dyfentery fubfided in October, but the fever continued. It appeared in the country, as well as town; and was ufually conquered by the ufe of alkaline remedies. Many of the patients had a yellow fkin and the predominant fymptoms of the yellow fever of our cities. In one inftance, this difeafe put on' the form of peftilence. A merchant, in a country village, where no fufpicion of infection could be entertained, was feized with a malignant fever; he lingered till the 36th day, and died highly putrid. His nurfe was feized and died; after death appeared livid fpots on the body A fervant alfo took the difeafe and died. The nurfe communicated the difeafe to three perfons in the family where fhe lay ill.

This laft inftance is decifive evidence that the peftilential yellow fever not only originates in our country, but in villages, in the 44th degree of latitude, a more temperate climate than that of New-York and Philadelphia.

In the winter fucceeding, the peftilential principle ftill exhibited its effects. The fever continued to prevail, being ufhered in with naufea, vomiting and chills fucceeded by heat; but it was generally accompanied with a fore throat and fcarlet efflorefcence. It prevailed in almoft every town in the county.

Dr Barker's letter, Med Repof vol 2 147

The year 1798 was remarkable for the moft general prevalence of the plague of our climate, that has been known; and in fome cities, the difeafe was peculiarly malignant.

The preceding winter had been unufually long and cold—the May following was dry beyond what is recollected in any former years—June was remarkable for deluging rains, which occafioned floods in the Connecticut, Delaware and Sufquehannah rivers, which did no inconfiderable injury. Two or three of the firſt days of July were exceſſively hot, and ſucceeded by twenty days of very cool weather—then commenced a long period of the moſt fultry weather ever known in our climate, accompanied, in ſome places, with great rains.

Catarrhous fevers were frequent in the ſpring, the conſtant forerunners of autumnal ſickneſs. Bilious fevers alfo occurred, in a few cafes very early, indicating the predominant condition of the atmoſphere. In ſummer and autumn, the grafs-hoppers multiplied to ſuch a degree from Pennfylvania to New-England, as to devour vegetables, and effentially injure the paſtures and grafs fields.

The peſtilential fever in Philadelphia appeared early in the feaſon—a number of cafes in June, and ſtill more in July. In Auguſt early, the city was alarmed and foon deferted by at leaſt three fourths of its inhabitants. The difeafe was unufually mortal; and extended to the remoteſt parts of the city, where it had not formerly prevailed. Owing to this circumſtance, ſome families ſuffered, which had eſcaped in former years. The number of deaths amounted to about 3440. The difeafe, as ufual, abated with the appearance of froſt, but individuals were attacked with it, and carried off, in the midſt of the following winter.

It is alledged by fome perfons that the fever was introduced into Philadelphia by the ſhip Deborah, which arrived from Jeremie, and anchored near Race ſtreet wharf, on the 18th of July. It is admitted that perfons who went on board, foon after ſickened and died; and fo did others ficken and die, without going near that ſhip. The truth is, many cafes of the difeafe had occurred three or four weeks, *before her arrival*. The ſhip had loft people by fever on her paſſage and might be infected; and perfons vifiting her might receive that infection; but theſe facts do not reach the point. The epidemic *began* in all parts of the city, in fcattering cafes, *previous to the arrival of this fomes*, and had the ſhip never arrived, that epidemic would have ravaged the city. This is evident from the number of its precurfors.

This peſtilential fever carried off fifty-feven perfons in the village of Marcus Hook, where the firſt perſons ſeized were a ſhallop-man and others from Philadelphia. But many caſes occurred which could be traced to no infection. See Dr. Sayre's letter in Currie's Memoirs, p. 136. In Cheſter died 50 of the ſame fever.

At Wilmington, in the ſtate of Delaware, thirty miles from Philadelphia, the ſame diſeaſe raged with more than its ordinary mortality. Its victims amounted to 250. It appears that the diſeaſe was introduced by the fugitives from Philadelphia, and by watermen who ply between Wilmington and Philadelphia.

See Dr. Tilton's letter in Dr. Currie's Memoirs, p 138.

The fever alſo prevailed in New-Caſtle and at Duck creek in the ſame ſtate.

Letters from reſpectable phyſicians, in the public prints, have informed us that this diſeaſe prevailed alſo in ſome parts of New-Jerſey, as at Bridgetown and Woodbury; and eſpecially near the meadows on the borders of the Delaware. From careful examination, it was found that the diſeaſe muſt have originated where it exiſted; no intercourſe having been held with infected places. In ſome inſtances the fever was probably infectious.

At Norwalk in Connecticut ſeveral perſons died of the ſame diſtemper. The phyſicians are doubtful as to its origin; as ſome caſes may be traced to a diſeaſed perſon who had been in New-York. Three caſes however occurred at ſome miles diſtance from the heart of the town, in perſons who had not been in the leaſt expoſed to infection.

M. S letter from Dr. Betts.

In the firſt week of Auguſt, appeared a bilious fever in New-York, between Old ſlip and Coenties ſlip, in the ſtreet next to the water; a place remarked for great accumulations of filthy ſubſtances. By the exertions of the Health Commiſſioners, in covering theſe nuiſances with freſh earth, this alarming fever ſubſided in that neighborhood, and diſappeared by the 26th of that month.

But on the 12th, the peſtilential fever appeared in other parts of the city, and about the 20th, began to extend and aſſume a more formidable aſpect. The diſtrict of the city, ſubjected to its moſt deadly effects, was that ſection comprehended between

John-ſtreet and Beekman-ſtreet, particularly in Cliff-ſtreet and its neighborhood. The probable cauſe of this effect, was the fetid air from large quantities of ſpoiled beef, ſtored in the cellars in Pearl-ſtreet, on the windward ſide of this ſection. The cellars were filled with water by heavy rains, or were otherwiſe damp; which circumſtance, added to the extreme heat of the ſeaſon, occaſioned a greater loſs of ſalted proviſions, than perhaps was ever before known. To augment the effect, large quantities of pickle had been diſcharged, in the proceſs of re-packing beef not yet ſpoiled, but in a bad ſtate, which pickle had been carried by the gutters into a ſewer in Burling ſlip, from which iſſued a very offenſive ſmell *

About the laſt of Auguſt, the inhabitants of New-York were greatly alarmed; ſome removed from the eaſt to the weſt ſide of Broadway, a part of the city which has hitherto been exempted from the violent effects of the yellow fever; but a great proportion of the people deſerted the city. The diſeaſe was more malignant, than in its preceding viſits, and exhibited more frequently the bubo and carbuncle. It extended over two thirds of the city, and numbered with the dead about two thouſand of its inhabitants. I am informed the diſeaſe was leſs generally characterized with the inflammatory diatheſis, and that veneſection was leſs generally attended with ſalutary effects, than in former years.

This diſeaſe exhibited little infection, beyond the limits of its own amoſphere. In the hoſpital, at a little diſtance from the

* There is reaſon to believe, that ſalt, if not ſufficient to preſerve the article to which it is applied, renders it doubly noxious in a ſtate of putrefaction, and that a ſmall quantity of ſalt will accelerate the proceſs of putrefaction. From an experiment related to me by Mr. Moſes Brown of Providence, it is proved that a piece of fleſh, in pure water, will not putrefy as ſoon as in water, in which a few grains of ſalt have been diſſolved.

Do not the ſaline particles of the air, on the ſea coaſt, render the putrefaction of fleſh and vegetables more rapid, and the exhalations more deleterious, than perfectly freſh water? And is not this one cauſe, why peſtilential diſeaſes appear firſt, and are moſt general, in maritime places?

Dr Cogſwell informs me that a boat-man on Connecticut river, in the hot weather of 1798, contracted a violent fever of which he died, by ſleeping in an open boat, near a quantity of pickle which had leaked out of a barrel of ſalted proviſions. The diſeaſe was of a very malignant kind.

city, were admitted about 300 patients, ill with that difeafe; yet fixteen nurfes, feven wafherwomen, and the boatmen who conveyed the fick from the city to the hofpital, *all efcaped.* Dr. Douglafs, the attending phyfician, efcaped the difeafe, until October, when he vifited his friends and flept *in the city,* three days after which he was feized with the fever.

> See Letters from the Health-Office, by Dr. Bailey, whofe zeal, talents and induftry, in his employment, have rarely been equalled

The laft fact is very important towards correcting the popular errors refpecting the contagion of this fever. In the city perfons took the fever—in the hofpital they did not That is, the diftemper has an atmofphere, in which it is readily contracted— beyond that atmofphere, it is not infectious In other words, it is a *condition of the atmofphere,* and *not the effluvia from the fick,* which is to be dreaded.

Thus, in 1797, the fugitives and fick from Philadelphia did *not* fpread the fever in Wilmington—in 1798, they did. That is, in 1797 the atmofphere of Wilmington would not *generate* and *nurfe* the difeafe—in 1798, it would.

In Bofton, the difeafe began near the town dock and the neighboring wharves, in the month of June, but its moft violent effects were experienced on the fouth fide of Fort-Hill, an elevated part of the town and expofed to free air. This circumftance has occafioned no fmall furprife; but as the fever of 1796 began in that part of the town, perhaps we may find the caufe in the very extenfive flat, between Bofton and Dorchefter point, which is uncovered at low water; perhaps in the expofure of that hill to the direct rays of the fun, perhaps in the nature of the foil which is clay of a folid texture, and fitted to retain on its furface whatever impure fubftances are thrown from houfes.

The fever afterwards invaded the north part of the town, and a ftreet rear the pond; fuppofed to be excited by noxious exhalations Some parts of the town, which are low and filthy, efcaped the fever.

At firft it attacked the moft robuft young men, and the diathefis was highly inflammatory. Later in the feafon, it attacked persons of all ages and habits. At first it was not infectious, but in the later stages of its progress, it exhibited infection. It disappeared with the arrival of frost, after carrying off nearly 200 patients.

M S letter from Dr. Eliot.

See a full account of the disease in a letter from Dr. Rand, published by order of the Academy of Arts and Sciences. This gentleman observes that no infection appeared, except in places where the disease was originally contracted.*

Massachusetts Mercury, Feb. 8, 1799.

The same malady appeared in Portsmouth, New-Hampshire, with equal mortality, as far as it extended; but its progress was limited to one street near the water.

New-London, in Connecticut, is situated in a very healthy part of the country, on a harbor, whose shores as well as the surrounding lands, are dry and rocky—its population about 3000 inhabitants.

In the last week in August 1798, this town was suddenly invaded by the plague of our country, which began in the family of Mr. Bingham, keeper of the Union coffee-house. No vessels from the West Indies, no sick from other places, occur, in this instance, to help out popular credulity. The idea of importation is abandoned by the citizens of the town. The fever was very fatal within its atmosphere, which was confined to Bank street and its vicinity; a part of the city well built, clean and airy as any street in the town. Within a small space, were fifteen houses, inhabited by ninety-two persons—of which ninety were affected with the disease; thirty-three of this number died, and two only escaped the fever. The disease prevailed about eight weeks and destroyed eighty-one lives.

Printed account of the fever by Charles Holt

On enquiry I find that this disease in New-London had its precursors, in sporadic cases of the same fever, in the three preceding summers. In 1795, died Dr. Joseph W. Lee with all the symptoms of the yellow fever. Some instances occurred in

---

* That is, infection was attached to the *place*, rather than to the *persons* of the diseased—a fact which is true of every pestilence.

1796; and in 1797 died of the same, Matthew Grifwold, Efq. and foon after his mother; indicating the communication of infection. Yet in thefe years, it did not fpread and become epidemic. The peftilential period however was progreffing in that town, as appears by the bills of mortality; for the ordinary number of deaths does not exceed 60 in a healthy year; but in 1795, the number amounted to 86—in 1796, to 80—in 1797, to 101—in 1798, to 133. Here we obferve a great augmentation in the mortality of the town, feveral years before the crifis of peftilence, and efpecially in the year next preceding it. The importance of this fact towards a right underftanding of the caufes of epidemic peftilence, cannot be miftaken.

Confiderable quantities of falted fifh, which lay in certain ftores in New-London, and which had not been well cured with the ufual quantity of falt, became fetid and offenfive, altho not putrid, and affumed a red caft with a flimy feeling—it alfo loft its texture and firmnefs. This was opened and fpread in the ftreets for the purpofe of being dried; and from its offenfivenefs and vicinity to the place where the difeafe firft appeared, it is fuppofed to have been an exciting caufe of the fever. This opinion has doubtlefs fome foundation; but putrid fifh will not always occafion difeafe. It is probably true that the bad ftate of the fifh was partly owing to a previous bad ftate of the air; altho it afterwards became a *caufe* of a *worfe ftate* of the air.

What feems to put this beyond doubt, is, the unufual number of mufketoes, in the adjacent country, and the multitudes of flies of uncommon fize, exceeding what had been before obferved. With thefe phenomena before our eyes, we can be at no lofs to account for the peftilential fever of New-London.

The ufual lake and river fever prevailed in the fame feafon, in many of the interior parts of the country; as at Royalton in Vermont, on the Grand Ifles in Lake Champlain, at New-Milford in Connecticut, and in various parts of the ftate of New-York; in which places, it was attended with confiderable mortality. Sporadic cafes occurred in all parts, and in the healthieft fituations, of the country. In many places, intermittents and dyfentery were unufually violent and obftinate.

I have no account of the temperature of the weather in any part of Europe, during the fummer of 1798; except that in fome parts of Sweden, the firft months of the fummer were exceffively dry, as the month of May was in America.

A peftilential fever appeared in Italy in June; but I have no details of its progrefs. It is however to be obferved that this fever was preceded by a violent earthquake in fome part of the Tufcan territories, in the month of May, which did no fmall injury.

In autumn broke out a peftilential fever on the Baltic, in Dantzick or its vicinity. The government of Denmark, in confequence of official information of the prevalence of this difeafe, directed all fhips from Dantzick and the neighboring ports to be watched with vigilance, and appointed a committee of quarantine.

According to the report of a mafter of a veffel, there was an eruption in Teneriffe in the fummer of 1798, which lafted feveral weeks. This volcano had been quiet for 94 years.

In November and December, the peftilence in America was fucceeded as ufual by influenza, which was very prevalent in all parts of the country, and in the fouthern ftates attended with fome mortality. This was merely a change of the form of the epidemic.

The winter of 1798-9 was very long and fevere in both hemifpheres. In the United States, it began about the middle of November, with fnow, and a heavy fall of fnow on the 18th and 19th was followed by fevere cold that lafted till the fecond week in January. From this time, there was a relaxation of cold for about three weeks, and the ice in Connecticut river gave way. But in February commenced fevere cold, which continued, for the moft part to the vernal equinox. April was alfo cold; fevere frofts occurred often, and checked vegetation. On the 2d and 8th of May were confiderable falls of fnow, followed by froft. On the morning of the 4th and 5th, we had ice at New-Haven as thick as window-glafs. Peaches bloffomed about the middle of May, and apples were not in full bloom, till the 22d. This long duration of cold exhaufted all the barns of hay and other fodder, and multitudes of cattle perifhed in various parts of the country.

In Europe, the winter was equally severe. The rivers in England, Germany, Holland and France were covered with solid ice, and at the breaking up of winter, the Rhine rose and burst its barriers, inundating many parts of Holland with terrible destruction. The severity of the winter was felt even in the south of Italy, and the French and Neapolitan troops suffered greatly from snow on the Appenine, in the vicinity of Naples. In Siberia, we are informed by the public prints, perished whole villages of men and cattle by the severity of the frost.

In America, the diseases of the winter were characterized by the predominant diathesis of the reigning epidemic constitution, a yellow skin and bilious discharges. An earthquake of considerable extent was felt in the Carolinas on the 12th of April. What will be the state of health in the ensuing summer, must be left to be determined by the event. The present pestilence has been long and severe and the citizens look with impatience, for the usual salubrious state of their atmosphere.

In August, about the time the pestilence began to show itself in New-York, immense numbers of flies died suddenly, and occasioned no small speculation and alarm. Some were found on the floors; others adhering to the ceilings of rooms, and what is singular, their bodies became white. A pestilential air usually generates flies in unusual numbers; but on this occasion, some sudden change in the elements, destroyed their lives. How little do we know of the powers of the elements, and the nature of the alterations in them which produce such astonishing effects. Will imported infection account for such phenomena?

This is the best statement of facts I have been able to make from sixteen months investigation. It is not improbable that some mistakes have occurred, which more time and more ample materials, would enable me to correct. But I trust that the substance of the statements is accurate, and that no error of consequence will be found to result from them, to impeach the general principles suggested in this work.

POSTSCRIPT.

Additional facts, collected on a journey which I made through the Northern States, while this volume was in the press.

IN the autumn of 1732 raged in New-York a malignant, infectious fever, of which died seventy persons in a few weeks.

M S of Mr Alexander.

In 1745 a malignant bilious fever prevailed in New-York, of which died an eminent phyfician of the city, Dr. Nicoll. By the defcription of the difeafe, given to me by a gentleman who was affected with it, there appears to be no queftion that it was the fame difeafe now called yellow fever.

About this time, for the year is not exactly known, a malignant epidemic difeafe laid wafte the Indian tribes. By the defcription of the fymptoms, as given by Indian traders, then among the tribes, and ftill living, it is certain this was the infectious yellow fever. In confequence of this diftemper, the Senecas removed their quarters two or three times, in a few years—it being a practice among the natives to abandon the place infected with this plague. The difeafe was confined to the Indians—the white people, living and trading with them, not being affected.

In 1746 the Mohegan tribe of Indians, between New-London and Norwich, was wafted by the fame malady. Dr. Tracy of Norwich now deceafed, was the only white man affected—he attended them as their phyfician. From Mr. Philemon Tracy, a fon of the doctor, who has taken the trouble to examin a Mohegan prieft, a man of good fenfe and integrity, who was himfelf affected by the diforder, I have the following account of this peftilence.—That it appeared in Auguft and prevailed till cold weather—that about one hundred of the tribe perifhed—that it was the year after the reduction of Cape Breton (of courfe in 1746—and Dr. Tracy's books confirm the dates mentioned by the Indian)—that the patient firſt complained of a ſevere pain in the head and back, which was followed by fever—in three or four days, the ſkin turned as yellow as gold, a vomiting of black matter took place and generally a bleeding at the noſe and mouth, which continued, till the patient died. Theſe are the words of the old Indian, as penned at the time by my informant.

It will be remarked that this was a local peſtilence, the fever being confined to a ſingle tribe of Indians and not prevailing in the neighboring towns. But it will be remarked alſo that this was the ſame year, it prevailed in Albany, when the bills of mortality were generally high.

I have aſcertained that the canker-worm, which lately ravaged the fruit trees in New-England, appeared as early as 1788 or 1789.

A fatal malignant diſeaſe raged among the tribes of the Mohawk Indians, about the year 1776, and reduced ſome of them to a few men.

From Dr. Wheeler of Redhook, on the Hudſon, I learn that the angina ſcarlatina appeared there in January 1789 and prevailed till April—it prevailed alſo in the two ſucceeding winters.

The influenza, in that year, firſt appeared there about the middle of October, and prevailed two months, among all ages and both ſexes. Catarrhal coughs have been prevalent every year, ſince that time. In the ſpring of 1793, angina ſcarlatina, mumps and catarrhal coughs prevailed till June, and diſappeared. Soon after commenced the remitting fever. In ſome caſes the paroxyſms invaded the patient in the form of madneſs.

The reader will note that in our interior country, the remitting fever of that diſtinguiſhed year, 1793, had nearly the ſame ſpring precurſors, as the yellow fever in Philadelphia.

The meaſles at Redhook in 1795, partook of the character of the preceding epidemic fevers; beginning with a highly inflammatory diatheſis, and ſometimes ending in typhus, with petechiæ, vibices and hemorrhagy. Pleuriſies had the ſame character.

At Brattleborough, on the Connecticut, a family by the name of Morgan were seized in 1791 with a fever of the typhus kind, and six of them died. Several persons who visited the family took the disease and died, and there its progress ended. The family resides in a healthy situation, near a small active stream of water; and no visible cause could be assigned for the origin of this distemper. These facts are taken from Dr. Hall of that town. It will be remembered that this was the year when autumnal diseases first put on the malignant aspect of our late pestilence, when the plague broke out in Egypt and the yellow fever in the West-Indies began to assume what Dr. Chisholm calls unusual symptoms.

Dr. Center of Newport informs me that in 1798 occurred in that place many cases of a bilious fever bearing some resemblance to the infectious fever; and one case of decided carbuncular and glandular plague, in a man of robust constitution. There is no pretence of foreign origin, in any of those cases.

From sundry gentlemen living in Chelsea, a village at the landing in Norwich, I learn that two or three cases of malignant bilious fever occurred there in 1798, marked with the usual symptoms of the infectious fever. Some of these cases could not possibly have been derived from infection. One of the patients might have contracted his disease at New-London.

Dr. Holyoke of Salem, in Massachusetts, informs me that in 1798, many cases of malignant bilious fever occurred in that town, which could not have been derived from infection.

From Dr. Woodruff and Dr. M'Clellan of Albany, I learn that several cases of malignant bilious fever appeared in that city, in 1798, marked with all the symptoms of the pestilence of our cities and which must have originated in that place. About one half who were seized, died.

The first case of influenza at Albany in 1789 is noted by Dr. M'Clellan to have occurred on the 30th of September. This was precisely the time of its appearance at Philadelphia, and a little after its first appearance at New-York. In the country, between New-York and Albany, it did not appear till a week or two later. These facts prove that this disease falls on distant places at the same time.

The scarlatina anginosa appeared at Albany in the winter and spring of 1793, about the time it did in New-York and Philadelphia.

In every part of our country, one remark has been made by physicians, that from the year 1792 or 3, intermittents and remittents have become more numerous and obstinate, and attended with unusual symptoms. In many places, these diseases have been multiplied in a ten fold ratio; elucidating the principles of the great Sydenham, relative to "Constitutions of Air," and demonstrating the existence of a general cause in the insensible properties of the atmosphere, to which we may and must ascribe the pestilence of our maritime towns.

In 1798 multitudes of dead pike were observed to float down the Mohawk and Hudson.

From Dr. Thatcher I learn that for some years past, an autumnal fever has prevailed in Plymouth, in Massachusetts, of the remitting kind, with low typhus symptoms. In winter it takes the type of the nervous fever. It was very prevalent in 1798 in that and a neighboring town.

From Dr. Smith of Hanover, in New-Hampshire, and Drs. Green and Trask of Windsor, in Vermont, I have obtained information respecting a very infectious fever which prevailed in those towns and the vicinity in 1798. This disease is described by Dr. Spalding in the Medical Repository, vol. 3. p. 5. It approaches nearly to the typhus mitior of Cullen, but the fiery red eye at the invasion seems to indicate its alliance to the infectious fever of our cities; and it resembles the disease known by the popular name of long fever.

This fever, in Windsor and Hanover, was preceded by dysentery of uncommon malignancy in 1797, which, in Windsor, was attended with an unusual inflammation of the lungs. The disease which preceded these epidemics was the scarlatina anginosa, which was very prevalent in 1796.

It is worthy of notice that in all parts of our country, the autumnal infectious fevers have had precursors in other epidemics, especially catarrhal complaints and anginas. I do not find an exception to this remark.

This fever at Windsor deserves further to be noticed for its infectious or contagious quality. It was far *less* fatal, but *more* infectious than the yellow fever of our cities. Nurses often took the disease, and when they returned to their dwellings in distant towns, rarely failed to communicate it to the whole family. This is a phenomenon rarely, perhaps never exhibited by the pestilence of our maritime towns, which has an atmosphere of its own out of which it is not communicated.

I have examined personally the positions of many of the towns where this fever and dysentery have been most prevalent, and I find no where any marsh that can rationally be supposed to originate these distempers. In general the towns are situated on a basis of clay, between high ridges of land or mountains, where the heat of the sun is greatly concentrated, and on the margin of rivers. To this description, there are some exceptions as to the soil; some towns being on sand or gravel. The neighborhood of fresh streams of water cannot be admitted as a cause of these fevers—nothing being more salubrious than such streams. But I am persuaded from careful observation, that, under a pestilential constitution of air, great heat is the immediate exciting cause of autumnal fevers, in situations not exposed to marsh effluvia.

With respect to the origin of the pestilential fever in Portsmouth, in 1798, the facts are as follow.

A laboring man, who was given to liquor, received his wages on Saturday evening. He was seized with the malignant fever, and died on the next Wednesday. While he lay ill, a vessel arrived which had lost a man or two by the fever on her voyage, but no person was ill on board, at the time of her arrival. Some of the persons who afterwards died of the fever, had been on board of that vessel; but whether they took the disease from infection or not, cannot be known. The first case occurred *before* the arrival. This is an agreed point. I have these facts from two of the principal gentlemen of that town, one of them a respectable physician; the other, the person who paid the wages to the man who first died. All my enquiries have been made at the sources of correct information; and I find every where *popular reports* are false or incorrect. Yet popular reports are received as truth by many physicians and writers, and are made the basis of false and pernicious theories, both in America and Europe.

The fever in Portsmouth was limited in its progress to the northern part of the town. In the southern part, at the same time, prevailed a malignant dysentery, which was as mortal as the fever in the northern part. The line of division was drawn by a wide street or square on which stands the court-house. The scarlet fever had been prevalent in the town for two years preceding.

In 1799, the present summer, many persons have taken the pestilential fever from vessels arrived from the West-Indies; but in most, or all cases, the fever has become extinct, without any considerable mortality. In Boston, the mortality was limited to two or three persons.

The case at Newburyport was singular. A vessel went and returned from the West-Indies, without a case of malignant fever, but as she arrived at the mouth of the river Merrimack, 18 days from St. Thomas's, a boy was seized with the fever, and afterwards one or two others. Several persons took the disease and died; but people left the vicinity, and the disorder became extinct. This was a fever generated on board of the vessel.

The beginning of the summer of 1799, tho late, was favorable to vegetation, and the first crops were good. Wheat, which had been blasted, for several preceding years, in the eastern states, was excellent.

But in July commenced a most distressing drouth, in all the northern states; and particularly in the middle states, and the interior country, by which the maize, buck-wheat and potatoes were greatly injured. In some parts of the state of New-York, the maize was totally destroyed.

Over the eastern states, a species of caterpillar of small size appeared in unparalleled numbers, covering the wild cherry-tree, the apple, the willow, the ash, and the hickory. In some parts, a large caterpillar, with variegated colors, stripped the black oak of all its leaves. Grass-hoppers were as numerous as the blades of grass, and in some places, injured greatly the grass and other vegetables. But especially to be noted were the small toads of the color described by Fernelius, "Coloris cineritii" like ashes; of the size of a filbert, and in numbers not to be estimated. These were numerous also in 1798. They answer the description of those which medical writers of former ages observed to they appeared and difappeared, is not exactly known—they were moſt generally obſerved in July.

In the ſpring prevailed influenza or catarrhal fevers ; in ſome places cynanche maligna ; and generally rheumatic complaints, and ſlight ulcerations of the throat. In many places, the fevers of winter were characterized with a yellow ſkin and bilious diſcharges. All theſe marked the continuance of a peſtilential atmoſphere.

The plague ſhowed itſelf early, in ſcattered caſes, in Philadelphia ; but diſappeared, to the unſpeakable joy of the inhabitants. Alas ! When ſuch caſes appear in July, and eſpecially if other diſeaſes in winter and ſpring manifeſt ſymptoms of the prevailing epidemic, it is hardly poſſible that our cities ſhould eſcape a peſtilential fever in autumn. This terrible ſcourge renewed its ravages in Philadelphia and New-York ; and in various parts of our country, bilious fevers appeared with malignant ſymptoms.

At Hartford, on the Connecticut, appeared the malignant fever in Auguſt, to the ſurpriſe of the inhabitants and of the ſtate. People who have no juſt ideas of the nature and origin of this diſeaſe, attempted to find the cauſe in ſome veſſel from the Weſt-Indies ; but being diſappointed, reſorted to a ſmall coaſting veſſel. On examination it appears, that this veſſel was uſed as a market boat between Connecticut river and New-York —the maſter had died in June, but of what diſeaſe, I am not able to learn. Another maſter took poſſeſſion of her, and finding her very dirty, with the remains of various vegetables, he overhauled her and gave her a thorough cleanſing. He took in at New-York a cargo of ſalt, and ſailed to New-Haven, where the veſſel lay ſome time, about the middle of July. Here the ſalt was purchaſed by a merchant of Hartford, and the veſſel ordered round to that place, where ſhe arrived and diſcharged her cargo, in the beginning of Auguſt. From the time the veſſel left New-York, to the time of diſcharging the ſalt, muſt have been from four to ſix weeks. After leaving Hartford, and going down the river, the maſter and mate of this veſſel were ſeized with the fever and died. Inſtead therefore of being *imported*, the fever was *exported*.

Some attempts were made to trace all the firſt caſes of the fever to that veſſel ; but it does not appear that more than one person who had the difeafe, was ever on board ; and it is *proved* that moft of the perfons affected were never near that veffel and never vifited the fick. It is proved further that of ten or twelve perfons employed in unloading the veflel, not one was ever affected by the malady. Yet even in this cafe, the filly tale of importation is fwallowed with eagernefs by the advocates of that doctrin.

I confefs myfelf weary and afhamed of refuting fuch groundlefs opinions and furmifes ; but it is a tafk which truth and juftice and public happinefs demand. The truth is, the fpot where this fever arofe, is low ground, retaining water to ftagnate after the fpring floods—built upon in a crouded irregular manner—extremely filthy—penetrated by a creek which has been dried and neglected, and become the refervoir of every unclean thing —in the vicinity is a flaughter-houfe, where loads of garbage contribute to render the air foul and noxious. Let any man walk over the ground and examin it with care, as I have done fince the fever, and he will be convinced that no imported fomes was neceffary, in that place, to breed a peftilence.

But one of the ftrongeft arguments to prove the domeftic origin of the malady, is, what people rarely confider. Numerous fevers of the remitting kind, and typhus mitior, have originated on the fame ground, for feveral years paft ; and in 1798, two cafes of malignant yellow fever—one of which terminated in three days. Thefe fevers marked the predominant ftate of that local atmofphere, and decide the queftion of domeftic origin.

On the 15th of July a tremendous hail ftorm paffed over Connecticut from the weftward, attended with violent wind and thunder. The ftones and pieces of ice were of various fizes, from that of a walnut to that of a hen's egg. In Gofhen, Cornwall, New-Hartford, &c. on the weft, and Lebanon, Franklin, &c. on the eaft of the Connecticut, the grafs, corn and every green thing was injured or deftroyed ; glafs was broken, trees galled, and fmall animals killed. The champain country on the Connecticut was lefs injured. This ftorm, unexampled in Connecticut, refembles numberlefs hail ftorms defcribed in hiftory, as the precurfors and companions of peftilence.

END of the FIRST VOLUME.

CPSIA information can be obtained
at www.ICGtesting.com
Printed in the USA
BVHW04s1036080718
521071BV00005B/92/P